Safe Eating

SAFE
EATING

A practical four-point program to reduce
your intake of toxins and increase
your tolerance of unavoidable toxins
—because what you don't know *can* hurt you.

Dr. Patrick Quillin

PATRICK QUILLIN, PH. D., R.D.

M. EVANS AND COMPANY, INC.,
NEW YORK

Library of Congress Cataloging-in-Publication Data

Quillin, Patrick.

   Safe Eating : a practical four-point program to reduce your intake
of toxins and increase your tolerance of unavoidable toxins—because
what you don't know can hurt you / Patrick Quillin.
     p.   cm.
   Includes bibliographical references and index.
   ISBN 0-87131-619-6 : $19.95
   1. Nutritionally induced diseases—Prevention. 2. Food
contamination—Health aspects. 3. Nutrition. I. Title.
RC622.Q55   1990
613.2—dc20   90-42603
                                                        CIP

To my brother, Frank, for teaching so many people
so much about life without ever sounding
like a teacher. Wish you could have stayed longer.

Table of contents

Acknowledgments

There may be one name on the cover, but there are hundreds of people who were vital to this project. Let's have a round of applause for my versatile, helpful, and supportive wife, Noreen; for my friend and agent, Harold Roth, who got the book started; for the diligent efforts of my professional clipping service and research associate, Jack Quinn; for George DeKay and Richard Kislik at M. Evans for their support of this project. Let's have a standing ovation for the thousands of unassuming research scientists whose patient and brilliant efforts unravel nature's secrets for the betterment of all.

Safe Eating

Introduction

"**S**o just exactly what *are* we supposed to eat!" shouted an angry young mother from the back of the room. More and more people were asking the tough questions: "You tell us how important nutrition is, then you tell us what to eat. But isn't that food laced with poisons?" Maybe so. I needed some answers. Not just for the thousands of people that I lecture to, but for myself.

We all eat. Most of us enjoy eating. It can be one of life's regular pleasures. Yet a steady stream of reports over the past decade have warned about the hazards of eating and drinking. "Eating and drinking has become a death-defying act," commented one seminar participant. Many of us choose to take certain risks: ride motorcycles, use skateboards, drive without seat belts, smoke, drink, climb ladders, use power tools, etc., but these are voluntary risks. Risks from tainted food and water are involuntary. Amid this hysteria, many people have just gone back to their old habits of coffee and doughnuts with the attitude, "Since all of this food is bad for me, I might as well eat what I want."

I got into the field of nutrition to help people, to show them that through healthy nutrition, they can take charge of their own destiny and avoid the common ailments that plague Americans. And now, many of these "healthy" foods had been implicated in the expanding ring of "dangerous" foods. My formal training in nutrition was being turned upside down.

This is a book of hope that matters will improve; of fear that we may have permanently spoiled some parts of the earth; of anger at the greed and incompetency that allowed our food-pollution issue to disintegrate into a crisis; of disbelief at the illogical approach of pesticides; and of amazement at the incredible tenacity of the human body.

Although we are the most agriculturally productive nation in the history of the world, we have mindlessly tainted our valuable food and water supply—but there is hope. I started this project with a sense of duty, and resignation, that the facts would support the pessimistic theory about many foods being dangerous to your health. However, after many interviews with experts and after reading thousands of scientific papers on the subject, my conclusions are more positive than I had anticipated: we can protect ourselves with reasonable guidelines. Most of us will live to tell our grandchildren about the insanely polluted times of the later twentieth century.

Please do not mistake my optimism for escapism. We do have a serious problem. We dump over 1.2 billion pounds of pesticides on American food, water, and soil annually. We dump another ninety billion pounds of toxic wastes in our 55,000 toxic-waste sites, most of which ends up in the water supply, much of which is then pumped on food crops. Thousands of water wells across the country have been closed in the last decade, and thousands more are still used even though they are tainted with hazardous chemicals. Half of all antibiotics produced in this country are routinely fed to domestic animals to encourage faster weight gain; most domestic animals are also fed hormones and drugs, herbicides and pesticides. Up to 270 million cases of food poisoning each year result in over 9,000 deaths from microbes on tainted food. Lead in the air, water, and food supply has boosted lead levels in the bodies of Americans to 500 times what they were 350 years ago.[1] The prestigious National Research Council found that pesticide residues on our food may cause an extra one million Americans to contract cancer over the next seventy years.

Our food supply is so tainted that the Food and Drug Administration has developed an "acceptable daily intake" (ADI) guide of various pollutants in our food and water supply. In many areas, fish, once the quintessential symbol of nourishment, are now repositories of pollutants.

The ironic twist here is that most pollutants continue to concentrate as they move up the food chain, until the ultimate carnivorous predator (man) eats and stores the highest concentrations of all. There is more at work here than the scientific principle of "bioaccumulation"—we are also witnessing a lesson in "as you sow, so shall you reap." Hopefully, we can learn from our mistakes.

Don't be too discouraged. There is a way out of this mess. In addition to the obvious need for better regulations and monitoring of the food and water supply, nature provides us with some ingenious food substances and nutrients to protect us against pollutants. And fortunately, humans are far from being "virgins" on the issue of poison intake: for millions of years humans have been refining the detoxification pathways in the body, so that most of us can eat and drink marginally safe food and still live to tell about it. Our immune system is equally impressive at capturing stray chemicals and cancer cells in the body.

By age sixty-five, most Americans will have eaten about 100,000 pounds of food, give or take a ton. For better or for worse, the quality and quantity of your food will have a major impact on your health, vitality, disease resistance, alertness, and longevity. When 3,583 Americans were asked to name the one thing that is most important in life, 5 percent answered wealth while 50 percent answered health.[2]—what good is wealth without health?—but our American health is dismal compared to what it should be. Experts estimate that 30 to 90 percent of our cancer and at least 20 percent of many other health woes are due to polluted food and water.

You picked up this book because you are understandably concerned about the safety of our food and water supply. You are not alone. In a Food Marketing Institute phone survey of over one thousand shoppers, 77 percent considered chemical residues on our foods to be a *serious* hazard, while another 18 percent considered this to be something of a hazard.[3] Over 80 percent of Americans want politicians to clean up the environment—regardless of the cost. All of this says that we want a clean environment and clean food, which we don't have right now. In our hurry to develop technological wizardry, we have forgotten to responsibly dump our toxic trash in safe ways. We also have become dazzled with the fleeting effectiveness of pesticides and forgotten the wisdom of nature (Integrated Pest Management) to produce clean plant and animal food.

This is a pragmatic book which shows you ways to protect yourself and your family against the significant risks of unsafe food and water. It shows you how to eat and drink on the planet earth, with your friends and even in restaurants, and still maintain a high level of safety, using easy, practical, inexpensive, flexible, and scientifically proven methods. Most importantly, following these principles will allow you to sleep better at night because you have cut your health risks dramatically.

You are to be congratulated for your interest in this subject. Naivete is dangerous. It is the uneducated consumer who is more likely to suffer the effects of tainted food. Once you know the "game plan," it is easy to avoid the major pitfalls. What you don't know can definitely hurt you.

This book is written for lay people with no scientific background. Any complex language is explained or omitted. For the purpose of simplicity, I have often lumped many of the poisons that are intentionally used on our food under the banner of "pesticides," although there are specific names for poisons that kill weeds (herbicides), rodents (rodenticides), fungi (fungicides), and nematode worms (nematocides), etc. "Bugs" and "insects" are the terms I use for various pests, including worms, beetles, grasshoppers, mites, spiders, boll weevils, aphids, and other creatures that attempt to share our bountiful food harvest. We want to keep matters simple and not get bogged down in complicated terminology.

Why should you believe me? I am a registered dietician with nine years of teaching university-level nutrition. I hold bachelor's, master's, and doctorate degrees in the field; have years of experience with Scripps Clinic and the La Costa Spa; am the author of three other books on nutrition; and have a computer modem hookup to the National Library of Medicine. This book is full of the latest information and most of my statements are not common knowledge (see the Notes and Bibliography sections).

Now, a "road map" of this book to get you started. Part 1 discusses the good news. Not only are matters beginning to improve in this field, but humans have some impressive detoxification and immune systems that have allowed us to neutralize a limited amount of toxins and cancer cells in the body. Fortify yourself with these encouraging facts. You will need their positive message to carry you through the bad news. Part 2 outlines the problem of not only our tainted food and water supply, but our widespread pollution and the general government apathy on the subject. Part 3 provides the solution, which is a practical guide showing you how to *reduce your intake* of toxins and *increase your tolerance* of unavoidable toxins through certain foods, nutrients, mental attitudes and exercises.

Since following the program in this book may necessitate changing your lifestyle, I have included an appendix with some resources to help you in that transition. You will find consumer action groups to join, places to write for more information, and how to get politically involved. There are also companies who sell Integrated Pest Management information and supplies, fruit trees and organic food by mail, and more. The companies are listed for *your betterment,* not mine or theirs. I have no vested interest in any of these companies.

If used properly, this guide could be the beginning of a healthy and safe lifestyle for you and your family. You can now enjoy peace of mind knowing that you are doing as much as is realistically possible to protect yourself. Hopefully, you can also spare some of your time to get involved in cleaning up our pollution problem.

I fervently hope that you live as long as you want and never want as long as you live.

PART ONE

Some Good News: the Sky is not Falling . . . Yet

1

Fuel for the Optimist

> "The way things are going,
> you feel like a fool when buying
> a five year calendar.
> ROBERT ORBEN

*T*here are a multitude of reasons to be pessimistic about the food safety issue, but overall this is an optimistic book because it shows that you can do something to protect yourself. I see hope where others see despair. There are good reasons to foresee a cleaner food supply and a healthier America. This chapter is dedicated to the optimist in all of us that desperately wants to envision a brighter tomorrow, a better world for our children, reasons to go on—and the steps being taken to achieve these goals.

YOU CAN DO SOMETHING.

Helplessness can be a crippling emotion. You are not helpless in the food safety issue. There are many steps you can take to protect yourself and your family from tainted food, and also political efforts you can make to accelerate the cleanup of the food and water supply.

We have enough food. Although America's food supply is not equally distributed and is not always wisely used, we *do* have enough food—unlike many developing nations where even tainted food would be preferable to no food at all. With its rich soil, advanced agricultural methods, ideal growing climate, and genetically groomed plant species, America can be considered a cornucopia. Making our abundant food supply clean and safe is entirely within our reach.

Side benefits of a healthier lifestyle. You may be reading this book simply to avoid the minefield of dangerous food in your grocery store; yet as a side benefit of following the recommendations in this book, you will probably find yourself feeling better, with more energy, and avoiding many common ailments.

The same nutrients that help to bolster your body's defenses against poisons also improve other biochemical functions of the body. For example, by lowering your fat intake, which is a major carrier of pollutants, you not only protect your body against poisons but also lower your risk of heart disease, hypertension, obesity, cancer, arthritis, and other major diseases that are linked to fat consumption.

Consumer awareness. Just a few decades ago, not many consumers were aware of the effects of pesticides or growth hormones. Today, consumers have lost their naive reliance on governmental protection—unfortunately creating one more area of life to worry about. However, by becoming educated we can gain a sense of self reliance and confidence in knowing that we are taking charge of our lives. Knowledgeable consumers know that they must be intimately involved in the process of lawmaking to steer the food industry in the right direction.

A Harris poll in 1987 found that 96 percent of consumers were, to some extent, concerned about pesticide residues in their food supply.[1] Ninety-three percent reported that they were also concerned about hormones and antibiotics in their food. In a separate survey, 75 percent of the 1,285 people polled said that pesticides were excessively used in fresh produce. Ninety-six percent of these people were also concerned about the use of wax coatings on fresh produce. Because of this nearly unanimous public concern, people are getting involved in the safety of their food supply, which the way it should be. It took dozens of depressing headlines and thousands of martyrs before the public became irate enough to do something about food safety—a painful lesson with positive results.

Humans are tough creatures. Are there poisons in our food supply? Plenty of them! Nonetheless, humans have survived for millions of years because we could eat various poisons, including naturally occurring pesticides, and render these poisons nontoxic. Healthy, well-nourished, nonpregnant humans have an awesome capacity to survive poisons in the food, air, and water supply; and also to destroy cancer cells that get started by poisons. Yet there is a finite limit to our detoxification systems, and many people are at or beyond that threshold due to our tainted food supply.

You can make a difference. With 235 million other Americans to contend with, many of us tend to feel lost in the crowd. What difference does one opinion make? The food safety issue has proven that your vote and opinion count. Congress and the Environmental Protection Agency have been reluctant to ban or regulate many chemicals used in agriculture and food processing, yet the people have spoken and changed that inertia problem. Democracy works.

Two-thirds of the voters in New York and New Jersey endorsed major costly environmental cleanup acts. In Massachusetts, similar measures passed with 73 percent of the votes. Californians approved their Safe Drinking Water and Toxic Enforcement Initiative (requiring 264 known carcinogens in their food and water supply to be labeled as such) with 63 percent of the votes, although this bill had become a political wrestling match between the governor (heavily supported by the chemical industry) and consumer action groups. It took a law suit in the state Supreme Court to wrangle cooperation out of the governor. Industry is not taking a passive stance on this issue, either: d-Con company, a manufacturer of household pesticides, has filed a legal challenge to this toxic-cleanup bill, saying that a state cannot restrict something approved by the federal government (EPA).

Another bill was recently introduced into the California legislature that would gradually ban the use of cancer-causing pesticides.[2] Although the bill has virtually no chance of passing due to opposition by the agriculture industry, the proposal many end up as a ballot initiative for the voters to decide.

The people have finally sent a clear message into the political and business arena: we will no longer tolerate contaminants in our food, air, and water supply. Although the wheels of democracy grind slowly, they do work.

Increasing governmental protection. Granted, our government food inspection program is riddled with fault, but it is better than no program at all. The Government Accounting Office and the National Academy of Sciences, both congressional advisory bodies, have shown us how to improve our antiquated food protection system. Progress is being made, much of it due to your insistence.

The government is beginning to consider our food and water supply sacred, as indicated in the Beech Nut Foods case. Beech Nut is the second-largest American manufacturer of baby foods. Over a five-year period, the company knowingly sold "a chemical cocktail" that was supposed to be "100 percent pure apple juice" for infants. Just a few years ago, this issue might have been ignored by governmental regulators, but in 1986 Beech Nut and its top two corporate officials were indicted on 215 criminal counts, fined a total of over $8 million, and the two men were sentenced to a year in prison. This is over six times higher than any previous fine levied by the FDA. Bad publicity caused sales at Beech Nut to fall by 8 percent (off $10.8 million) the next year, sending a warning to the food industry: we will not tolerate a tainted food supply.

Sustainable agriculture. Driven to desperation, many consumers needed but could not find "clean" produce in their local grocery stores, making "organic" farming a viable option.

Although organic produce only accounts for about 3 percent of the total produce sold in the U.S., growers cannot keep pace with demand, and many now earn a decent living ($50,000 to $80,000) doing what they love and providing a necessary product. Without all the scary scientific studies about pesticides and hormones, organic farmers would still be little more than amateurs, barely eking out an existence. Due to the health risks of much commercial produce, organic growers have joined forces, weeded out the unfit, set quality standards, perfected their techniques, and lowered costs to the consumer.

Consumer action groups. In the 1960's, a Harvard Law School graduate wrote a book condemning an American car manufacturer for unsafe design. Both the book, *Unsafe At Any Speed,* and the author, Ralph Nader, became household names—and so the first consumer action group was born. People soon learned that such groups could be incredibly effective at doing what elected representatives are supposed to do: work for their constituents. Without the efforts of such groups as the Natural Resources Defense Council, the Center for Science in the Public Interest, and many others (see Appendix), there would still be precious little consumer awareness of the dangers in our food supply. Though we all may have lost some confidence in our elected officials, we have gained considerable confidence in supporting consumer action groups that parallel our interests in life.

Environmental sensitivity. For decades a few persistent voices have been warning us about polluting the planet earth, but politicians and voters were reluctant to spend the money to provide proper waste-disposal facilities; and no one wanted to risk upsetting corporate America with costly environmental regulations. We reached near-apocalyptic levels of pollution before anything was done. Unfortunately, humans have a tendency to ignore all but the most urgent issues: while fire prevention tends to be a non-issue, fire fighting gets top priority. This mentality is almost a stereotype among humans, but perhaps the food pollution issue will change such attitudes.

Polls now find that 80 percent of Americans want our nation cleaned up, regardless of the cost. We have turned too much of our precious land and water reserves into cesspools of poisons. We have finally realized that you cannot dump toxins irresponsibly without eventually having to eat and drink those pollutants, and that dousing our crops with a rain of poisons only creates pesticide-resistant bugs, kills off friendly predatory bugs—and we get to eat the pesticide residues. The more than 1.2 billion pounds of pesticides and ninety billion pounds of hazardous wastes dumped annually in America have been taking a serious toll not only on human health, but also on other life-forms. A 1989 Gallup survey found that Americans consider a clean environment to be just behind not smoking in relative importance for a healthy life.

John Muir, the famous naturalist who helped to establish our national park system, noted: "When you look at Nature, you see that everything is hitched together in some way."

Protecting American children. Americans have become understandably jaded about dangers in our society. Adults take their chances at everything from freeways to muggers to tainted booze—but we draw the line when it comes to protecting our children. Not until the childhood leukemia rate was suspiciously high in Woburn, Massachusetts, did the people begin to act against industrial polluters of their water supply. Once again, another clear message went out to the politicians and business people: "We are serious about protecting our children!"

THE ALAR INCIDENT

The Alar incident shines brightly as an example of how the American public has been able to do in months what Congress could not do in decades. It could be called the "Watergate of the food industry," a major turning point for the bulk of consumers, a watershed year for farmers who realized the wrath of angry Americans.

Alar (chemical name: Daminozide) has been used on fresh produce for over twenty years. Although classified as a pesticide, Alar is actually a growth regulator that will prevent fruit from falling off the trees before harvest time, increase storage life, enhance color, reduce the occurrence of bruises and scars, and produce a less bitter core. Approximately 75 percent of the 825,000 pounds of Alar used annually was applied to red apples, 12 percent to peanuts, and the remaining fraction used on cherries, nectarines, peaches, etc. Although Alar on apples has only cosmetic and commercial value, it has significant health risks—especially for children.

Alar is sprayed on the crop early in the season during flowering time, thus becoming a systemic poison that cannot be washed off. Since 1978, there has been scientific evidence that Alar and its by-product (UDMH) increased the risk of cancer, and consumer action groups had petitioned the EPA and FDA to do something. Although the EPA attempted to ban Alar in 1985, heavy resistance from the manufacturer (Uniroyal) squelched that movement when Ralph Nader and company were denied a trial in the Supreme Court to force the EPA to act against Alar.

In February of 1989, the EPA concluded that Alar had an "inescapable and direct link" to cancer, yet it would take eighteen months of regulatory hearings to ban Alar. However, in March of that year a non-profit consumer action group, the Natural Resources Defense Council (NRDC), showed evidence that Alar could alone cause cancer in up to 6,200 children in the U.S., also stating that 90 percent of children's cancer risk from pesticides was due to Alar. The EPA sheepishly pointed out that there are also sixty-six other approved pesticides that are known carcinogens, with fungicides, rather than Alar, actually leading the list.

The public reacted fiercely. Several large school districts banned apples in their cafeterias. Mott's and Tree Top, the largest apple processors in the country, along with several major grocery chains, announced that they would no longer accept Alar-treated apples.

Some scientists think that there is no safe level of Alar intake, especially in children. The problem is that children consume more Alar-treated products than adults: infants consume seven times more Alar than the population at large, while children under age twelve consume twice the nation's norm. Also, children have a reduced ability to detoxify poisons and control cancer cells through their immature immune system.

The numbers varied wildly. While the NRDC claimed that one in 4,200 exposed children might get cancer, the EPA interpreted the same studies to mean one in 20,000 children would get cancer, and the manufacturer claimed there was no risk at all unless a person consumed 28,000 pounds of Alar-treated apples every day for seventy years. While the NRDC claimed that 32 percent of the previous year's apple crop was treated with Alar, the EPA said the number was 4 percent and later revised their estimate to 15 percent—yet a government survey found Alar traces in 85 percent of baby apple juice, 93 percent of adult apple juice, 96 percent of cherry pie filling, and 99 percent of peanut butter.

The Alar incident eventually cost the apple industry about $100 million with a 20 percent dip in sales for that year. The USDA subsidized some of this loss by spending $15 million to buy and distribute the unwanted Alar apples to low-income people.

Although the manufacturer of Alar, Uniroyal, never admitted any adverse health effects from their product, the demand for Alar dipped to near zero and Uniroyal voluntarily ceased production in June of 1989.

The moral of the story: *you* can make a difference.

CHAPTER 2
Humans Are Tough Creatures

*I*n H.G. Wells's classic novel, *War of the Worlds,* Martians landed on earth and began devastating all forms of human resistance. Suddenly, their giant spiderlike war machines came toppling down to the ground. As the story relates, the Martians were so advanced that they had long since purged bacteria and other infectious organisms from their world: after generations of living in a totally sterile environment, their protective immune systems had atrophied. Once on the planet Earth, the Martians were exposed to our teeming sea of germs. Though the Martians may have won the war on the outside, they lost the critical war on the inside as they had no "soldiers" to defend their bodies against the impurities of the planet Earth. The story leaves us with the impression that although humans may not be the brightest creatures in the galaxy, we are tough to kill.

Life is not perfect today, nor has it ever been. The only reason that humans have survived this long is because we have been able to detoxify most of the common lethal substances in our environment. When you read about the frightening levels of pollution we are drinking, eating, and breathing, you may ask the obvious question: "If so many of us are consuming so many lethal poisons, then why aren't we all dead?"—because of our immune and detoxification systems, that's why. This chapter provides foundational material to help you understand how optimal nutrition can encourage healthy immune and detox systems.

Some animals and most plants make their own naturally occurring "pesticides" to discourage predators, so the only way humans can derive the nutritional benefit from many foods is to detoxify the inherent poisons. The only way that we could survive amid predatory microbes was to have an efficient internal army waiting to subdue any invaders. And, since the ongoing process of cell reproduction involves inevitable mistakes, we needed to have that internal army willing to destroy defective (cancerous) cells before they could grow into a serious problem.

We are a tough species. According to the *Guinness Book of Records*, various humans have survived: six years of burial in a bomb shelter; a 21,000-foot fall without a parachute; car crashes at two hundred miles per hour; six-month marathon dances; being fired 175 feet from a cannon; and being set adrift for 133 days alone on a raft in the ocean. Chain-smoking malnourished alcoholics may take decades to perform their slow ritual of suicide. In 1848, Phineas Gage survived a freakish accident in which a large metal rod was fired through the center of his brain. He finally died thirteen years later of an epileptic seizure.[1] Grigori Rasputin was a Russian monk who survived repeated foiled attempts on his life, involving guns, knives, and poisons. In a recent incident in Wisconsin, liquid ammonia leaked into milk that was consumed by school children. Although over five hundred children drank dangerous amounts of a poison, only twenty suffered nausea and a burning sensation, while there were no hospitalizations or deaths.[2] Humans have survived this long because we could tolerate repeated bouts of malnutrition and exposure to toxins.

THE AMES TEST

As a biochemist doing research at the University of California at Berkeley, Bruce Ames was motivated by Rachel Carson's book, *Silent Spring,* to look at the ingredients in a package of potato chips, and he thought, "No one really knows if these chemicals are safe." It used to take years and hundreds of thousands of dollars to determine the safety of chemicals through mice studies, hence few were done. But through a combination of brilliance and laziness, Ames found that he could determine whether a chemical was carcinogenic (cancer causing) or mutagenic (DNA altering and hence may cause cancer) by adding it to a dish full of bacteria. This new method was quicker than conventional toxicology studies with animals, and seemingly quite reliable. Since then, more than five thousand different substances have been tested in three thousand laboratories throughout the world via the famous Ames test.

Environmentalists rallied around Ames as he proved their suspicions: that many products of industrial America caused cancer. In 1971, Dr. Ames wrote a scientific paper which stated that even one molecule of a carcinogen may trigger cancer in the body. Yet Ames started finding that *many* things were carcinogenic, including a wide variety of naturally occuring products. Bracken fern, a food commonly consumed by grazing cattle, is loaded with carcinogens that may even be more potent than DDT. Comfrey, the herb tea with various touted cures, is equally lethal. While cabbage and broccoli may help to reduce the incidence of intestinal cancer through the presence of indoles, this same family of plants contains a substance similar to dioxin (ingredient of Agent Orange) that makes up 5 to 10 percent of their weight. About half of all the chemicals tested, both natural and synthetic, may cause cancer since they are mutagenic in the Ames test.

EDB was a fumigant that was widely used on grains and fruit before being banned by the EPA. According to Ames, the average intake of EDB was less lethal than eating one mushroom per day or a peanut butter sandwich.[3] Environmentalists have abandoned his camp in droves. Many of his scientific peers have criticized Ames for producing writings applauded only by the major polluting industries.

The real importance of Dr. Ames' work is showing that humans have been exposed to an intimidating array of poisons since the beginning of time. Because of this exposure, we had to develop systems to neutralize a variety of toxins and to squelch cancer and microbe growths. Eliminating toxins is not possible in 20th century industrial America. However, we can rev up our detoxifying and immune systems for maximum protection. More on that later in part three.

By gathering hundreds of scientific studies and comparing the LD-50 (lethal dose required to kill 50 percent of the animals), and other data, Dr. Ames and his colleagues at the University of California at Berkeley have developed an intriguing ranking of poisons and their relative risks. Not all poisons have the same toxicity. Some are worse than others. For instance, aflatoxins from peanuts are 27 times more carcinogenic than DDT. The following HERP (Human Exposure/Rodent Potency) index is data extrapolated from lab animals, but provides a model that shows relative toxicity of various common chemicals in our food, air, and water. The lower the number, the lower the risk. For example, the hydrazines in mushrooms (HERP of 0.1) may be 100 times more carcinogenic than the chloroform (from chlorine) in tap water (HERP of 0.001).

A STEADY DIET OF POISONS FOR SIXTY MILLION YEARS

In the "back to earth" movement of the 1960s and '70s, people developed the general concept: "If it's natural, then it must be good for you." That ain't necessarily so. From rattlesnake venom to the paralyzing herb curare, many natural ingredients can be quite lethal. Anise (licorice flavor), apples, basil, cantaloupe, carrots, cinnamon, cloves, fennel, grapefruit, honeydew, kale, nutmeg, orange juice, pineapple, raspberries, tarragon, and turnips all contain small amounts of their own potent pesticides which could be considered lethal by laboratory standards. Yet, most humans do not get cancer. Why? Because we have an intricate network of detoxification enzymes to neutralize many of the poisons that enter our system.

Figure 2A: Ranking possible carcinogenic hazards; the higher the number, the greater the risk. Source: Ames, B. N., et al., Science, 236 (1987) 271–280.

RANKING	SOURCE
.2	PCBs (residues in diet): PCBs were once used in oil for transformers
.3	DOE/DOT (residues in diet): DDE is a by-product of pesticide DDT
1	Tap water (1 quart a day): contains chloroform, a by-product of chlorination.
3	Cooked bacon (about 15 slices a day): contains dimethylnitrosamine, a preservative by-product
4	Contaminated well water (1 quart a day): e.g. Silicon Valley well, contains trichloroethylene
8	Swimming pool (1 hour a day): a child's exposure to chloroform by swallowing chlorinated water
18	Electricity: both at home and in the workplace
30	Peanut butter (2 tablespoons a day): contains aflatoxin, a mold
30	Comfrey tea (1 cup a day): contains symphytine, a natural pesticide
60	Diet cola (12 ounces a day): contains saccharin
67	Background radiation: at sea level, excluding radon
100	Raw mushroom (1 a day): contains hydrazines, natural pesticides
100	Dried basil (3/4 of a teaspoon a day): contains estragole, a natural pesticide
300	Phenacetin (2 pills a day): ingredient in pain reliever
367	Home accidents: includes falls, fires, poisoning

600	Indoor air (14 hours a day): formaldehyde vapors emitted from furniture, carpets, and wall coverings
667	Air pollution: in the eastern United States
733	Police work
808	Auto accident
2,800	Beer (12 ounces a day): contains ethyl alcohol
4,700	Wine (8 ounces a day): contains ethyl alcohol
5,800	Formaldehyde (6 mg a day): worker's daily exposure
12,000	Cigarettes (1 pack a day)
16,000	Phenobarbitol (1 pill a day): a sleeping pill
140,000	EDS (150 mg a day): worker's maximum legal exposure

There are ten thousand more *naturally occurring* pesticides in our diet than *synthetic* ones, according to Dr. Ames.[4] This bad news comes as very good news indeed, because if we were entering the arena of twentieth-century pollution as "virgins," we would be in double jeopardy. As it is, we are seasoned veterans at neutralizing many different poisons.

Humans in general are tough, and people in Third World countries tend to be even tougher because they have to adapt to harsher conditions. Water and food from these countries is often so contaminated with lethal microbes that it can kill an outsider through dysentery, but the water doesn't seem to bother most of the locals. They have somehow developed the ability, or induced the enzymes, to detoxify the poisons in their food and water supply.

SURVIVING VERSUS THRIVING.

The law of evolution is: "survive to reproduce." Note that nothing in that statement includes happiness, optimal health, or long life. Just survival. And many people do survive, in spite of their circumstances. Although 210,000 people died in the atomic bombing of Hiroshima and Nagasaki at the end of World War II, over 300,000 peopled survived these horrific events. Many survivors developed health problems later, but they lived through a "ground zero" nuclear blast. However, humans may be tough to kill (surviving), yet any more than a modicum of poisons can seriously detract from a healthy life (thriving).

Tenacious life. Humans are far from the most tenacious creatures on this planet. Anyone who has tried in vain to poison rodents out of their house will testify to the tenacity of rats and mice. In one study, scientists fed a group of mice the maximum sublethal amount of 120 different carcinogenic chemicals. After two years of such toxic exposure, only eleven of the chemicals caused cancer in the mice.[5] Sheep have developed the ability to neutralize the deadly poison cyanide that is found in some grazing plants. Vultures can neutralize the lethal bacteria anthrax and other poisons in decaying meat. Seventeen different insect species are now resistant to all five categories of chemical pesticides. (The Colorado potato beetle has developed resistance to *all* chemicals used against it.)[6] And the ultimate tenacious creature is the scorpion, which seems to be unharmed by nuclear blasts in the New Mexico desert.

Probing for poisons. We have four basic sensors on our tongue for food detection: sour, sweet, salt, and bitter. Sour and bitter often indicate a nonnutritious or even poisonous food. Sweet indicates the presence of simple carbohydrate, which is a primary bodily fuel. Salt indicates the presence of sodium, an essential mineral to balance the high potassium intake of our ancestors' semivegetarian lifestyle. By design, the taste sensors on the tongue provide a critical clue as to whether the food is useful, useless, or poisonous. We are not unlike insects groping their way through a treacherous food supply, with our tongues as the equivalent of the insects' probing antennae. Unfortunately, many natural and synthetic poisons are not detected by the tongue.

Useful, useless, or poisonous? Since plants cannot bite back or run away, many of them produce their own poisons as a deterrent to predators. For millions of years, humans have been consuming these naturally occurring "pesticides," many of which cause cancer in lab animals and bacteria colonies.[7] Celery, parsnips, figs, and parsley contain a deadly chemical (psoralens) that could cause cancer;[8] bioflavonoids are a group of vitaminlike compounds that are not considered essential, but may be helpful[9]—and may also cause cancer when consumed in excess; vitamin A in normal amounts (2000 to 25,000 i.u. per day) sustains health, but in excess amounts can cause birth defects; selenium is essential in small amounts but lethal in excess. Many nutrition scientists now feel that even arsenic, though deadly in more than trace amounts, may be essential to human health. Apparently humans have not only developed the ability to tolerate many toxins, but in some cases the poisons have become an essential nutrient.

Carbinol, a substance found in broccoli, cabbage, cauliflower, and related vegetables, is similar in both structure and action to dioxin[10], the feared ingredient in Agent Orange used to defoliate jungles in Vietnam. Here is the ironic twist: when carbinol is given to animals before aflatoxins (another even more potent carcinogen), the cancer rate goes down. It seems that a small continuous intake of certain "poisons" in the diet induces enzymes to detoxify other poisons, like priming the pump. This "induction" system works like a vaccination, in which a small amount of a dangerous bacteria is injected into the body to induce the immune system into action. Essentially, the cancer-protective effect in certain plants may come not only from beneficial agents (like vitamins, fiber, and indoles) but also by stimulating our detoxification system; not unlike the theory "a hair of the dog that bit you."

In the past four hundred years, mankind has seen a global exchange of table crops, which means that many of the naturally occurring toxins in our diet are relatively new. Kiwis, potatoes, chocolate, avocados, pepper, string beans, corn, citrus, and tomatoes all contain potent pesticides. Since Americans are an eclectic blend of ethnic backgrounds and few of us have the evolutionary advantage of long-term adaptation to these foods, one might be concerned. But fortunately, most detox systems in the body are inducible, meaning that you can encourage their efficiency just by regularly using them; and versatile, meaning that you don't need a specific detox enzyme for each poison.

A double-edged sword. The problem in prosperous America is that many people experience long term subclinical malnutrition (which "starves" their detox and immune systems) coupled with dangerous intake of pollutants. The result is that many people suffer ill health, while the majority of people merely survive, limping along with malnourished bodies full of toxins.
The point of this section is:

> Don't think you can avoid poisons. That is not possible.
> In most healthy, well nourished adults, a small amount of most poisons can be safely neutralized.
> You *can* make reasonable efforts to minimize your intake of poisons.
> You can enhance your protective detox and immune systems that allow you to neutralize poisons and purge cancer cells.

LIFE IN AMERICA THE POLLUTED

Vultures and scorpions aren't the only creatures who desperately need their detox systems intact. Humans are exposed to a plethora of toxins on a daily basis. For example, Jane tries to lead a fairly healthy lifestyle, which involves:

> Decaffeinated coffee. One of the caffeine extraction methods leaves behind a known carcinogen. Methylxanthines in coffee are suspected of causing

birth defects, behavioral disorders, and cancer in some people.

Doughnuts. These contain few nutrients and many questionable ingredients, like bleached and brominated flour.

Orange juice. The peel retains lots of lethal pesticide residues.

Fabric whitener. Her crisp dress shirt contains a likely carcinogen which can be absorbed by the skin.

Newspaper. The ink contains toxic trace minerals that can be absorbed by the skin.

Television. Electromagnetic radiation from TV can be harmful.

Air-conditioning. Fluorocarbons, which can be quite deadly, leak into the room.

Breathing. High levels of radon gas, the second leading cause of lung cancer in the U.S., have been detected in many American homes.

Driving. Breathing carbon monoxide and lead fumes from nearby cars.

Walking. The sun's rays can cause skin cancer and cataracts.

Breathing. Secondhand cigarette smoke from her office mates, two of whom are continuously coughing and sending out thousands of exotic viruses looking for a new host.

Working. Her downtown office is a "war zone" of microwaves from FM transmitting towers, which have been suspect of causing harm to some sensitive people.

Eating. Lunch consists of a salad, with its pesticide residues and naturally occurring toxins, and a diet soft drink—the safety of aspartame and other chemical additives is questionable.

Happy hour after work. Not only is alcohol itself a toxin, but there are seventy different pesticides and herbicides used in the growing of grapes. Phenols, tyramines, and urethane are a few of the other likely toxins in wine. The high-fat cheese and meats at happy hour can create carcinogenic by-products in the colon.

Exercise. By increasing the intake of oxygen, you seriously increase the oxidative free radicals in the body. The damage can be blunted by antioxidant nutrients.

The point here is not to scare you, but to show you that avoiding poisons is impossible. We can only hope to minimize our intake, allowing our protective systems to defend us from rational levels of toxins. The "factory warranty" on your detox and immune systems has two major specifications:

1. Don't overload the system with excess poisons, especially the exotic unmanageable poisons.
2. Provide the system with optimal amounts of raw materials to work at peak efficiency.

Dr. Ames speculates that 35 to 70 percent of our cancer is brought on by undernourished detox and immune systems, while another 20 percent is caused by pollution other than alcohol and tobacco consumption. Hence, harm from pollutants is a double-edged sword: you get hurt by consuming too many toxins, but you can also be hurt by not properly feeding the detox systems in the body.

YOUR BODY'S DETOX CHEMISTRY LAB

You have an impressive array of detox chemicals within your body that allows you to survive a continuous bombardment of poisons and pathogens. Poisons (xenobiotics) enter your body through the food and water supply, the skin (which screens out most, but not all, substances), the lungs, and even the eyes.[11] The body may immediately try to excrete the poison through the urine, feces, sweat, or exhale it from the lungs; or it may try to defuse the toxicity through changing the chemical structure of the poison.[12] Bodily secretions, including mother's milk, are other avenues of venting a poison. Some poisons are more difficult to neutralize than others and may end up being deposited somewhere in the body. In some instances, the detox system is simply overwhelmed with the volume of poisons to process, in which case many of these lingering poisons end up sabotaging the body.

There are a number of known enzyme systems that detoxify substances in the body, including catalase, superoxide dismutase (SOD), glutathione peroxidase (GSH), microsomal oxygenase, UDP-glucuronic acid, mixed-function oxidase, cytochrome P450, cyclo oxygenase, aldehyde oxygenase and others.[13] Many of these enzyme systems are headquartered in the liver, hence liver-crippling conditions, like alcoholism cirrhosis, can hamper the detox systems. Other detox agents include antioxidants like vitamins E, C, and beta-carotene, which are given the assignment of binding up destructive free radicals. There are some other surprising antioxidants in the human body which can have a dubious impact on health: while uric acid is a potent internally produced antioxidant, too much uric acid in the blood causes the excrutiating pain of gout. People who are prone to gout may have antioxidant protection almost comparable to a continuous intravenous infusion of vitamin C.

Most of these enzyme systems are dependent on an optimal supply of nutrients in order to function at peak efficiency. For instance, GSH is directly dependent on selenium, vitamin E, and sulfur-bearing amino acids (like cysteine or glutathione) for its activity. Many detoxification systems in the average malnourished American operate at suboptimal performance, and almost all drugs and alcohol can lower the body's ability to neutralize toxins. It is ironic that one of the problems in using chemotherapy agents to treat cancer is figuring out how to immobilize the cytochrome P450 system that desperately wants to detoxify the lethal chemotherapy agent.

As part of our detoxification system, we have a series of

Figure 2B. The Pathway of Poisons Entering the Body

POISON EXPOSURE	ABSORBED *via*	PROCESSED *via*
	lungs	reduction
	GI tract	oxidation
	food	conjugation
	water	
	skin	
	STORED in	EXCRETED in
	fat tissue	urine
	liver	bile/feces
	blood	lung
	bone	secretions (i.e.
	other	breastmilk)
		sweat

enzymes that repair broken components on the crucial DNA molecule. This systems gets a daily workout, even in the most health-oriented person. Our precious DNA carries the "blueprints" to build and repair a healthy body. Yet the DNA is subject to attack from internally produced poisons, such as hydrogen peroxide, and ingested poisons from both natural and synthetic sources. Even the ultraviolet radiation from the sun can induce DNA changes in the eyes and skin which can lead to cancer. There is a repair crew, called DNA polymerase, that rolls along the DNA molecule like a train down a railroad track, finding and repairing any broken rails or ties. By measuring the number of such points, researchers find that each cell in the body may have to repair its own DNA molecule up to ten thousand times each day![14] Imagine being up on your roof in a hurricane, trying to replace and nail down ten thousand roof shingles each day as they are being ripped off by the incessant storm. That is what your body does internally all day and every day.

And yet, in spite of being exposed to literally pounds of poisons per year, most Americans die of heart disease caused by stress, poor diet, and sedentary lifestyle—not from poisons. While tobacco is a known carcinogen and the single most preventable health risk in America, the majority of smokers still die from a non-smoking-related disorder. Credit these staggering facts to your detox system. Where would you be without it!

YOUR IMMUNE DEFENSE DEPARTMENT

In addition to a complex array of chemicals to detoxify poisons, we also have an immune system that swiftly and mercilessly hunts down invading microbes, dead cells, cancerous cells, and other debris. Research in this area has been hotly pursued because the success of treating AIDS, allergies, arthritis, lupus, chronic fatigue syndrome, and even organ transplants are all predicated on understanding the immune system.

Some of the more recognized warriors in the immune system include:

- Specialized "green beret" units of immunoglobulin antibodies G, A, M, E, and D, which recognize specific viral or bacterial invaders, bind to them, and self destruct.
- Captains, like T-lymphocytes, who direct the battle against the invaders
- Chemicals, such as interferon and interleukin, fired by cytotoxic T-cells to kill microbes and tumors
- Buglers to sound the "charge" (helpers) and "retreat" (suppressors) to make sure that the battle does not cause damage to your host tissues
- A tenacious crew of special forces, T-cells, to stalk down the enemy and inject a lethal mixture into the unwelcome parasite
- Pac-Man gobblers, like neutrophils, to devour invaders
- A cleanup crew, including macrophages, who rally to the site of the battle to digest any remaining debris

Figure 2C. Your Immune Defense Network

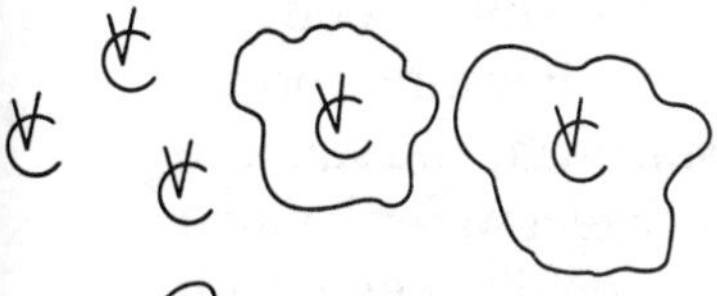

A virus or cancer cell tries to reproduce itself before the immune systems destroys it. (Two have already taken over host cells.)

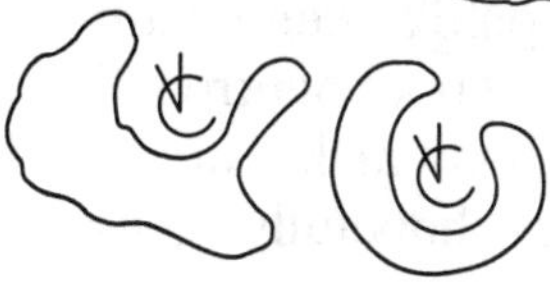

Macrophages recognize the foreign threat and begin to gobble up the invaders.

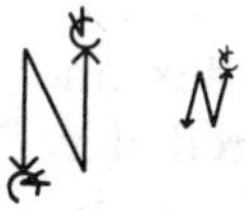

Natural killer cells are drawn into the battle when they detect the interleukins released from macrophages.

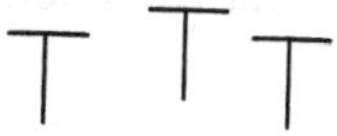

Helper T-cells are captains of the battle and will call for help from antibodies and cytotoxic T-cells.

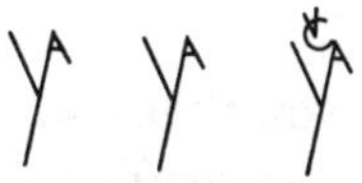

Antibodies are Y-shaped proteins that are formed by B-cells from the bone tissue. Antibodies recognize specific virus or bacteria, bind to them, and neutralize them.

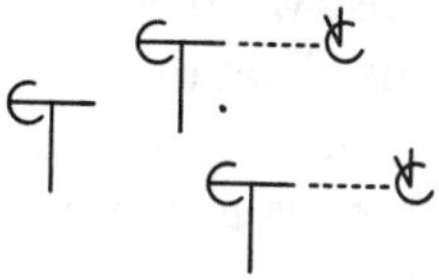

Cytotoxic T-cells fire lethal proteins at the invaders.

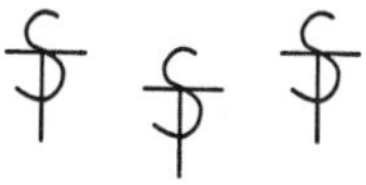

Once the battle appears to be under control, suppressor T-cells gear down the immune system to avoid host cell damage, as happens in autoimmune diseases.

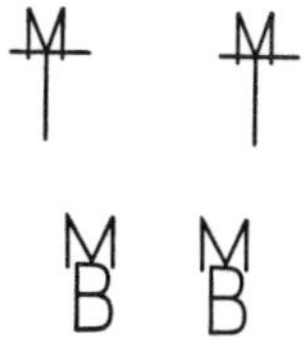

Memory T-cells and B-cells take "snapshots" of the dead invaders and then permanently circulate in the bloodstream so that, the next time, these particular invaders can be swiftly recognized and destroyed.

Neutrophils, for example, are manufactured in the bone marrow and constitute about 65 percent of your total white blood cell count. Somehow, these find out about any invading forces, adhere to the blood vessel walls near the skirmish, and squeeze through the cells of the blood vessel walls, like a water balloon being pushed through a mail slot. The neutrophils then engulf the invader, inject digestive enzymes into it, and both neutrophil and invader are destroyed. Fortunately, your body makes about 100 billion neutrophils daily, so the loss hopefully goes unnoticed.

Your immune defense department is a complex and well-orchestrated armed force that is constantly on "red alert." The job of the immune system is to mop up any cells or chemicals that are not supposed to be there. Hence, a healthy immune system can dramatically improve your defense against the effects of polluted food and water.

WITH A LITTLE HELP FROM YOUR FRIENDS

The thrust of this chapter has been to show you that you are not alone in this war against polluted food and water. Through our time-tested detoxifying and immune systems, we have an enviable capacity to neutralize many potent toxins. That doesn't mean that you should ignore the pollution issue, but it does take some of the pressure off. Later chapters will show you how to minimize your intake of poisons and maximize your own natural defense systems.

PART TWO
The Problem

CHAPTER 3

What Food Pollutants Do to Our Health

"May you make lots of money and spend it all on doctor bills."
Famous old curse

*I*n a recent public opinion poll, 3,583 Americans were asked: "Given only one choice, what is the most important thing in life: to be famous, powerful, wealthy, creative, or healthy?" The response was surprising: 1 percent wanted power and 5 percent wanted wealth, with 55 percent choosing health as their top priority in life.[1] But many Americans do not have that elusive health. As a matter of fact, a Yale professor has provided evidence that we are even less healthy than our primitive nomadic ancestors.[2] Cancer, heart disease, diabetes, osteoporosis, Alzheimer's disease, mental illness, criminality, drug abuse, infertility, and leukemia are at record high levels today while none of these conditions were common before "civilization" and its inherent chemical pollution.

Disease is usually the product of a clash between an environmental insult (such as pollution) and a genetic weakness. For example, fair-skinned people are more at risk for skin cancer when they lie in a sunny climate and are exposed to excessive sunlight, whereas those who stay in northern latitudes, where their ancestors evolved, do not usually have this problem. The sun, however, is a relatively avoidable environmental insult, while food and water pollution is unavoidable. Although some people seem to have nearly impregnable detox systems, most of us will experience a diverse array of health problems when we are exposed to excessive poisons. Has our wealth and technology brought with it a Pandora's box of ill health? Does food and water pollution have anything to do with our dismal health picture? Unless we can provide evidence that pollutants are instigating a measurable rise in health problems, all of the hysteria surrounding the food pollution issue is for naught. But irrefutable proof can be elusive.

CONCLUSIVE VERSUS CIRCUMSTANTIAL EVIDENCE.

Scientists have a tendency to be skeptics: "Prove it to me" could be their bumper stickers. If you walked into a room where one person was holding a smoking gun and there was a dead body on the ground, you would have a decent chance of proving "cause and effect," but seldom is anything in the health field so clearly defined. Seamless arguments in science are rare.

Our legal system must prove "beyond a reasonable doubt" that the suspect is guilty. The burden of proof rests on the prosecution, which is a challenge in even the most obvious cases. Unfortunately, pesticides have also been considered "innocent until proven guilty."[3] I say "unfortunately" not to deny the beauty of our constitution that protects us from unjust incarceration, but because it has taken decades and literally millions of innocent victims to accumulate the evidence necessary to start restricting pesticides. Food pollutants are indeed exacting a heavy toll on the health of Americans.

Circumstantial evidence is admissable in the courts, but rarely acceptable in health science, because it does not prove cause and effect. The largest nuclear waste processing station in the world is in northern England, and although children in the nearby town have ten times the national leukemia rate, a company spokesperson for the plant claims that no one has proved "cause and effect" linking the facility with the disease. The tobacco industry can still pay scientists to pedantically argue against the evidence that tobacco is harmful to health. It took two decades and thousands of martyrs before the Department of Defense started caring for the veterans who were poisoned by the defoliant Agent Orange (dioxin) in the jungles of Vietnam. The most industrialized and polluted regions of American also have the highest cancer rates,[4] which suggests, but does not prove, that pollutants cause cancer. Such is the problem of providing conclusive evidence that A is causing B.

CHILDREN AS CANARIES IN THE MINE

If robbers broke into your home, would you use your children as a shield against their bullets? If you were forced to walk through a minefield, would you insist that your children walked ahead of you? That's exactly the kind of thing we are doing in the game of roulette we're playing with our tainted food supply. Why are children the most vulnerable of all age groups to pollutants?

Children are growing. Growth involves an increase in cell numbers (hyperplasia) and/or an increase in cell size (hypertrophy). Hyperplasia is an intricate high-speed biological process that can easily be disrupted, just as a bullet train moving at 165 miles per hour is more subject to derailment than a slow-moving freight train. This "derailment" can lead to cancer or birth defects.

An example of the vulnerability of growing infants is found in Fetal Alcohol Syndrome and Thalidomide babies. Both alcohol and Thalidomide are drugs that are relatively harmless to adults, but even small quantities can derail the high-speed construction phases of prenatal growth. When alcohol, Thalidomide, and other poisons are consumed during pregnancy, birth defects are likely. Many food poisons can cause cancer, depressed immunity, or behavioral disorders in children; but the same poison would be relatively harmless in adults.

Some of the harm done to children can be irremedial. Lead toxicity in the developing brain can create permanently lowered intellect or behavioral disorders.[5] A major category of pesticides (organophosphates) can also permanently retard mental development.[6] Through our indiscriminate use of poisons on the food supply, we may be drastically increasing the numbers of children who will grow up to be incompetent and criminal people.

Children have immature immune and detoxification systems. Children are physically and mentally unable to defend themselves against the world. That's why they rely on their parents. Internally, children are equally immature and unprepared. The same underdeveloped immune system that allows kids to be victims of many infections will also allow more harm to be done when kids consume poisons because their detox and immune systems are equally vulnerable. Both systems become more effective as we mature, so adults are much more able to tolerate toxins than are children. A recent bill has been introduced into the California state legislature to force pesticide residues to be safe for children, not just for the more resilient adults.

Children eat more tainted food. A ten-year-old child needs about the same number of calories as an adult who weighs twice as much. An infant eats three times as much food on a body-weight basis as his or her parents, due to the extraordinary fuel requirements for growth. Therefore kids effectively eat two to three times the amount of food than the level on which the government using adult body weights calculates your "acceptable daily intake" (ADI) of poisons.

This means that kids eat more foods that contain high levels of pesticide residues. While fruit comprises only 20 percent of the adult diet, 34 percent of the preschooler's diet is fruit. The 1987 FDA food monitoring program found that half of all fruit samples had detectable levels of pesticides. (Keep in mind that normal FDA testing procedures will not detect 60 percent of the pesticides that are used.) A toddler consumes thirty-one times more apple juice and eight times more fruit than the average adult woman, while the preschooler consumes eighteen times more apple juice than Mother.[7] A preschooler consumes fourteen times more cranberries, six times more grapes, five times more apples and oranges, and four times more strawberries than the EPA estimates used to formulate the ADI.

This disproportionate consumption pattern is reflected in children's intake of pesticides, which leaves our children well outside of the already lenient EPA pesticide standards. The net effect is that toddlers consume eight times more mancozeb, fifteen times more azinphos-methyl, and eighteen times more UDMH (three of the most dangerous pesticides in use) than an adult woman. While the EPA considers one extra case of cancer in one million people to be acceptable, 238 children out of one million may get cancer just from exposure to Alar alone. If a young child were exposed to the maximum legal levels of EBDC (a carcinogenic fungicide used on one-third of our fruits and vegetables), that exposure alone might cause one thousand out of one million children to get cancer. We are literally following our children through a minefield. They are the most likely to get hurt.

Miners used to bring canaries into the mines because the more sensitive canary would die when the oxygen level was too low or toxic fume levels were too high. Are we using our children as "canaries?"

PEOPLE MOST VULNERABLE

If you gathered together a group from every strata of the American population, not everyone would have the same ability to learn baseball or recuperate from a brawl. Just as we have different external talents, we all have different internal talents. Some people are more tenacious than others, and poisons do not affect everyone in the same degree. People that are more at risk from pollutants include the following:

Infants, children, and pregnant and lactating women are all undergoing the magical but vulnerable stages of rapid cellular growth. This process can be easily derailed by chemical pollution. In some cases, the derailment is permanent, as illustrated by birth defects.

Older adults often have a compromised immune system which puts them at much greater risk for ailments from poisons in the food supply. As we age, the average person's ability to squelch tumor growth declines greatly. Another factor working against the older adult is the cumulative effect of pollutants. By age sixty-five, the average American has consumed about 100,000 pounds of food. Pesticide residues that were not a problem in a vibrant healthy thirty-five-year-old may become a serious problem in an ailing seventy-year-old who now has twice the level of accumulated poisons in their body.

Sick people *or those using drugs* often have a depressed immune or liver function, making them more exposed to the effects of food pollutants. Most foreign substances, including alcohol, tobacco, and prescription and "recreational" drugs, all blunt the immune system. Actually, lowered white blood cell count (depressed immune system) is the most obvious and common indicator of pesticide poisoning.

Genetically vulnerable people have quirks in their immune and detoxification systems which make them uniquely vulnerable to poisons. A conservative guess is that at least 2.5 percent of the population are genetically vulnerable to poisons: 5.8 million Americans who are likely to suffer from the government's "safe" levels of pesticide residues.

Psychological and physical stress has been shown to lower the immune system, which can then elevate the chance of harm from polluted foods.

Malnutrition is common in many Americans. Although we do not have widespread clinical malnutrition (i.e., scurvy, rickets, pellagra), we do have many people limping along with subclinical malnutrition. Decades of eating a marginal diet will lower the efficiency of all systems, including the immune and detoxification systems.

Those who suffer from poisoned food are very much like leaves falling from a tree in an autumn breeze. The strongly attached leaves (like healthy adults) stubbornly cling to the tree, while the poorly attached leaves (like the sick, young, old, and malnourished) fall off. As the winds get stronger and the attachments get weaker, more leaves fall. Similarly, as our tainted food and water problem worsens, there will be more needless victims of unconscionable pollution.

MAXIMUM RISK AND LEVEL OF EXPOSURE

The amount of harm done by a pollutant is directly proportional to the amount of poison being consumed—The more alcohol, the worse the hangover; the more heroin, the greater the symptoms of withdrawal. Often, the people who get the greatest exposure to a poison are those who work with poisons in agriculture or industry. These workers have, in effect, become our lab rats, getting heavy doses which allow us some insight into the symptoms that may appear at our milder intake levels.

Scientists at NIOSH (National Institute for Occupational Safety and Health) have found that chemical-plant workers who use benzene at even one-tenth the federally permissible level still have an increased risk for leukemia.[8] In another study, Shell Oil employees working around benzene had twice the normal incidence of leukemia, although a company memo told the employees that there was no current danger in these findings.[9] Benzene is a common pollutant in the water supply.

We learn a great deal about the toxicity symptoms of a pesticide from those people who get the greatest exposure: agricultural workers. Most pesticides have a dose-dependent response, which means that if you are exposed to less pesticides, you will have less symptoms, but will still be affected. The problems suffered by farm workers are quite relevant to you, since you are exposed to the same chemicals in smaller quantities; just as, though you may have had less alcohol than the heavy drinker next to you, your hangover will have similar but less acute effects.

Although life on the farm used to be synonymous with health and vitality, things have changed in our chemical age. Farmers today spray poisons from tractors and airplanes, mix the irrigation water with pesticides (called chemigation), inject gaseous

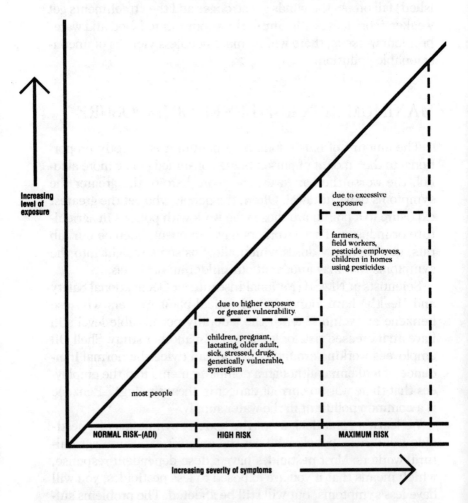

Increasing level of exposure

due to excessive exposure

farmers, field workers, pesticide employees, children in homes using pesticides

due to higher exposure or greater vulnerability

children, pregnant, lactating, older adult, sick, stressed, drugs, genetically vulnerable, synergism

most people

NORMAL RISK–(ADI)   HIGH RISK   MAXIMUM RISK

Increasing severity of symptoms

Figure 3A. Continuum of Health Effects from Poison Exposure

pesticides into the soil, drop pesticide pellets on the soil, dip their domestic animals in pesticides, and add pesticides to the feed. Commercial farming is truly hazardous work today.

Cancer. Seven of the ten states with the highest percentage of men employed in agriculture also have the highest leukemia rates.[10] In a 1986 study involving Kansas farmers, those who used certain herbicides for more than twenty days had a six-fold increase in their risk of cancer (non-Hodgkin's lymphoma).[11] The farmers who actually mixed or applied the herbicides had an eight-fold increase in cancer risk. The herbicide they were using was dioxin (Agent Orange), which was used to defoliate jungles in Vietnam until the National Academy of Sciences condemned it as being too inhumane even for warfare. Dr. Diane Courtney of the Environmental Protection Agency calls dioxin "by far the most toxic chemical known to mankind."[12] That's odd. We won't use dioxin on our enemies, but we will use it on ourselves and our food supply. Much of the herbicide runoff that does not soak into the ground ends up in the nearby water supply.

Another study found that farmers who work with pesticides have a high risk of contracting cancer,[13] and there are dozens of other studies from around the world showing that farmers and fieldworkers are at much higher risk than other people for cancer of the lymph tissue (lymphoma, non-Hodgkin's lymphoma), bone (leukemia, multiple myeloma), testicles, gastrointestinal tract, liver, pancreas, lungs, and brain.[14] Cancer risk in farming has understandably alarmed the farm state of Iowa, where three out of four Iowans would like to see less chemicals used on their fair land.[15]

You don't have to be a field hand standing out under a crop duster to be exposed to such toxic levels of pesticides. Children living near agricultural areas are also at great risk. McFarland and Earlimart, California, have five and twelve times the national average for childhood cancers. Nearby Rosamond has six times the norm for childhood cancer with five of their nine cancer cases involving rare forms of brain cancer, medullablastoma. Although investigators found twenty-three toxic waste sites containing everything from lead to dioxin near Rosamond, they could not conclusively prove a "cause and effect" link. Once again, no "smoking gun."

Children don't even have to live near a farm to be exposed to carcinogenic levels of pesticides and herbicides. Children living in homes where household and garden pesticides were used had a seven-fold increase in the risk for leukemia.[16] A study of eighty-four children with brain cancer in Baltimore showed that insecticide use in the home seriously elevated their risk.[17] Five children in one hospital in Ohio showed up with cancer of the nervous system, neuroblastoma: all five mothers of these children had been exposed to the pesticide chlordane.[18] Nine insecticide-exposed children from Mississippi, Arkansas, and Tennessee all showed up at the same hospital, all with colon cancer, which is very rare in children.[19] Investigators looked at 309 cases of childhood leukemia versus 618 healthy controls, which showed there was a major increase in the leukemia risk if the mother of the victim worked in either agriculture or the chemical industry.[20]

Infertility. In one study, men who worked around pesticides were found to have a 600 percent increase in the incidence of sterility. Two of the sterile workers had not been near the soil fumigant DBCP for over nine years, and both had fathered children prior to their exposure to DBCP—which has now contaminated over 2,400 wells in California alone.

Birth defects. In a California study, children born to agricultural workers had a thirteen-fold increase in the rate of deformed limbs.[21] McFarland's cancer rate is accompanied by a much higher incidence for low birth weight babies and fetal mortality.[22] Although the organophosphate insecticides that attack the nervous system have not been shown to cause birth defects in lab animals, they do retard the growth and longevity of the offspring of exposed animals.[23] Most of the 42 million pounds of herbicides used annually on U.S. farms are quite teratogenic (causing birth defects).[24] Admiral Zumwalt was the military commander who ordered the use of the herbicide dioxin to defoliate the jungles of

Vietnam. Zumwalt's son was in a gun boat that was sprayed with dioxin. Zumwalt's son developed cancer, and his grandson had serious birth defects.

The miscarriage rate for female farm workers is seven times the national average. Each year over 344,000 pounds of the pesticide captan, similar in structure to Thalidomide, are used on grapes. The offspring of farm workers and Thalidomide babies have something in common: a high risk for being born without arms or legs.

Not all studies have found a link between pesticide exposure and high incidence of birth defects, but this may be due to the fact that most defective fetuses will spontaneously abort in a miscarriage. (Female farm workers in the U.S. and India suffer a much higher than normal miscarriage rate.)[25]

Nervous disorders. A major category of pesticides (organophosphates) is derived from the internationally banned nerve gas developed during World War I, yet less than 10 percent of all pesticides have been tested for their effect on the nervous system (a pesticide fails the test only if it induces paralysis in chickens). Twelve pesticide workers in Texas were found with nerve disorders that were totally caused by their pesticide exposure: Four had multiple sclerosis (an untreatable condition in which the "insulation" is being dissolved off the nerve cells), two had psychiatric problems, and three had encephalitis (inflammation of the brain).

Many pesticides induce a commonly diagnosed long term paralysis called pesticide-induced delayed neurotoxicity (PIDN). Leptophos is an organophosphate that was used on Egyptian cotton fields, and which killed thousands of nearby water buffalo. If a pesticide can kill a one-ton water buffalo, what can it do to a 30-pound child, or a 200-pound adult?

These same "nerve gas" pesticides have been shown to induce anxiety, difficulty in concentrating, memory deficits, and other more subtle problems.[26] A follow-up study of farm workers who were occupationally poisoned by organophosphates found that 33 of the 117 people still had visual disturbances and other problems three years after exposure. One mental patient who was administered organophosphates in the pre-human-rights days of the 1950s permanently lapsed into psychosis. A 1964 report from the Federal Aviation Administration showed that crop duster pilots exhibited reduced flying performance, memory loss, depression, and even symptoms of schizophrenia up to a year afterward.[27]

General ill health. Richard Wiles of the National Academy of Sciences has evidence that the nation's 472,000 field workers are in serious jeopardy from exposure to farm chemicals.[28] Of the Texas farm workers surveyed, 78 percent had chronic skin rashes, 56 percent had liver and kidney abnormalities, and 54 percent suffered from problems in their chest cavity. More than 300,000 farm workers are made ill each year from pesticide exposure with the rate doubling over the last ten years, probably due to increased dosages being used to combat pesticide-resistance bugs. In California alone, there are about 3,000 reported cases annually of pesticide-poisoned agricultural workers, with another 15,000 cases in urban areas.[29] Remember, many of these field workers are migrants who do not seek medical attention unless their health problem is very serious.

State health officials are desperately trying to decide on a "safe" waiting period before agricultural workers can reenter a sprayed field. The pesticide Zolone, which is so dangerous that it may be banned soon, was so potent that University of California experts recommended a thirty-five-day waiting period, while state officials set the wait at seven days. Seventy-eight farm workers then had to be hospitalized after entering a "safe" field.

General symptoms of acute pesticide poisoning may include headache, blurred vision, nausea and vomiting, pulmonary edema (fluid in the lungs), changes in heart rate, muscle weakness, respiratory paralysis, mental confusion, convulsions, coma, and possibly death. These symptoms, suffered by the residents of Bhopal, India, in 1984 when a chemical plant exploded and blew toxins on the town, are also experienced by at least 300,000 American farm workers each year. Milder versions of these symptoms are, no doubt, suffered by millions of American consumers each year due to excessive pesticide residues on the food supply.

HIGH RISK AND EXPOSURE

This category includes people who consume more than the ADI for pesticides or other toxins. Victims of this category often think they are eating a healthy diet high in fish and fresh produce, but tainted food can make an allegedly healthy diet quite dangerous.

Picnics over the Fourth of July weekend in 1985 took on a macabre aspect as 1,350 people on the west coast were poisoned with watermelon that contained Aldicarb. The victims' symptoms included nausea, diarrhea, seizures, blurred vision, and irregular heartbeat. There were several puzzling questions in this episode:

> How did the Aldicarb get on the watermelon? Aldicarb is a mite killer that cannot be legally applied to watermelon.
>
> Why didn't the FDA's screening procedure protect the public from these ten million tainted melons?
>
> After lab tests were run on the confiscated melons, the most provocative question of all was raised. Since the Aldicarb residue levels were well below the residue amount that could be detected in routine FDA screening tests, what other harm is being done by "acceptable" or "undetectable" levels of pesticides?

The answers to these and many other pesticide-related questions are blowing in the wind, or lying in some hospital bed.

A five-year study in Florida found that regions which were heavily sprayed with pesticides had a higher incidence of birth defects among the region's *residents,* not just the agricultural workers. California has been battling the medfly insect with aerial sprayings of malathion in urban areas. A study conducted by the University of Southern California and the Kaiser Research Institute found an increase in birth defects among women who were doused in the San Francisco Bay area, but the increase was not "statistically significant." Once again, no "smoking gun."

NORMAL RISK AND EXPOSURE: ACCEPTABLE DAILY INTAKE

Does a small amount of pollution do just a little harm? Or no harm at all? Or considerable harm in a minority of vulnerable people? Or does a small intake of poison over several decades become cumulative, thus causing considerable impact on health in later years? No one really knows. Most U.S. adults normally fall into this category.

We know that heavy exposure to food pollution causes blatant problems, but does this mean that less exposure is acceptable? I think not. You will see later that many statistics show health in America to be deteriorating, and that many of our health problems are milder versions of the symptoms found in the "Maximum Exposure" section just discussed. Food pollution may be a major contributing factor to many puzzling ailments in America.

A PROFILE OF AMERICAN HEALTH

Some experts will paint a rosy portrait of American health, with reassuring statistics that the death rate from heart disease and cancer are beginning to decline. All is well in Camelot, they will tell you. However, there are some deeply disturbing health statistics that many experts feel are related to our pollution issue.

Before the Great Depression (1929) Americans spent 3.5 percent of our gross national product (GNP) on health care. After Medicare was firmly established (1975), we were spending 9.3 percent of our GNP on health care. In 1989, Americans spent $600 billion, or 11.5 percent of our GNP, on health care.[30] By comparison, most other advanced nations spend about 3 to 6 percent of their GNP on health care, usually with better overall health results.

Among the twenty industrialized nations who keep the best records, the U.S. has the worst infant mortality rate, being twice as high as Japan's.[31] Meanwhile, such underdeveloped nations as Mexico, Sri Lanka, Venezuela, and the Philippines also have a higher neonatal survival rate than the U.S.[32]

One-third of our children and 98 percent of all older adults are taking prescription medicines. Fifty-eight million Americans have high blood pressure, with 39 million of these people being

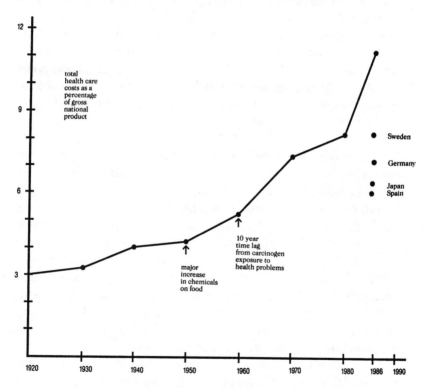

Figure 3B. Skyrocketing Health Care Costs (source: Universal Almanac, p.217, Andrews & McMeel, Kansas City, 1989)

under age sixty-five.[33] In spite of massive expenditures on health care for the elderly, the life expectancy of a sixty-five-year-old man is still the same as it was at the turn of the century.[34] Both in 1990 and today, that sixty-five-year-old man is expected to live another thirteen years.

Statistically speaking, the "average" American is overweight; has six colds per year; wears glasses; is continuously plagued with constipation, lethargy, and mild depression; gets dentures by age forty-five; gets sick sometime in their sixties; and dies sometime in their seventies of heart disease or cancer. Also, 97 percent of all Americans have measurable levels of organochlorine pesticides (like DDT) in their fatty tissue.[35] That is "normal." That is also unenviable.

We have among the highest rates in the world for many "diseases of civilization," those rare in underdeveloped countries. No doubt there are complex factors that create a disease. Food pollution is not the only cause. Yet much of our major health problems as well as some of our puzzling rare diseases can be linked to food and water pollution.

Cancer. Some experts will tell you that the death rate from certain types of cancer is falling in America and that we finally have this ogre under control. Not so, says Harvard researcher Dr. John Bailar, who presents convincing statistics that we have "lost the war" against cancer.[36] Even after adjusting for the aging population, Dr. Bailar finds that cancer incidence has increased by 8.5 percent, while mortality rate has increased by 8.7 percent since 1962. About 985,000 new cancer cases each year are discovered, with 477,000 deaths. Of the 235 million Americans living right now, 74 million will eventually get cancer.[37] Cancer now accounts for 22 percent of all deaths in the U.S., with the annual medical bill for cancer running at $23 billion.[38]

The epidemic proportions of breast and colon cancer in America have been closely linked with our pollution intake.[39] According to the most conservative estimate by the National Cancer Institute, what we eat or don't eat causes one-third of all cancer in this country. Other estimates have predicted that proper nutrition could prevent 90 percent of all cancer; which means that somewhere between 325,000 and 886,000 cases each year could be prevented simply by following the precepts in this book.

Dr. Samuel Epstein, a noted research physician from the University of Illinois and Harvard Medical School, has provided substantial evidence that our cancer epidemic is largely due to chemical pollution.[40] One gets the queasy feeling that the nearly one million cancer patients each year in this country are considered unavoidable "sacrificial lambs" by the powers that be in politics, agriculture, and industry.

Bladder cancer has been linked to the consumption of nitrates (from fertilizer runoff) in the water supply.[41] Chlorine in the water supply also substantially elevates the risk for cancer.[42] One out of four bladder cancer cases in nonsmokers is probably caused by chlorine from drinking water.[43] Major studies in Chile, England, Colombia, and Canada have found a definite link between the consumption of nitrates and cancer of the stomach.[44] Globally, the intake of aflatoxins, which are a deadly chemical from a plant mold, have been strongly linked to liver cancer.

Since the advent of the chemical age after World War II, most developed countries around the world have experienced a gradual increase in the incidence of most types of cancer,[45] while cancer in many parts of Africa and Asia is low; which gives us a clue that cancer is not an unavoidable fact of life. Although some experts claim that our rising tide of cancer is due to the aging American population, who are more vulnerable, figure 3C shows you that age alone does not account for our horrendous cancer rate.

The National Academy of Sciences says that up to one million Americans per generation will get cancer from pesticide exposure alone.[46] The EPA admits that sixty-six of the three-hundred food-approved pesticides are likely carcinogens and has rated food pesticide residues as the number three environmental risk for cancer, just behind toxic chemicals in the workplace and radon in the home.

Some agricultural and industrial states, like New Jersey, Ohio,

Pennsylvania, and Texas, are suffering from a disproportionately high cancer rate.[47] For example, an average of 202 out of 100,000 Americans each year die from cancer, but New Jersey has a cancer death rate of 227, which is nearly twice that of the most cancer-free state, Utah. Not surprisingly, New Jersey is

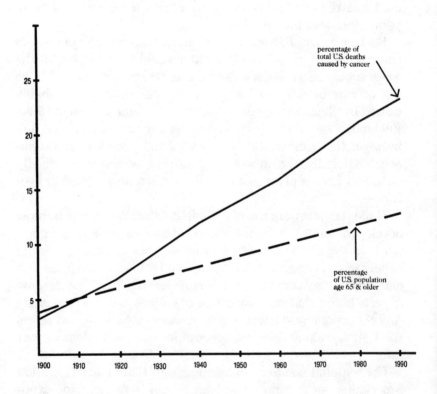

Figure 3C. Increasing Incidence of Cancer
(source: Universal Almanac, p.225, Andrews & McMeel, Kansas City, 1989)

home to ten of the fifty worst toxic waste sites in the country. You don't get cancer just by living near carcinogens. You have to eat, drink, and breathe the pollutants for them to do any damage.

Since most experts agree that cancer risk increases with age,[48] then why is cancer the number two cause of death in American children?[49] Although the *death rate* from leukemia has dropped since 1960, the *incidence* of childhood leukemia has continued to "mysteriously" climb since World War II.[50] Of the 26,900 Americans who will get leukemia this year, 24,700 will be adults, 2,200 will be children,and a combined total of 18,100 will die. Most experts agree that the majority of leukemia is caused by exposure to radiation and chemical carcinogens in the food, air, and water supply.

Scientists know that hormones and steroids increase the risk for cancer. Recently, there has been a flurry of evidence showing that growth-hormone therapy in children markedly increases the risk for leukemia.[51] Although the amount of growth hormones used to stimulate animal growth is supposed to be low, there is very little monitoring of this hormone use by the FDA.

Since it takes years or decades of exposure to a carcinogen to bring about cancer, our cancer rate will probably continue to escalate until about twenty years *after* we begin to clean up our pollution problem.

Mental illness. The brain was once thought to be a sturdy organ that functioned well in spite of low nutrient intake or pollution exposure. That is no longer considered true. It may be quite the contrary; that the brain is the first organ to experience symptoms of malnutrition or pollution toxicity. The same pesticides that were based on nerve gas and designed to attack the nervous systems of insects will cause behavioral disorders in humans.[52] The major pesticide groups of organophosphates and carbamates inhibit the transmission of a very important chemical in the brain, acetylcholine, which can lead to irritability, dizziness, tremors, and convulsions.[53] Organochlorines (like dioxin and DDT) also affect the nervous system.

While 90 percent of all fumigants are considered carcinogenic, most of them can also cause nervous-system depression. Although less than 10 percent of pesticides have been tested on animals for their effect on the nervous system, only paralysis is considered a "negative reaction." Most experiments find that younger animals are more sensitive to neurotoxic effects than older animals; yet older mature chickens are the most common test animal for neurotoxicity in pesticides. At least 17 percent of American preschoolers, or three million children, are exposed to levels of pesticide residues that can cause nerve damage.

The President's Commission on Mental Health estimated in 1979 that one out of four people passing you on the street was suffering from some form of mental illness.[54] More recently, a survey of 18,500 American adults conducted by the National Institute of Mental Health found that one-third of all Americans suffer from some form of mental illness, which puts mental illness above high blood pressure for being the most common disorder in this country. There was a 400 percent increase in episodes of mental health treatment from 1955 to 1977.[55] Mental illness causes more hospital days than any other condition in America.

Hyperactivity, a condition unknown in 1950, now afflicts 10 to 20 percent of our school children.[56] Since 1950, the teenage suicide rate has increased by 500 percent. There are 15 million alcoholics, 50 million tobacco addicts, and at least 20 million other drug addicts in American. In certain metropolitan areas, up to one out of three babies are born as cocaine addicts. Nineteen million Americans suffer from severe anxiety, another 14 million are plagued with severe depression, and at least 7 million are schizophrenic.

Each year 12 million children are arrested for non-traffic crimes, like rape, robbery, and murder. On any given day in America, over one million adults are on probation or parole from prison, while another 600,000 rot in jail. We cannot build our prisons fast enough. There aren't enough teachers in special education to meet the needs of the millions of learning handicapped American children.

None of these numbers can include the inestimable rate of wife and child abuse in this country, nor can numbers accurately depict the tears, pain, suffering, and wasted potential of millions of people due to mental illness.

Alzheimer's disease is a frightening and untreatable condition in which the mind deteriorates. Alzheimer's is not only the most common form of senility in America's older adults, but it is also appearing in increasing numbers among people thirty to fifty years of age. A new study finds that Alzheimer's is twice as common as experts had estimated, with 3 percent of people aged sixty-five to seventy-four, and half of all Americans over age eighty-five, having the disease.[57] Aluminum, a major ingredient in some antacid medications and also added as a humectant (drying agent) in most dry packaged food in America, is found in high amounts in the brains of Alzheimer's victims.[58] Alzheimer's may also be due to lipid peroxidation, or "rusting," of the fatty tissue in the brain, which can be slowed with adequate intake of antioxidants.

Food additives and naturally occurring food ingredients can cause problems with the nervous system. Red wine contains tyramines and phenolic compounds that can cause migraine headaches in some individuals.[59] Headaches are on the increase, with many people having ten to twelve headaches per year at a nationwide cost, in lost work time and medical help, of $10 billion. There are at least 500,000 Americans who experience serious asthma attacks when consuming the food additive sulfite, used as a preservative on many produce items. Sulfites probably affect both the muscular and nervous system in some people. A researcher at the Massachusetts Institute of Technology has found that a high intake of the artificial sweetener aspartame can cause everything from headaches to epileptic-type seizures in some sensitive individuals.[60]

Lead. Of all the pollution issues discussed throughout this book, lead is perhaps the most devastating. A researcher at Texas A&M University has found that lab animals who are exposed to typical American levels of lead poisoning experience stress, irritability, jangled nerves—and turn to alcohol for comfort.[61] Perhaps our greatest pollution problem (heavy metals) could be linked to our high rate of alcoholism and drug addiction. Cadmium-exposed test animals preferred alcohol over water, while the cadmium-free control group preferred water over alcohol. Cadmium, which has been shown to cause hypertension in test animals, is found in polluted water and in trace amounts in canned food.

A recent report from the U.S. Public Health Service finds that between three and four million American children are suffering developmental lags and reduced intelligence due to lead poisoning from our food, air, and water. Over 400,000 babies are born each year with their nervous systems already damaged by lead poisoning. Forty percent of U.S. children have lead levels in their blood that predict intellect stunting, and children with higher levels of lead are four times more likely to have IQ scores below 80 (retarded) and seven times more likely to suffer learning disorders, like hyperactivity[62] (while 5 percent of low-lead children were geniuses—IQ above 125—none of the high-lead kids were geniuses.) And lead stunts physical growth, too.[63]

The better we understand lead, the more fearsome it becomes. Prior to 1981, the upper limit of acceptable lead levels in the blood was considered to be 100 micrograms per deciliter (mcg/dl). Although the Center for Disease Control now considers 30 mcg/dl to be the level at which mental impairment probably begins, most scientists agree that toxicity in children starts well below 25 mcg/dl,[64] with the newest data showing that 4 mcg/dl could cause mental impairment. Eighty-eight percent of all U.S. children and 77 percent of American adults have blood lead levels at or above 10 mcg/dl, which the EPA experts consider a likely "threshold" level for toxicity symptoms.[65]

Lead toxicity can erode emotions, behavior (including hyperactivity and criminality),[66] intellect, reaction time, kidney functions,[67] hearing,[68] vitamin D metabolism (resulting in calcium and magnesium disorders), iron status, muscle tone, create anemia and interfere with various amino acids and enzymes. Let's ponder just one of these points: The greater the lead levels in the body, the worse the hearing ability in children. Psychologists have found that criminals and poor school performers have a disproportionately high rate of hearing problems, which leads to problems in school, which often times triggers a life of crime.

Although lead is a particularly nasty poison in the nervous system of young humans, lead also affects other ages and other parts of the body. Lead is a major contributor to high blood pressure in adults, behavioral disorders in all ages, and even criminal acts.

Where do we get our lead? From food, air, and water. Forty million Americans now drink tap water that is too high in lead, according to new standards set by the EPA. By 1985, lead levels in the air from leaded gas exhaust had dropped by 80 percent to a mere 20,000 metric tons per year. Yet this level is still high enough to instigate hypertension in 123,000 people each year.

Children absorb two to five times more lead than adults. Iron or zinc deficiencies, which are common in growing children, can accelerate the effects of lead toxicity. The body has a difficult time purging itself of lead. Chelation therapy can greatly accelerate lead excretion. Lead pollution has truly become a plague upon our land, and especially our children.

Hypertension. High blood pressure is found in 58 million Americans and causes the death of 149,000 people annually. Millions of others are paralyzed or disabled through strokes.

Arthritis. Up to fifty million Americans have some degree of arthritis, which is 250 percent higher than the world average. Twenty million Americans must take medication for arthritis, and four million are disabled by it.[69] One common cause of arthritis is food allergies, which may be caused by an unhealthy immune system.[70]

Heart disease. Researchers compared the health statistics in two similar villages in Hungary, with the primary difference being that one village used more pesticides than the other. Residents of the high-pesticide village were more likely to have circulatory, respiratory, or stomach disease; *and* they had a higher suicide rate.[71] Fifteen million Americans have heart disease and 973,000 each year die from it. Although fat, fiber, stress, smoking, and exercise are major risk factors in heart disease, food allergies have also been found to induce heart disease.[72]

Allergies and Immune Problems. Just two decades ago, the subject of allergies was consider quackery or hypochondria. Today at least 8 percent[73] and possibly up to 24 percent of Americans suffer from food allergies.[74] A food allergy is basically caused by an erratic immune system that begins attacking the host's tissue, and it is well known that most xenobiotics (poisons) affect the immune system.

I have helped many people through food allergy counseling. Some of these people are allergic to so many foods that you wonder how they could still be alive. Pollutants could be a major factor in provoking this abnormal immune response, as many physicians have found great success with patients by minimizing their toxin intake, which eliminates food allergies and clears up a disparate collection of symptoms.[75] Although pesticides are not tested for their impact on the immune system in order to achieve EPA approval, some recent studies find that pesticides *do* damage certain components of the immune system.[76]

Food allergies can cause major behavioral changes, migraine headaches, and a long list of seemingly unrelated conditions. Some health problems may be due to a domino effect: poisons alter the normal functions of the immune system, which precipitates allergies, which cause all sorts of problems.

Reproductive failure . . . Silent Nursery. Joseph Bellina, M.D., Ph.D., of the prestigious Omega Clinic in New Orleans, finds that 16 to 20 percent of American couples are infertile.[77] Dr. Bellina feels that pollution is taking a staggering toll on the fertility of Americans. The rate of infertility among women age twenty to twenty-four has tripled in the last twenty years.[78] The sperm count from young healthy men has declined dramatically in the past forty years. Recall that Rachel Carson in her classic *Silent Spring* forewarned of reproductive failure in birds due to pesticide exposure.

Since 1970, there has been a mild (2.7 percent) to significant

(17.5 percent) rise in the incidence of most birth defects, especially involving heart defects.[79] About a year after a major toxic spill was reported in the San Francisco Bay area, a nearby hospital experienced a fifteen-fold rise in the birth of infants with a rare heart defect.[80] Newborn infants who weigh less than 2,500 grams, or about 5 ½ pounds, have a much higher risk for death and disease. While the rate of slightly smaller babies (less than 2,500 grams) has been improving, the incidence of very small babies (less than 1,500 grams) has been increasing since 1970.

Gastrointestinal problems. Food-borne infections cause 69 million to 275 million cases of GI problems each year in America, according to FDA microbiologists. The U.S. Center for Disease Control estimates that nine thousand Americans die each year from food-borne infections.[81] Actually, many experts predict that our widespread and unnecessary use of antibiotics in food will eventually incite an epidemic that could make all other issues in this book pale by comparison.

Other problems. Nationwide, fungal infections have tripled in the last five years. Tuberculosis is on the upswing after decades of dormancy. In May of 1988, researchers found hundreds of dead seals washed ashore in northern European coastal areas. The seals had died from a herpes virus that was likely induced by pollution in the seals' water. Epstein-Barr syndrome (also called Chronic Fatigue Syndrome) is a disease caused by a virus that, for some reason, depresses the immune system so that it cannot purge the body of a pesky virus. The virus creates constant fatigue and other debilitating problems, and is on the rise in this country.

Acquired Immune Deficiency Syndrome (AIDS) is a relative newcomer to the medical world. First diagnosed in 1980, only about one-third of those people who are exposed to the HIV virus actually contract AIDS. We know that drug users, who blunt their immune systems through poison intake, are much more at risk for AIDS. Legionnaire's Disease first struck a convention of

American Legion members in Philadelphia in 1976. Twenty nine of the 200 people affected died.

Lupus erythematosus is an immune disorder in which the connective tissue—the glue that holds the body together—begins to mysteriously decay. Lupus is on the incline and no expert can tell you what causes it or how to treat it. Is it merely coincidence that these bizarre conditions surfaced in the most polluted era in history?

There are a number of freakish diseases that may relate to food pollution. Over a seven-year period in Puerto Rico, over three thousand children experienced premature and abnormal sexual development.[82] Seventeen-month-old female infants would begin to menstruate, while five-year-old girls were developing breasts. The physicians treating these cases found that the cure was to take meat and poultry out of the diet. Although hormones in meat and poultry are supposed to be low risk due to the trace amounts used, ignorant or greedy animal growers probably instigated this epidemic.

Then there are exotic nerve diseases with no known cause or cure that may be related to long term ingestion of food and water poisons. Lou Gehrig was a famous baseball player raised in New York City. His mother often fed him fish that was caught in the nearby Hudson River, which even in the earlier part of this century was an obvious cesspool. Gehrig died in 1941 from a strange condition in which the nerve tissue in the muscle, spinal cord, and brain region just starts to deteriorate for no known reason. The disease is now called amyotrophic lateral sclerosis, or Lou Gehrig disease, and still baffles medical researchers. Could decades of consuming poisons erupt into this unexplainable condition?

None of this sounds like Camelot to me. Granted, some of our problems are due to stress. But was it less stressful in America during the Civil War or the Great Depression? Some of our problems may be due to the erosion of the family structure. But which comes first: eroding mental health or eroding family structure?

Obviously, something is very wrong with the health of our very rich nation as we continue to wallow in our high-tech poisons. Some of the studies detailed in this chapter provide conclusive evidence against food and water pollutants. However, most of the evidence is circumstantial. The burden of proof rests on the defenseless public. Oftentimes, the proof doesn't gather until the bodies begin to fall. For many people, it is already too late.

CHAPTER 4

Pesticides: The Fallen Angel

*I*n the beginning, it seemed like pesticides must have been delivered to mankind by angels who drifted away on gossamer wings. Prior to World War II, crop losses averaged 30 percent worldwide and 18 percent in America, but pesticides which then consisted of arsenic, heavy metal sprays, nicotine (from the tobacco plant), and cyanide—all of which are expensive and extremely lethal to humans—were rarely used.

Then came "the gift." Although DDT (dichloro-diphenyl-trichloroethane) was discovered in 1874, its insecticidal properties were not recognized until 1939. Dr. Paul Müller of Switzerland was awarded the Nobel prize in 1948 for his DDT work.[1] DDT was instantly hailed as a cure for disease, pestilence, and famine from crop loss. Soldiers coming home from World War II were fumigated with DDT, killing the lice without any apparent harm to the men, and DDT prevented millions of deaths from lice-borne typhus following the war and virtually eliminated malaria from many parts of the world.

Farmers and health officials saw DDT and its chemical cousins (chlorinated hydrocarbons) as "magic bullets" against pestilence and disease. U.S. production of pesticides increased from less than 0.5 million pounds in 1951 to 1.5 billion pounds in 1980.[2] Farmers began reporting record harvests with each succeeding year, and America quickly became the most agriculturally productive nation in the history of the world. Farmers, consisting of only 2 percent of the population, could support the remaining 98 percent in sublime style.

America grew enough food last year to feed us well, get half of us overweight, waste enough food to feed another 50 million people daily, ship enough food overseas to somewhat offset our horrendous trade imbalance, and keep a one-year supply of food in government surplus bins—all while paying many farmers subsidies not to grow food. Although it was large-scale mechanized farming that was more responsible for our record harvest, pesticides were given some of the credit.

Then reality set in. Although pesticide use has increased tenfold in the last four decades, crop loss from pests has more than doubled.[3] American farmers now lose 37 percent of their crop to pests.[4] Initially the bugs were devastated by DDT but they quickly developed a chemical resistance. Recall the chapter on "tough humans" and the chemical detox systems humans possess, and consider that we are amateurs at detoxification when compared to many insects and pests. By 1963 the World Health Organization's twenty-one-year $2-billion spraying program had worked so well that there were only seventeen cases of malaria in Sri Lanka (then Ceylon) that year—however, once chemical resistance had begun, malaria incidence bolted up to more than one million cases in Sri Lanka in 1968.[5] According to the World Resources Institute, fifty-one of the sixty malaria-carrying mosquito species are now immune to DDT.[6] Score: bugs 1, humans 0.

In 1976 only seven species of insects were resistant to all five categories of pesticides. Now there are seventeen insect species, including house flies, cockroaches, and mosquitoes, that are resistant to nearly any chemical thrown at them. From 1970 to 1980 the number of insect species that were chemically resistant jumped from 224 to 428. There are also 150 plant pathogens and 50 weed species that are resistant to pesticides and herbicides. The ultimate chemically resistant bug is the Colorado potato beetle, which is now immune to any chemical sprayed on it. It gargles with DDT, bathes in dioxin, and mainlines EDB. You cannot kill it with chemicals. Enter the chemist's nightmare.

BULLETPROOF BUGS

Imagine spraying a field with a pesticide. Of the one million bugs that are hit, all but one die. That one bug is a genetic mutant, in the sense that it has some abnormal biochemistry that can detoxify DDT. Obviously, this once-useless trait has now become an enviable survival skill. The bug passes on its unique characteristic of chemical resistance to its many offspring and, since the chemically-resistant bug does not have to compete for its food supply, since all of its buddies are now dead, reproduction accelerates at a staggering rate. You now have a situation where the bugs are relatively immune to the poisons heaped upon them, while the pesticides keep killing the friendly predatory creatures that normally would eat the bugs. Big mistake.

Insects have a life span ranging from weeks to months and they have hundreds to thousands of offspring: compare that to humans who have two to four children in a seventy-year life span. Scientists have speculated that if conditions were ideal for the bugs and if only two insects (one male, one female) from each species were left on the planet earth, it would take about one month for the bugs to breed and eat to their current level of trillions of insects. Ironically, the genetic roll of the dice heavily favors the insects developing chemical resistance while humans suffer from their own poisons.

There is a certain amount of time required for insects to develop chemical resistance by continuously rolling the genetic dice—kind of like winning the lottery—but it took the bugs only 6.3 years to beat DDT. Now 450 species of insects are resistant to DDT. Fungicides are no exception. In three to five years, a fungus species can beat a fungicide. Not only does a chemically-resistant bug become immune to one pesticide, but it holds a distinct advantage in developing some means of detoxifying the next chemical used on it. Hence, we are unintentionally encouraging the survival of "bulletproof bugs" that can develop chemical immunity from pesticides faster than the chemist can create new poisons. Most insects today can beat a pesticide in one season. Game, set, and match to the bugs.

Meanwhile, the chemists have been falling behind. Between 1980 and 1985, no new pesticides were introduced at all. One

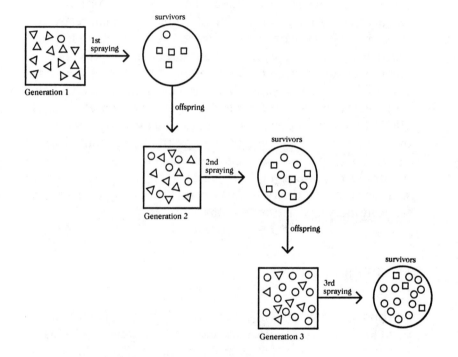

○ = *pesticide resistant insect*
△ = *not pesticide resistant*
□ = *not pesticide resistant but avoided pesticide*

Figure 4A. How Pesticides Increase the Numbers of Pesticide-Resistant Insects

reason is that costs have soared; the new group of pesticides (pyrethroids) cost one hundred times more than DDT to develop, while the most effective of our current pesticides (deltamethrin) cost more than 1,300 times as much. Research, testing, and approval for a new pesticide costs about $20 million to $45 million today.

The immediate solution, according to the pesticide salesmen, is to use more pesticides. There are numerous examples of how this strategy can backfire. The cotton industry in Central America got a major boost with pesticides until chemical resistance set in: in 1950, only two species needed pesticide control; within ten years, there were eight different insect species that needed chemical control, because crop-destroying bugs that were once controlled by natural predators were now unmolested. Initially, there were five applications per growing season of pesticides. By 1960, it took twenty-eight pesticide applications to stem the tide of insect crop damage, and by then pesticides accounted for 50 percent of all production costs. In some of the worst cotton scenarios, farmers are using sixty pesticide applications per season with as much as thirty to forty pounds applied per acre. The fields literally squish from poisons.

NO PROFIT LEFT

Although a few strident environmentalists were preaching the need for efficient cars decades ago, it wasn't until the OPEC oil nations tripled the price of crude oil in 1972 that Americans began thinking about economy cars. Change in America often must be motivated by the true engine of our capitalistic system: money.

Enter the ultimate threat to the survival of pesticides: cost effectiveness. The farmer can no longer afford to drench the bugs in poisons. Dr. Robert Metcalf of the University of Illinois, a recognized authority on pesticides, has summarized how pesticides may allow a farmer to evolve from a subsistence farmer to a vendor on the world marketplace, but end up unable to feed his family.

1. *Subsistence phase.* Yields are low. The farmer cannot enter the world marketplace. Natural controls and luck dictate the harvest. Rarely is IPM practiced in Third World farming.
2. *Exploitation phase.* Initial pesticide use results in massive increase in harvests. Pesticides are used whether needed or not.
3. *Crisis phase.* Insects develop pesticide resistance. Insects that were once harmless now enter the arena as adversaries. Higher doses are needed, which greatly increases production costs.
4. *No longer profitable* to grow the crop due to pesticide cost. Pesticide residues exceed the legal limit. Soil is saturated with pesticides. Biological controls are gone. Collapse of the program is imminent.
5. *Integrated control phase.* Utilize ecological factors, including integrated pest management, that is, low-input sustainable agriculture or organic farming.[7]

Most American farmers are somewhere between phases 3 and 4. Some have already reached phase 4, as exemplified in the fertile Imperial Valley, near San Diego. The local farmers wanted to fully exploit their cheap irrigation water and free sunshine to produce three separate cotton harvests each year. They immediately encountered problems with a pink bollworm common to cotton crops, and brought in an agricultural expert from the University of California to give them advice. He told them to rotate crops and allow the land to lie fallow every so often. They cordially thanked him, escorted him to the county line, and began blasting the bugs with every conceivable pesticide. Twenty years later, the farmers surrendered to the bugs and followed the advice of the agricultural expert, because farming was no longer cost effective. The only people making money on farming at that point were the pesticide manufactures.

POISONING NATURE

In 1962, a biologist by the name of Rachel Carson published her well documented indictment of pesticides, *Silent Spring*. She had found that pesticides had a pernicious effect on all forms of life, and that DDT was causing death and infertility among many creatures. Both Carson and her bold publisher were threatened with lawsuits and called Communists by the main manufacturer of DDT, and it was to be another ten years before the use of DDT was restricted. A 1984 study by the Natural Resources Defense Council found that DDT was still the most commonly detected pesticide residue on fresh produce; meaning that either DDT persists in the soil even longer than expected—or that it is still being used. Bird and wildlife populations in many farming areas have been decimated by pesticides.

Many pesticides do not break down easily and will linger for decades in the soil. U.S. soil absorbs 100 million pounds annually of the pesticide toxaphene. In a test plot of land, scientists found that thirty-four months after ceasing any toxaphene application, 66 percent of the original concentration was still in the soil, and there was a significant reduction in the turnip crop in this field. New data shows us that the soil is not a sieve allowing pesticides to filter through, but more of a chemical sponge, storing much of the pesticides applied.[8] These soil pesticides eventually leach into drinking water, contaminate food crops, and reduce harvests. Although BHC, DDT, and dieldrin are extremely toxic pesticides that have been banned in the U.S. for over a decade, these pesticides are still found on many fresh produce items. The only way to purge the soil of their presence is to wait five to ten years for gradual chemical decomposition, or to scoop up the soil and incinerate the pesticides at 1500 degrees F., at a cost of $500 to $1000 per cubic meter of soil.

Although we dump over 1.2 billion pounds of pesticides annually on U.S. soil, less than half of the chemicals even hit the right *field,* and less than 2 percent of applied pesticides actually hit the bugs. Pesticides can easily drift fifty miles from the application site, with one reported case of a Texas dust storm eventually dropping pesticides in Ohio.[9] About 25 percent of all pesticides in this country are applied with crop dusters. Since the wind takes away much of the pesticide from aerial drops, and even a good pilot must be fifty feet off the ground, pesticide applications from planes will add an extra 30 percent to the amount of pesticides that are actually needed. Much of this ends up on the neighbor's property, or in the drinking water (pesticides are the number one cause of drinking water contamination). Our current misuse of pesticides is like blasting away with a shotgun at a fly in your house—you are much more likely to hurt a family member than the fly.

BIOACCUMULATION

Not only do various pesticides harm "nontarget" populations, like birds, but pesticides accumulate in the environment until they are eaten by humans. Pesticide residues can now be detected in every crevice on this planet, from all human fatty tissue and all human milk to the polar ice caps.

In Clear Lake, California, health officials applied DDT at a concentration of 20 parts per billion to the lake to control the larvae of gnats, which bothered residents and affected tourism. Within a few months, the larger fish in the lake had DDT concentrations 10,000 times higher (now at 2 million ppb) than the amount originally applied to the lake.

Bioaccumulation occurs as algae absorb some of the DDT from the water. Then small fish, minnow, and insects eat the algae, which are eaten by smaller fish, which are eaten by larger fish. Since most pesticides are stored in fatty tissue, each rung on this biological ladder has a higher concentration of poisons. The largest carnivorous fish, favorites on the dinner table, literally become chemical reservoirs of DDT.

Bioaccumulation occurs on land as well as in the water. The plants that are sprayed with pesticides are then fed to grazing animals, which are fed to humans—a literal example of "as you sow, so shall you reap."

THE COST OF PESTICIDES

We spend $4.1 billion per year to buy pesticides; and only $1.2 billion to do a marginal job of monitoring well water for pesticide residue, with the social and environmental cost of pesticides running about $1 billion per year. Since our health care costs are at $600 billion per year, and if only 1 percent (a very conservative estimate) of our health woes are due to pesticides, then they are costing us $6 billion annually. No one can put a monetary value on the loss of human and animal life due to pesticide exposure.

THE MYTH OF THE SELECTIVE POISON

Allegedly, pesticides are supposed to kill "target organisms" like bugs. Actually, most forms of life share common pathways of biochemistry. Insects extract energy from food and transmit nerve impulses in similar ways to humans. Therefore, a poison targeted for the bugs is potentially lethal to humans, too. Chemotherapy for cancer is another "selective toxin" which attacks host and tumor cells with nearly equal toxicity. Many pesticides are as harmful to "nontarget populations" as they are to "target" populations, yet humans lack the chemical resistance of bugs, so we are actually worse off than insects.

A WHOLE LOT OF POISON

Our production of pesticides and herbicides is mind boggling. In 1936 there were thirty pesticides registered for use in the U.S.—by 1971, there were nine hundred. The world now produces 4.5 billion pounds of pesticides per year, which figures out to slightly less than one pound per person per year. Of the seven million chemicals currently registered with the American Chemical Society, over 15,000 are pesticides, not all of which are approved for use in the U.S.[10] Today we have 1,200 active pesticide ingredients that are formulated into 35,000 different EPA-registered pesticide products. There are an additional one thousand "inert" ingredients used to dilute and assist in spraying pesticides. Although the EPA admits that at least one hundred of these approved inert ingredients may cause cancer, skin rashes, or central nervous disorders, "inerts" are unregulated by the EPA or FDA.

Of the 1.1 billion pounds of pesticides produced in the U.S. in 1983, 36 percent was exported. In that same year, the U.S. used over 2.45 billion pounds of pesticides, of which herbicides and rot retardants on wood comprise about 40 percent of the total world supply. Much of these pesticides are used in greenhouses, to fumigate domestic homes, and to treat wood. Even so, 370 million acres of American land, or about 16 percent of our country, are being sprayed with pesticides, with an average of 3.7 pounds of pesticides per acre.[11] Many of the pesticides manufactured in this country are banned from use in the U.S., but are sold to other countries, who often use them on food crops that are sold back to us. Since DDT is banned, the FDA no longer tests produce for DDT, even though it is produced in this country and could easily, though illegally, be obtained.

While 80 percent of all pesticides used in America are for agriculture, the remaining 20 percent are for home and garden use. Annual sales figures are $4.1 billion for pesticides and $2 billion for herbicides. That's a lot of poison we are dumping onto this fragile earth. It might be easier to swallow if we were getting results, but the truth is that crop loss in Third World countries where pesticides are relatively unavailable is around 33 percent, while drenching our land in poison has our crop-loss figure at 37 percent.

ALTERNATIVES: INTEGRATED PEST MANAGEMENT (IPM)

Although pesticides initially seemed like the perfect quick fix, they soon fell from grace. Is there an alternative? Earl Butz, former secretary of agriculture, once said that we could cut back pesticide use as soon as we decide which fifty million Americans are going to starve. Not so. Actually, a recent 450-page technical manual by the National Academy of Sciences has found that IPM is not just a *viable* alternative to chemical farming, but a *preferable* alternative. A 1979 report by the Office of Technology Assessment of the U.S. Congress concluded that biological controls on a national scale could reduce pesticide use by 75 percent and cut harvest loss by 50 percent. For example, red scale is a blight on citrus crops that costs $200 per acre to chemically control but only $20 per acre to biologically control.

One of the earliest examples of biological controls (Low Input Sustainable Agriculture, or LISA) occurred in 1888 when California imported the vedalia lady beetle to feed on the cottony-cushion scale, a pest that threatened to wipe out the state's citrus crop. Since then, the cottony-cushion scale has remained innocuous, making only minor comebacks when pesticides were overused. In the 1940s, California introduced a $750,000 program using a beetle (Chrysolina) to control a weed that was toxic to cattle. Savings from the program have been more than $100 million, a 133-fold return on investment. Because of the extreme care that scientists have used in screening natural enemies before release, the environmental cost of IPM has been near zero.

At least 327 natural enemies have been successfully introduced throughout the world to alleviate pest problems that could not be treated with chemical poisoning. IPM is cost effective: according to a report prepared by the World Bank, the benefit-to-cost ratio of IPM is about 100 to 1. According to a Cornell University study, the benefit-to-cost ratio of pesticides is about 4 to 1.

There are many examples of IPM that are being used around the U.S. Soybean farmers release a parasitic wasp to control the devastation of the Mexican bean beetle—the wasps kill the beetles and the harsh winter kills the wasps. The soybean thrives without bathing in poison. In pilot programs, IPM cut pesticide use on cotton by 88 percent, on sorghum by 41 percent, and on peanuts by 81 percent. Cook County (Chicago), Illinois, has been using IPM since 1977, with great success and lowered costs, to keep down mosquito populations. Marin County, California, found that IPM cut spraying by 90 percent and reduced insect numbers.

In many instances, IPM is the only hope. Chemical cotton farming has produced twenty-five species of cotton pests in thirty-six different countries that are chemically resistant. Even after drenching boll weevils and pink bollworms in poison, harvested cotton acreage in a Texas region declined from 105,000 in 1970 to only 50,000 by 1975. Five years after Texas A&M University developed an IPM approach, the harvested acreage of cotton was up to 236,500. The farmers net benefit was $29 million annually from higher profits and lower production costs.

There are other scientific methods of reducing crop loss to pests without resorting to pesticides: rotating crops, fallow fields every few years, planting mixed varieties of crops (genetic variations can slow the onslaught of insects), using chemical sprays only when pests are most vulnerable, and using special plants with host resistance. There are many IPM manuals that can help encourage a scientific approach to sustainable agriculture. Some resources are listed in the appendix. For more on IPM farming, see the "organic" section in the chapter on lowering your intake of toxins.

In spite of all these encouraging results, less than 5 percent of our nation's 100,000 farms use IPM. The chemical treadmill is difficult to dismount. Farmers have a low-profit transition period of one to three years that they must endure in order to make the switch from chemical to IPM farming. Annually, the federal government spends $25 billion on farm subsidies and another $600 million on agriculture research, yet the budget for IPM/LISA farming in 1989 was a paltry $4.5 *million*. Although the EPA, USDA, and National Science Foundation jointly funded a seventeen-university IPM study in the 1970s, the 1980s saw these programs cut. Without some type of government tax incentive or subsidy, it will be difficult for farmers to convert to IPM. Even if you disregard the cost to nature and human health, IPM is the *only* sustainable form of agriculture: excessive pesticide use is a suicidal dead-end road.

Daniel Webster made a deal with the Devil, for a limited period of prosperity in return for his soul. Pesticides have been like a deal with the devil. Hopefully, we can extract ourselves from this deal, like Daniel Webster did.

CHAPTER 5
Our Widespread Pollution

*O*ur food pollution problem is nothing more than a reflection of our overall pollution problem. Since we recklessly spill garbage into our land, air, and water, why should food be spared such a fate? This chapter shows that we need to have an overall change in attitude in order to clean up our food pollution problem.

Pollution is not new. Humans have an extensive track record of being rather cavalier about their waste products. Lead pollution from lead-lined water ducts may have accelerated the downfall of the Roman Empire. Migratory American Indians used to pack up their wigwams and move on when "evil spirits" infested their village, usually due to fecal contamination of drinking water. In eighteenth-century London, three million inhabitants tossed their garbage and excrement out the window onto the narrow unpaved streets below; the river Thames became a thick swamp of human excrement and garbage. A suffocating cloud of coal smoke hung over most large European and American cities throughout the industrial revolution. The Mad Hatter syndrome, caricatured in Lewis Carroll's *Alice's Adventures in Wonderland,* was caused by mercury poisoning from rubbing mercury into wool felt to make hats stand up.

Pollution is not new. We have the same attitude about our garbage as we have had for centuries. But the high-tech effluvia of the twentieth century has elevated the stakes considerably. Pesticides, PCB, and acid rain are more subtle but probably more devastating pollutants than coal dust in the air and green foamy rivers.

Pollution relates intimately to the theme of safe eating because our food is contaminated with a variety of agents. Some of them are voluntarily applied in agriculture, like pesticides, fungicides and herbicides; some are used in rearing animals, like antibiotics and hormones; some are used in food processing, like food additives; some are unfortunate by-products of poor food storage and hygiene, like aflatoxins and salmonella; and some exist as a result of our ubiquitous twentieth-century pollution, like benzene, PCB, and lead. This chapter explains the nature and severity of the problem and what you can do about it.

A LIGHT AT THE END OF THE TUNNEL?

On the surface it may seem like the pollution crisis is beginning to abate:

- the air quality has begun to improve in many American cities[1]
- both the Columbia River and Lake Erie have returned from the "dead"
- environmental awareness has spread from the Birkenstock crowd to the wing tips, high heels, and tennis shoes crowd
- the residues of DDT and PCBs are beginning to dwindle in human tissue
- Congress has passed several superfund cleanup acts.

All of these indicators could mean we are through the worst of it. But we're not.

Since World War II, 50,000 new chemicals have been introduced into our environment. Each year, American dumps 90 billion pounds of toxic waste into our 55,000 toxic waste sites around the country, and up to 90 percent, or 81 billion pounds, of this is being irresponsibly dumped onto the land and water.[2] If you add in air pollution, then roughly six hundred pounds of toxic waste are being produced annually for every man, woman, and child in this country. On a daily basis, the U.S. spews 32 billion gallons of toxic chemicals and sewage into the sea.[3] Of the seven million chemicals currently registered with the American Chemical Society, there are 60,000 in active use in the U.S. and another 6,000 new chemicals introduced weekly.[4] It costs the national toxicology program $1.8 million to thoroughly test one chemical for safety (and half of the 175 chemicals tested so far cause cancer).

In 1975, my retiring physics professor told our class: "The solution to pollution is dilution." A clever rhyme, but a dangerous misconception that has lived for decades among scientists. People kept thinking that if you dumped the toxin into a massive river, or the ocean, or the atmosphere, then it would become diluted enough that it could not harm anyone. The theory could apply if a thousand people lived on earth, but not with five billion people and the colossal amounts of toxins being produced. Eventually the toxins reached saturation point.

There is a 3,000-square-mile "dead zone" located off the mouth of the Mississippi River, probably due to pollutant runoff from the agricultural and industrial midwest. In June of 1988, five hundred dead fish mysteriously washed ashore in the east San Francisco Bay region; not-so-surprisingly, in April of 1989 officials discovered an illegal toxic dumping site with 75,000 gallons perched on a river that empties into the east San Francisco Bay. In the summer of 1987, 750 dolphins died on the shores of New Jersey, their skin peeling off in sheets and their breathing labored as they neared death. The only possible explanation for such an unusual epidemic is pollution. In May of 1988, researchers counted hundreds of dead seals washed ashore in north European waters; they had died of a herpes virus that does not affect seals unless their immune system is devastated with pollutants. The river Rhine in Europe was defiled in November of 1986 with 30 tons of agricultural chemicals and 440 pounds of mercury compounds that were accidentally spilled into the river at Basel, Switzerland, by Sandoz Pharmaceuticals.[5] Experts fear that the upper Rhine is now biologically dead.

In April of 1989, departing from their normally staid bureaucratic jargon, the EPA released figures on pollution in America, calling our output of toxins: "staggering." It included 9.7 billion pounds of toxins dumped into streams and other bodies of water, 2.7 billion pounds into the air, and 3.2 billion pounds injected deep into the ground. The Surgeon General in 1980 called our toxic mess "an environmental emergency," while the EPA called it "a ticking time bomb primed to go off."

Scientists now find evidence of a "toxic wind," in which the vapors from volatile chemicals are picked up by major weather fronts and carried into the jet stream where they can be evenly dispersed throughout the earth. Furans and dioxin, two of industry's more notorious toxins, have been found in the mud of a small pristine lake near the upper reaches of Lake Superior.[6] Although these chemicals could not possibly have been physically dumped there, the wind has brought them from other spots in the country. So our food pollution problem is no more than the tip of the iceberg regarding our overall pollution problem. We need a change of heart for our food, water, and earth to be healthy again.

PCB: CHEMICAL WARFARE ON OURSELVES

Just one example will help to illustrate how serious and widespread the pollution problem is and how indiscriminant garbage disposal inevitably affects human health through the food and water supply. PCBs (polychlorinated biphenyls) were discovered in 1927 by Theodore Swann, who then sold the process to the Monsanto company. Initially, the list of PCB advantages would have made a carnival huckster blush with envy. PCB conducts heat well, refuses to dissolve in water, burns only at very high temperatures, and resists corrosive chemicals. Because of these valuable properties, it was used in everything from transformers, power capacitors, adhesives, washable wall coverings, upholstering material, flameproofers, and even early versions of carbonless copy paper. However, PCB is much more toxic and persistent in the environment than DDT, chlordane, and dieldrin. Less than 10 percent of ingested PCB is excreted, which is remarkable since the body is usually quite adept at expelling poisons. When burned, PCB becomes even more lethal.

Since 1930, 1.25 billion pounds of the stuff have been manufactured for use in this country. About half of that is still in use. Ninety percent of the remaining half was dumped into bays and landfill sites. Due to its strong affinity to fat soluble particles, PCB lodges in fatty tissue in food and humans.

The symptoms of acute PCB toxicity were discovered in 1968 when residents of the Japanese island Kyushu unwittingly ate large amounts of PCB-tainted rice oil. About 1,300 people complained of rashes, headaches, loss of libido, nausea, diarrhea, hair loss, fatigue, numbness, and menstrual disturbances—and these people were only briefly exposed to high doses of PCB. Of the thirteen children born to these PCB-exposed people, one was stillborn, four were small for gestational age, ten had unusually dark skin pigmentation, four had pigmented gums, nine had visual problems (conjunctivitus), and eight had neonatal jaundice.[7] The incidence of neonatal jaundice has gone up considerably in recent years, for no explained reason. Years later, the infants of this disaster who were breastfed showed measurable impairment in their nerve and muscle abilities, such as coordination and intellect.[8]

Researchers at the University of Wisconsin fed monkeys PCB levels that would approximate the upper end of human consumption. The offspring of these monkeys were developmentally impaired and some died at an early age. Upon autopsy, Dr. James Allen found many abnormalities in the lymph system, bone marrow, thymus, and other areas.[9]

Although the toxic effects of PCB were observed as early as

1943, when people who worked around PCB developed skin lesions and liver damage, it was not until the 1976 Toxic Substances Control Act that PCB was banned from further production in this country. Today, every person and every corner on earth, including the polar ice caps, contains measurable levels of PCB.

In adults PCB may cause cancer and elevated fat levels in the blood,[10] yet the real hazard is to the newborn infant. The body regards breast milk as an avenue of excretion for pollutants, especially fat soluble ones like PCB. The average level of PCB in human milk is seven times higher than the amount permitted in cow's milk by the FDA, and it is about ten times what the FDA recommends as an acceptable daily intake of PCB for infants. All mother's milk now contains PCB.[11]

What to do? Do not eat more than one fish per year from the tainted waters of the Great Lakes and northeastern U.S. If a woman is exposed to considerable amounts of PCB, she should not breast-feed since the risks outweigh the benefits. Women should not lose weight during pregnancy, since mobilizing fat stores brings PCB rushing out of adipose tissue and into the bloodstream to affect the developing fetus. Most importantly, minimize fat intake, which is where PCB hides.

HOW MUCH WILL IT COST TO CLEAN UP OUR MESS?

There are 378,000 waste sites that may require immediate action, says Congress. Proposed federal cleanup bills are $10 billion for the next five years,[12] but that may just keep the situation from getting out of control. One toxic dump site near Los Angeles (Stringfellow) has an EPA-estimated cleanup bill of $812 million.[13] The Office of Technology Assessment, a research arm of Congress, has counted more than 10,000 hazardous waste sites that pose a serious threat to public health and should be given top priority in cleanup efforts. The bill? $100 billion, or about $1000 per U.S. household. We also have a calamity of nuclear wastes ready to spew forth from our fifteen major nuclear defense facilities. Under the guise of "defending national security" the departments of Energy and Defense have violated federal laws for the past ten years and dumped untold amounts of radioactive and toxic wastes into rivers and crude landfill sites. The bill to clean up that mess is another $100 billion. We have 30,000 tons of lethal nerve gas that will cost $3.5 billion to incinerate.[14] Just to overhaul existing municipal sewage treatment plants will cost over $76 billion. Since Congress passed the Clean Water Act of 1977, federal, state, and local agencies have spent over $100 billion to upgrade existing sewage treatment plants. Yet, according to the EPA, another $400 billion will have to be spent by the year 2000 in order to have all cities comply with the 1977 law.[15]

This pollution ends up in our food and water supply. North America's largest estuary, the Chesapeake Bay, has experienced a significant drop in fish and oyster harvests, with PCB and heavy metals being detected in the remaining fish. Carp caught near St. Louis contained four times the FDA's "action" level of chlordane, a potent pesticide. Health officials warn that fish caught in the Great Lakes, the world's largest collection of fresh water, are unsafe for consumption due to PCB levels.

Pollutants can linger for a very long time. Even though DDT and dieldrin were banned over fifteen years ago, they are still detected on fresh produce.[16] Asbestos, lead, and other heavy metals are immortal pollutants. Once in the food and water supply, they are nearly impossible to remove, except by humans who consume them and store them in their tissues.

WHO ARE THE POLLUTERS?

Everyone. Although 75 percent of pesticides are used in agriculture, over half a billion pounds of pesticides and herbicides are used in American homes. Herbicide use on lawns is rampant. Of hazardous industrial wastes, 34 percent are organic chemicals (crude oil and its many by-products) and 38 percent are primary metals (lead, zinc, arsenic).

Not only are industry, agriculture, and private citizens at fault; a recent report from the Government Accounting Office found that the worst polluter of all is the federal government. [17] This study examined 150 major U.S. facilities and found that 10 percent of industrial plants were polluters, while 20 percent of federal facilities were polluters. The study went on to say that 40 percent of all violating federal facilities were noncompliant for more than a year. The GAO also criticized the EPA for not taking effective measures against anyone, especially the government itself. How can we expect industry to comply with the vague laws on the books when the government itself is the worst offender of all?

WHO IS GOING TO CLEAN IT UP?

Even when the people demand a cleaner environment, as voters have in many states, the cleanup efforts are sometimes astonishingly slow. An overwhelming two-thirds of California voters told the state officials to "clean up" in Proposition 65 passed in 1986. While California had 300 toxic waste sites listed as "critical," state officials have only cleaned up 43 of the 126 sites they had promised by a 1988 deadline, in spite of tripling the staff and doubling their budget. [18]

You can't expect city governments to be prosecuting polluters when cities are among the worst offenders. The Boston sewage-treatment facility is euphemistically called a "primary" system, which means that it dumps raw sewage into their own harbor. Just a few years ago, a bold pair of Marines vowed to swim the length of the Mississippi River—within a week, both had to be hospitalized for toxin exposure. New York City's fourteen sewage-treatment facilities still don't meet EPA standards, and New York Harbor is a rich stew of sewage, chemical, and industrial contaminants.

We are doing more than wreaking havoc on our delicate planet: we are poisoning ourselves and making the future for our children look grim indeed. Pollutants are persistent; it may take decades or centuries to clean up some of our major aquifers. Pollutants have a delayed reaction in the body; it takes years to decades for major problems like cancer to surface once we are exposed to toxins.

GOOD NEWS

We *are* changing our ways. New public opinion polls show that Americans have given environmental issues top priority, ranking them above crime, drugs, AIDS, the economy, war, and communism.[19] Robert Stavins, an environmental economist at Harvard University, argues that "the era of identifying smokestack villains has passed." We have discovered the enemy—and it is us. And we are changing.

Recycling has become a popular issue. Eighty percent of Seattle homes participate in the county recycling program. Manufactures and consumers are looking at alternatives to the 16 billion disposable diapers that we bury in landfill sites each year. There are many heartwarming stories in the newspapers of people who have shouldered the burden and become unpaid "lifeguards" of the environment. Against all odds, the once-doomed Chesapeake ospreys are making a comeback.[20] Pollsters now predict that elections in the 1990s will be strongly based on ecology issues. Now that we have recognized the need for responsible disposal of our wastes, we are en route toward a cleaner food and water supply.

CHAPTER 6

Should We Call It "Government In Action" or "Government Inaction"?

*I*f you think your food supply is dangerous today, then take a ride back in a time machine to a Chicago meat packing plant circa 1900. Working conditions for these newly arrived immigrants were atrocious. So, too, was the hygiene and quality control of meat production. Hair, rat turds, diseased carcasses, bones, and other unmentionables went into the production of sausage, bologna, and liverwurst. Hygiene was an unpracticed luxury. Upton Sinclair described this tale of horror in his book, *The Jungle*, in an attempt to bring improved working conditions for the laborers. Instead, his readers became outraged at the poor sanitation in their meat production. The ruckus raised in response to this book led to the passage of the 1906 Pure Food and Drug Act, an impotent but important first law to safeguard our food supply.

The purpose of this chapter is to show that the government does make some efforts to inspect foods and maintain a certain minimal standard of safety. The American food supply is certainly the most bountiful in the world—even the most remote corners of the United States now have fresh produce on a year round basis—and we also have one of the safest food supplies in the world. However, being one of the best in a field of mediocrity and incompetence is no great honor, like boasting that you are the best ice skater in Fiji. In Tibet, you will find the "chef" chopping food on a wooden doorstep next to the yak dung; in the Philippines, a common fishing method is to poison entire lagoons with arsenic, so the fish are laden with poison.

Throughout much of the underdeveloped nations, the farmer's market sells produce right next to open containers of pesticides, which have no labels nor any warnings. Farmers bring the pesticides home in food containers. In Iraq, the water supply is often tainted with poisons and feces. In Central and South America, DDT and other American-banned pesticides are liberally applied to many crops with no standards of safety and no worker protection. Keep in mind that, in spite of the many failings of the federal government to protect your food and water supply, it could be much worse if you lived in another country or another era.

EVEN THE GOVERNMENT ADMITS THAT OUR SYSTEM NEEDS IMPROVEMENT

While we have become used to the continuous criticism that private and consumer groups heap on the government, it is not often that the government criticizes itself. A report issued by the Government Accounting Office, a watchdog agency of Congress, stated ". . . we believe the Federal Government can do a better job in protecting the public from potentially hazardous pesticides in the food it consumes . . . some foods coming from various countries are not being tested for any pesticides at all."[1]

It is always easier to be the critic than the doer; but the government track record of protecting our food and water supply borders on criminal negligence. Recall the scene in *The Wizard of Oz* where Dorothy and her friends are cowering before the flaming figure of the mighty wizard, and Toto the dog pulls back the curtain to reveal the flimflam professor. His response? "Pay no attention to that man behind the curtain!" The government is asking for an equal blindness on our part. You will see the strengths and weaknesses of our governmental protection in the coming pages.

THE GOOD OLD DAYS?

"The prime essence of the good old days is a poor memory."

Mark Twain

Up until 1906, anyone could sell anything to anyone else with anything in the container and no label of ingredients, and with any claims they cared to make. "Take no prisoners" marketing, you might call it. Cattle with anthrax, tuberculosis, and cancer ended up on the dinner table. Meat was laced with formaldehyde (embalming fluid) and boric acid (used in cockroach poison today) as "preservatives." Coumarin, the principle artificial vanilla flavor used then, was so effective at blocking normal blood clotting that it is now medically used as an anticoagulant for heart disease patients. Alum is now used medically to constrict wounds and also is full of aluminum which can cause Alzheimer's disease; it was once used to whiten old and decaying flour.[2] Lead and copper were used to pigment food. "Good-old-fashioned" root beer was flavored with safrole from the sassafras root, which was later shown to cause liver cancer. Tuberculosis victims were sold elixirs of chloroform (once used as an anesthetic) and alcohol with the vague promises of a cure. Although the 1906 law had no enforceable "teeth," it did serve fair warning to the charlatans that things were changing.

Were it not for food decay and predatory bugs, food safety would be a non-subject. But food does rot and, if left unchecked, bugs will devour a good portion of the harvest. Until this century, there was no refrigeration and only primitive means of preserving food through drying, smoking, and salting. In 1492, Columbus really set out in search of food additives. The Spice Islands of the Pacific held a treasure that royalty was willing to pay handsomely for: something to hide the nauseating flavor of rotting food. I bring up this issue for two important reasons which may bring some limited comfort to you:

1. Food safety has always been a problem for humans.
2. Since our ancestors have been eating questionable food for centuries, we have developed a limited

ability to tolerate poisons and bacterial infections in the food.

Governmental food inspection programs. Governments have a short and rather mediocre track record at protecting the public from contaminated food and water. Probably the earliest effort at safeguarding the food supply came from Judaic law, found in the 3,700-year-old Torah, which outlined methods for humane slaughter of animals and inspection for "broken" or defective organs.[3] The great civilizations of Rome and Athens both conducted government-authorized inspections of the wine-making process. Since no one inspected their food supply, you can tell where their priorities lay. By the thirteenth century, King Henry III of England specified punishments for adulteration of foodstuffs. That law was later extended in 1634 with penalties for "any musty or corrupted meal, which may be to the hurte and infection of man's body." By 1830, two significant books had been published in Europe on the subject of food contamination.

By 1902, American food was highly suspect. There was no refrigeration, no laws, few scruples, and, with chemistry and food technology at a primitive level, some very inappropriate substances were used in food. Dr. John Wiley, director of the Department of Agriculture's Bureau of Chemistry, undertook the rudimentary beginnings of toxicology. He gathered a dozen healthy young male "volunteers" to serve as his poison squad. The men were fed large quantities of various common food additives: borax, benzoic acid, formaldehyde, salicylates (aspirin), and sulfites, with notes being made regarding changes in the men's appetite and digestion. Around the same time, England conducted a study using children as their test subjects. Vomiting, skin irritations, and total hair loss were among the symptoms reported. Lab animals soon replaced the students and children as test subjects. The science of modern toxicology was born. Then the real guessing began.

GOVERNMENT BUREAUS THAT INSPECT OUR FOOD AND WATER SUPPLY

The Food and Drug Administration (FDA) was created with the 1906 Food, Drug, and Cosmetics Act. The FDA is charged with monitoring the safety of food additives, fresh produce, and other foods. Meat and poultry inspection is under the jurisdiction of the Department of Agriculture (USDA) in the Food Safety Inspection Service (FSIS).[4]

The Environmental Protection Agency (EPA) was created in 1970 by Congress and charged with making sure that the public comes to no harm from the use of pesticides. That responsibility has always been and still is impossible. The EPA also monitors the water supply throughout the nation.

There are other federal agencies that work tangentially to protect the food supply, but these are the big three. Truth in advertising is regulated by both the Federal Trade Commission (FTC) and the U.S. Postal Inspector. Considering their tight budget and limited workforce, these agencies do a decent job of safeguarding the food and water supply. Although our food supply is definitely tainted and risky, it could be much worse without the basic skeleton of governmental protection.

FOOD INSPECTION PROGRAM

Americans consume over 290 billion pounds of food annually, with 25 percent of our fruit and 6 percent of our vegetables being imported into the country. Lab samples are taken from about 1 percent of all produce shipments. Between 1979 and 1985, the FDA analyzed over 100,000 different produce samples and found that about 4 percent contained pesticide residues above acceptable levels. Imported produce had twice the violation rate (6.1 percent) in comparison to domestic produce (2.9 percent). However, the standard laboratory tests used by the FDA do not detect over 60 percent of all pesticides used. Using more advanced lab methods, the Natural Resources Defense Council conducted a survey of pesticide residue on fresh produce sold in the San Francisco area and found that 44 percent of the seventy-one fruits and vegetables tested contained nineteen different pesticides. Although the majority of these residues were at levels below EPA tolerances, it does point out the pervasiveness of pesticide residues in our fresh produce.

Allegedly, even your meat and poultry is monitored for pesticide residues; but, unfortunately, the FDA does not use "state of the art" lab techniques to inspect for pesticides. Of the roughly 400 approved pesticides, 227 are considered "potential risks" by the FSIS. Of these 227 potentially harmful pesticides, only 40 (18 %) can be detected by the multiresidue lab tests that are used. Of the ten most lethal pesticides (including carcinogenic fungicides like mancozeb) that FSIS would like to monitor, *none* can be detected by the lab tests used.[5] Even when meat shipments were found to be violating federal laws, no investigation ensued in 79 percent of the cases. Time lags are so extensive that usually the questionable food items have already been consumed.

FEDERAL LAWS TO PROTECT THE FOOD AND WATER SUPPLY

1906: Food, Drug, and Cosmetics Act: established guidelines for safe food, drugs, cosmetics, additives, and medical devices. Amended or updated in 1938, 1958, 1960, 1962, and 1968.

1946: Agricultural Marketing Act: provides for quality grading and inspection of fish; authority for this law was later transferred to the Department of Commerce in 1971. Fish inspection was and still is a voluntary program.

1948: Federal Insecticide, Fungicide, and Rodenticide Act (FIFRA): gave FDA authority over pesticides. Amended in 1972, 1975, 1978, and 1988.

1958: Food Additives Amendment: includes the famous Delaney (from Congressman Delaney of New York) clause, section 409: "No additive shall be deemed to be safe if it is found to induce cancer when ingested by man or animal." After several lawsuits and petitions, the FDA later decided to "reinterpret" this clause to allow for more lenient use of carcinogens, such as pesticides. Hence, food additives must meet more stringent guidelines than pesticides. This amendment also contained the GRAS list (Generally Regarded as Safe) of food additives which were "grandfathered" in without any safety studies required. This list grew from an initial two hundred in 1958 to six hundred by 1969.

1960: Color Additives Amendment: requires that all color additives be shown to be safe before their use is permitted.

1967: Federal Meat Inspection Act: gave USDA authority over food, feed, color additives, and pesticide residues.

1968: Poultry Products Inspection Act: same as above.

1969: Concern over the safety of cyclamates led to a review of the GRAS list.[6] A gathering of elite scientists (Federation of American Societies for Experimental Biology) was asked to review the data on the GRAS list and make recommendations. Of the 415 additives reviewed, 305 were considered safe and the remaining 110 were considered to need further study. No additives were banned via this review.

1970: Egg Products Inspection Act: same as above.

1970: Creation of EPA. In charge of ensuring clean air, water, and some aspects of food purity, such as pesticide safety.

1974: Safe Drinking Water Act: gives EPA authority over drinking water contaminants. Amended in

1986 with goals set down to accelerate the glacier-like progress thus far shown by the EPA, described by Senator Durenberger of Minnesota as "miserable, discouraging, disturbing . . ."[7] (See "Lethargy" section below.)

1988: FIFRA seriously amended: assesses chemical companies $150 million over nine years (a half-cent tax on every dollar of pesticide sales) to safety test the many pesticides which have no such standards. No longer forces the the EPA to buy any banned pesticides, which was impossible on the EPA's budget. Authorizes $110 million in federal funds to be spent over the next nine years to review the safety of pesticides.

There have also been a number of environmental protection laws passed which were supposed to dovetail with food and water protection.

1952: Dangerous Cargo Act: Department of Transportation and U.S. Coast Guard to oversee the management of shipping toxic substances by water.

1954: Atomic Energy Act: the National Research Council asked to advise on radioactive substances.

1960: Federal Hazardous Substances Act: regulates toxic household products. Amended in 1981.

1970: Occupational Safety and Health Act: created the Occupational Safety and Health Administration (OSHA) to oversee toxic chemicals in the workplace. OSHA was basically neutered throughout the 1980s.

1970: Poison Prevention Packaging Act: regulates the packaging of hazardous household products. Amended 1981.

1970: Clean Air Act: regulates air pollution. Ignored by both government and industry. New, similar, law passed in 1989 with twenty-year plan (through year 2009) for cleaning up the air.

1972: Hazardous Materials Transportation Act.

1972: Clean Water Act: amended 1977 and 1978.

1972: Marine Protection, Research, and Sanctuaries: regulates ocean dumping.

1972: Consumer Product Safety Act: regulates hazardous consumer products.

1973: Lead Based Paint Poison Prevention Act: prevents the use of lead-based paint in federally assisted housing projects. Amended 1976.

1976: Resource Conservation and Recovery Act: controls solid waste, including hazardous wastes.

1976: Toxic Substances Control Act: regulates hazardous chemicals.

1986: Superfund Amendments: controls hazardous substances, pollutants, and contaminants at waste sites.

1989: Clean Air Act: twenty-year plan to clean up the air.

As you can see, we have no shortage of laws and government bureaus to protect us; but we do have a serious lack of compliance with the laws. Many of these laws are purposely written to give them no "teeth." For instance, food processors do not have to notify the FDA when they find their own food products to be adulterated. The FDA does not have the authority of subpoena, to compel the production of documents or witnesses, nor does it have embargo or detainment authority. Even when the FDA finds a shipment of produce with excessive levels of pesticide residues, the product usually has been sold by then and no action is taken against the offending party. Many of these "consumer protection" laws have loopholes that you could drive an RV through. Sometimes, good laws are just ignored, such as the Delaney clause and the Clean Air Act.

In most instances the legislators mean well. They hear a public outcry and want to appease their constituents; but they also are attentive to the needs of big business lobbyists and campaign contributors.[8] End result: a stalemate leading to another study to placate the voters, or an impotent law being written. Actually, the main progress in the cleanup of our air, water, and food supply has occurred when the consumers and voters have become enraged at the injustice and gathered forces for action. The 1988 public uproar over Alar on apples is a good example of something that should have been done long ago, but was tabled by lethargic bureaucracies until the people acted in unison.

To be fair, even the minimal effort made by the government has been helpful. Lead pollution in the air has been cut by 96 percent over the past sixteen years due to laws taking lead out of gasoline and paint products.[9] Dangerous chemicals like PCB and DDT are beginning to subside in most areas. Several risky pesticides have been banned for use in this country. But lest you become too confident in this progress, let's show you the incredible series of guesses and mistakes used to provide "acceptable daily intake" levels of pollutants and pesticides. Fasten your seat belt.

HOW DOES A PESTICIDE BECOME APPROVED?

Generally, an independent laboratory paid by the pesticide manufacturer will expose groups of fifty male and fifty female lab animals to varying levels of the pesticide over the course of two years. At the end of that time, animal autopsies are conducted by pathologists (doctors experienced in detecting changes in tissue).

New pesticides must pass the following tests:

- chronic toxicity tests (long term low intake) in two different species of animals
- oncogenic tests (cancer) in two species
- teratogenic tests (birth defects) in two species
- reproductive toxicity tests in one specie
- mutagenicity (changes of cells) in three species

Once these studies have been conducted, the company must then supply the EPA with the obligatory mountain of documentation regarding:

- chemistry of the pesticide
- expected quantity of residues present in food based on field trials
- lab analytical procedures used for obtaining residue data
- residues in animal feed derived from crop by-products
- toxicity data on parent compound, any major impurities, degradation products, or metabolites.[10]

More realistically, about 80 percent of federally approved pesticides have not been fully tested according to law. Most pesticides are in use thanks to the "grandfather" clause of 1986, meaning: "If it hasn't been blatantly toxic by now, then continue its use."

It is becoming increasingly difficult and expensive for a pesticide to be approved. The burden of proof once rested on the government to prove beyond a reasonable doubt that the pesticide was lethal before it could be removed. Today, the burden of proof rests on the manufacturer to prove that the substance is safe. In 1976, it cost $6 million in tests to get a pesticide approved. Today, it costs over $30 million. More than twenty-six pesticides have been cancelled by the EPA over the past few years.[11]

Yet there are many pesticides with the misleading label "EPA approved" that are quite dangerous. According to a 1984 report from the National Academy of Sciences, "Toxic Testing," scientists found that 71 to 80 percent of all pesticides sold in the U.S. had not been tested for cancer; 21 to 30 percent were not tested for genetic mutations; 51 to 60 percent were not tested for birth defects; and fully 90 percent had not been tested for adverse effects on the nervous system. And those that are tested and found to be harmful are often used on food crops anyway, due to "temporary" licenses.

ASSUMPTIONS MADE BY THE GOVERNMENT

In order to relate results from tests on lab animals to humans, there are some major "guesstimates" made by government agencies. No one can really criticize these guesses, because no one really has a more calculated method of creating guidelines. However, determining the ADI of a pesticide is based on a tenuous series of major assumptions:

That the lab test results were properly interpreted. In the study on the pesticide dicofol, there was a big argument whether the lesions produced in the animals were cancerous. It was decided that they weren't. Even the best pathologists will tell you that it can be difficult to separate cancerous from noncancerous lesions, and then to categorize the cancerous lesions as either benign (likely to get better) or malignant (likely to get worse). Lesions are okay on the lab animals doused with pesticides. Tumors are not okay. It can be difficult to tell the difference. if you think your weatherman is reaching for odds in forecasting the weather, step into a lab someday and get a real feeling for "subjective" decisions.

That no observable effect level (NOEL) means no actual effect. We know that humans can take decades to develop diseases such as cancer, heart disease, cataracts, Alzheimer's, or osteoporosis. These people may look healthy throughout the development of the disease, but a disease *is* making progress: you just can't see it or diagnose it. There may be subtle health problems developing in these rat and pesticide studies that parallel the subtle and not-so-subtle health problems that Americans are experiencing.

That the test lab is honest. One of the biggest labs, Industrial BioTest Labs of Northbrook, Illinois, was caught by the FBI fabricating lab data.[12] Yet the two hundred pesticides that were approved by the EPA based on BioTest's fictitious studies have not been retested, and ninety of these pesticides are still used on food crops.

That there is a safe level or threshold, of exposure. An example is alcohol intake. For nonpregnant adults, one drink (one ounce of liquor) seems to have no major effect on health. More than that amount raises the health risks considerably since there becomes a saturation of the enzymes responsible for neutralizing the alcohol toxin. A tiny bit is probably harmless, but more may cause damage.

However, more potent poisons may have no threshold. PCB and aflatoxin are two such likely chemicals. In a landmark study, the National Center for Toxicological Research used more than 24,000 mice and $12 million dollars over a four-year test to find out how valid these toxicology tests really are. This study, known as ED_{01} found that there was no threshold in the case of one chemical tested (2-acetyl-aminofluorene). Maybe even minute pesticide residues on our food may cause health problems in some sensitive individuals. Nobody knows for sure.

That humans are 10 to 10,000 times more sensitive to pesticides than the test animals.[13] The EPA takes the NOEL number and divides it by somewhere between 10 and 10,000 (up to the judgment of the federal agent involved) and calls that amount the Acceptable Daily Intake (ADI). From the animal studies, the researchers calculate a very important number, called Q star (Q^*, which means the number of people who are likely to be harmed by this substance. The Q^* of tomatoes, primarily due to the fungicide used on the outside, is 8.75×10^{-4}, which means that about nine out of 10,000 people will get cancer from eating this food regularly for a lifetime. You have an ADI for everything from DDT to PCB. The ADI is supposed to be a number that will allow no more than one additional case of cancer per million people. Note that word "additional," since we already have 22 percent of Americans dying from cancer, which is paradoxically considered "acceptable" and not related to tainted food and water. Any more than 22 percent is unacceptable. If you compare our cancer statistics to cleaner underdeveloped nations, even our 22 percent is entirely unacceptable.

Sometimes the EPA or FDA acceptable standard of a food poison is found to be dangerously high. That has been the case with lead, aflatoxins, and the banned pesticides DDT and dieldrin. A group of scientists from the EPA and the National Wildlife Federation have found that people consuming only one-fifth of the ADI for DDT and dieldrin in Great Lakes sport fish will have a markedly elevated risk for cancer.[14]

That we all eat the average American diet. By taking the ADI and spreading it out over an average diet for a year, the EPA decides how much of that pesticide can be used on the crops. Actually, you and I and Junior and Grandmother all eat very different amounts and types of food. That makes some people more at risk, others less. It then assumes that aerial spraying only drops a given amount of a pesticide on the plants and that farm workers (who are often illiterate and underpaid) will accurately dilute and disperse the pesticide.

That our only exposure to that chemical comes from our diet. Actually, many pesticides are also used in products found throughout the house. For example, captan is a pesticide that is also used in paints, mattresses, shower curtains, and shampoos. Skin contact and inhaling fumes can bring in more of a poison, which raises intake beyond the ADI. Although the EPA considers captan to be a "probable" carcinogen (the highest warning given by this agency), and instigated a special review on captan in 1987, no action has yet been taken.

That the combination of several pesticides in the diet is not compounding. Actually, researchers have found that synergism exists between poisons (that $1+1=3$). Asbestos workers who were also smokers had a much higher rate for lung cancer than would be expected by adding the two risks together. In another study, scientists found that rats who were fed one semidangerous food additive (either red dye #2, cyclamates, or an emulsifier) all survived the experiment. Then, a separate group of animals were fed both red dye #2 and cyclamates. They developed balding and scruffy fur. And when all three of these food additives were fed to another group of animals, they all died within two weeks.[15] The take-home lesson here is that the body may be able to tolerate small amounts of one poison, but many poisons may accentuate each other's toxicity. We know that occurs when people abuse drugs and alcohol together—and no one in America is consuming just one poison. The chances of synergistic action between two or more pesticides is quite high. Yet it is not economically feasible to ask the pesticide companies to prove that all combinations of pesticides are safe. It would be best if we could use safer alternatives, such as Integrated Pest Management.

That there is some relationship between the sickness and death of mice and men. Compared to mice, humans have 2,000 times more cells, live thirty-five times longer, and have lower metabolic and respiratory rates. Although extrapolation from animal studies is the best that science can do for now, conclusions from mice studies could be way off, in a positive or negative way.

That the risk and benefit of a pesticide's use can be calculated. Executive Order 12291, by President Reagan in 1981, required all federal agencies to weigh the risks and benefits of any pesticide before regulating or banning it. In order to do that, they had to place a dollar value on human life. OSHA chose $3.5 million for the value of one American, while the EPA's estimate ranges from $400,000 to $7 million. The National Highway Transportation Safety Administration uses $175,000 as their price tag on you, and the Federal Aviation Administration uses the figure $650,000. As you can see, different government bureaus put a different value on life. Was the life of Jesus worth only thirty pieces of silver? Metaphysics aside, these arbitrary assumptions stir up a sense of injustice in me.

BLATANT MISTAKES MADE BY THE GOVERNMENT

Although the above-mentioned assumptions may be questionable, no one really has a perfect answer to substitute for these guesses. Yet the examples below are obvious mistakes made by the government. Better data and reasoning is available to make our food supply safer. It just isn't being used.

Outdated dietary surveys. We now eat an extra sixteen pounds of vegetables and twenty-four pounds of fruit per year when compared to 1974, the arbitrary year chosen by the government to represent the standard American diet. Fresh produce is now a $228 billion per year business, with 98 percent of all consumers using the produce section of a grocery store as the main attraction. Grocery stores have doubled their shelf allowance and tripled the number of fresh produce items carried compared to a decade ago. Yet the EPA still uses our "pre-health movement" consumption levels to calculate the ADI. In 1974, the average *yearly* intake of fresh produce included one-half cantaloupe, one avocado, 1.5 cups of cooked summer squash, 2.5 tangerines, one mango, and 1.5 cups of brussels sprouts. If you eat more than this, then you are exceeding your ADI for many pesticides. Why hasn't the EPA updated their figures when everyone else has the latest information?

Average body weight. The EPA chose 132 pounds as the weight for the average person. Strictly based on weight, children are three to five times at greater risk because their smaller bodies cannot dilute the poisons as well. Also, children have a much higher metabolic rate due to their rapid growth, hence they eat even more on a per-weight basis than adults. Children are also more at risk because of undeveloped immune systems that do not provide adequate protection from poisons. While nearly all fungicides used are known to be carcinogenic, children age one to six are probably exposed to five to two hundred times the ADI for ten of the eighteen fungicides that are approved.

Letting the meat packers check their own meat. This is like having the fox guard the chicken coop. With budget cuts of $15 million per year, the USDA was forced to reassign half of its 2,200 inspectors who review the activities in 6,300 meat processing plants. Now meat packers hire their own inspectors—a company employee is supposed to tell the boss that he has to throw away some tainted carcasses and lower profits. The USDA will not protect employee inspectors who "blow the whistle" on their plant. In the 115 plants where this SIS (streamlined inspection system) has been tested, hygiene in 19 plants deteriorated. Those plants with previous bad track records are not supervised any more than the others.

Canadian meats will be randomly inspected and told which trucks need to report at the border, rather than checking all trucks crossing into the U.S. The results of this change? In two months of normal service during 1988, thirty-one loads of meat were rejected. In the first two months of this program in 1989, only sixteen loads were rejected. Are the Canadian packers suddenly more hygienic under the honor system, or are we eating more subpar meat?

This major reduction in inspection quality will save us the grand total of $2.6 million per year. When compared to our $2 trillion national debt and $550 million per Stealth plane, do we really want to save money by eating questionable food and sacrificing our health?

Bureaucratic chaos. The USDA is supposed to inspect meats, while the FDA is in charge of all other food inspection. A frozen pizza is considered a bakery item under FDA jurisdiction, unless it has large chunks of meat, which swings it over to the USDA, except for the fresh onions and mushrooms on it which are inspected by the FDA and EPA, maybe. You would think that a packaged hamburger would fall under the USDA, except that it is considered a sandwich, which is under the authority of the FDA. So who guards your fast food hamburger shops? None of the above. Your local (state, county, city) health inspector is in charge there. Confused? Who isn't?

Figure 6A: Acceptable Daily Intake (ADI) of Selected Toxins source: FDA, Residues in Food-1987

Pesticide	FAO/WHO ADI*	6–11 mo.	14–16 yr M[b]	60–65 yr F[b]
Acephate	3	0.0025	0.0031	0.0047
Aldoxycarb	5[c]	0.0002	0.0001	0.0002
BHC, alpha + beta	—[d]	0.0019	0.0017	0.0007
BHC, gamma (lindane)	10	0.0010	0.0018	0.0007
Captan	100	0.0194	0.0088	0.0244
Carbaryl	10	0.1550	0.0173	0.0227
Carbofuran, total	10[c]	0.0001	0.0001	0.0001
Chlordane, total	0.5[c]	0.0015	0.0018	0.0015
Chlorobenzilate	20	0.0090	0.0031	0.0026
Chlorothalonil	3(T)[e]	<0.0001	<0.0001	0.0001
Chlorpropham, total	—	0.1432	.2072	0.1189
Chlorpyrifos	10	0.0207	0.0065	0.0040
Chlorpyrifos-methyl	10	0.0054	0.0066	0.0036
2, 4-D	300	<0.0001	<0.0001	0.0001
DCPA	—	0.0015	0.0011	0.0019
DDT, total	20[c]	0.0348	0.0191	0.0104
Diazinon	2	0.0146	0.0123	0.0066
Dicloran	30	0.2767	0.0682	0.1793
Dicofol, total	25	0.0329	0.0103	0.0101
Dieldrin	0.1[c]	0.0101	0.0045	0.0040
Dimethoate	10	0.0092	0.0009	0.0024
Endosulfan, total	8[c](T)	0.0724	0.0206	0.0400
Endrin	0.2	<0.0001	<0.0001	0.0001
Ethion	6(T)	0.0168	0.0063	0.0070
Fenitrothion	3	0.0004	0.0005	0.0005
Folpet	10(T)	0.0078	0.0029	0.0096
Fonofos	—	<0.0001	<0.0001	<0.0001
Gardona	—	0.0002	<0.0001	0.0001
Heptachlor, total	0.5[c]	0.0030	0.0018	0.0009

Figure 6A: Cont.

Pesticide	FAO/WHO ADI*	Age/Sex Group		
		6–11 mo.	14–16 yr M[b]	60–65 yr F[b]
Hexachlorobenzene	—	0.0026	0.0018	0.0010
Iprodione	300	0.0064	0.0025	0.0038
Linuron	—	0.0010	0.0003	0.0004
Malathion	20	0.1395	0.1193	0.0710
Methamidophos	0.6	0.0092	0.0087	0.0215
Methiocarb	1[c]	—[f]	0.0004	0.0030
Methomyl	10(T)	0.0022	0.0029	0.0033
Methoxychlor, p, p[1]	100	0.0007	0.0005	0.0003
Mevinphos, total	1.5[c]	0.0126	0.0046	0.0139
Monocrotophos	0.6	<0.0001	<0.0001	<0.0001
Omethoate	0.3	0.0025	0.0011	0.0034
Parathion	5	0.0062	0.0007	0.0016
Parathion-methyl	20	0.0001	0.0001	<0.0001
Pentachlorophenol	—	0.0001	0.0002	0.0001
Permethrin, total	50[c]	0.0710	0.0300	0.0405
Perthane	—	0.0042	0.0016	0.0024
Phosalone	6	0.0808	0.0034	0.0040
Phosmet	20[c]	0.0078	0.0021	0.0049
Pirimiphos-methyl	10	0.0012	0.0016	0.0002
Quintozene, total	7[c]	0.0011	0.0011	0.0005
Sulfur	—	0.0025	0.0009	0.0031
Tecnazene	10	—[f]	<0.0001	<0.0001
Toxaphene	—	0.0101	0.0138	0.0099
Vinclozolin	40[c](T)	0.0121	0.0044	0.0145

[a]ADIs are usually expressed as mg/kg body wt/day but are expressed here as µg/kg body wt/day for ease of comparison. The ADIs cited here reflect revisions made in 1987.

[b]M = male, F = female.

[c]Includes other (related) chemicals.

[d]ADI not established.

[e]T = "temporary" ADI.

[f]No consumption of a food item containing this residue in this age/sex group.

Sometimes, the federal agencies decide to add their own "interpretation" of the law to adjust to the current presidential administration. The Delaney law states that no carcinogenic substance can be used as a food additive. Pesticides are added to food. However, the EPA and FDA decided to reinterpret the law and not to extend the Delaney clause to fresh produce. They used a "risk versus benefit" concept to allow for some carcinogens in our food supply. A consumer protection group, Public Citizen, sued the FDA over this flagrant violation of the law and won. Several food dyes may be banned due to this recent court victory.[16]

Sometimes, after endless studies and reports, the EPA would ban a pesticide, only to allow it on certain crops. For instance, chlorobenzilate was banned in 1979, except on citrus crops. EDB was banned in 1984, except on mangoes. The aldicarb-laced watermelon that made hundreds of people ill over the Fourth of July in 1985 is not sanctioned for use on watermelon. Aldicarb is so lethal that one drop of concentrated ingredient injected into an adult would cause death. If it is so deadly, why is it allowed on anything?

Minimal inspection of fresh produce. The FDA samples 1 percent of domestic fresh produce and 0.2 percent of imported produce consumed in this country.[17] For instance, in 1982, only fourteen oranges were sampled of the two billion pounds that were imported, which computes to one orange tested per 200 million pounds of oranges. Hardly what one could call effective screening.

Of the 17 billion pounds of bananas imported during 1983 through 1985, only 139 samples were taken, which is one banana per 122 million pounds. Bananas from ten of the fifty importing nations were never sampled at all. EBDC is a "probable" human carcinogen commonly used on tomatoes. Over an eight-and-a-half-year period in California (a main tomato growing state), the FDA did not test for EBDC at all. Hence, a grower is more likely to win the state lottery than be monitored by the FDA or EPA for illegal pesticide residues.

Antiquated inspection methods. Although more advanced lab techniques exist, the FDA uses lab methods that will detect only about 40 percent of all pesticides used. They cannot detect any of the ten worst pesticides, nor do they even bother to check for pesticides that are known to be used on foreign produce but are banned in this country. 80 percent of all violation shipments are consumed anyway.

When the USDA began its meat inspection program eighty years ago, the biggest known problems were anthrax or tuberculosis in the meat. Both are detected by "organoleptic" inspection—smelling and feeling the meat. Neither anthrax nor tuberculosis are common today—but salmonella infection is. In 1986, the USDA admitted that 37 percent of all approved chicken, 5 percent of all beef, and 12 percent of all ham is infected with salmonella.[18] Although scientific methods exist to detect bacterial infection, the USDA does not do this because they follow an eighty-year-old law. The National Academy of Sciences has issued a report with major recommendations to improve our meat inspection services.

Lethargy. In 1972 Congress rewrote the pesticide laws and charged the EPA with testing pesticides for safety. Although the act exempted six hundred different pesticide ingredients from immediate scrutiny, it required that these pesticides be reviewed for their safety by 1976. By 1986, fourteen years later, none of the chemicals had been tested, reviewed, or reevaluated![19] To date, seventeen years later, only one hundred pesticides have been reviewed for their safety, and only four have been completely tested for their health effects.[20] In 1987, Congress gave EPA another deadline: finish pesticide review by 1997. In view of the EPA's dismal track record, some states, like California, have taken it upon themselves to establish their own pesticide safety laws.

Of the fifty pesticides considered by the EPA to be the most dangerous, forty-three are still in use. It was the California State Department of Agriculture (not the EPA) who finally ordered the destruction of ten million suspect watermelons when hundreds of people became sick through aldicarb poisoning. Nearly four years later, the EPA was finally recommended that aldicarb be banned for use on potatoes and bananas because it poses a serious threat to the health of infants and children. However, they would still allow its use on ten other food crops. Alachlor (trade name Lasso) is the best selling pesticide in the U.S.: by 1981, there was enough evidence to convict alachlor of carcinogenicity. In 1985, Canada banned alachlor, but the EPA has done nothing on this issue. In 1977, the FDA proposed banning the food preservative BHT from the GRAS list. Nothing has been done since then.

What did the EPA do when they found that underground fuel tanks from a Hollywood studio had contaminated the ground water with a dangerous chemical, ethylbenzene? Nothing.[21] What did the EPA do when a paper mill in northern California was found to be polluting the Sacramento River with dioxin and causing toxic levels in sport fish? Nothing. What did the State Department of Health Services do? Issued an announcement that sport fishers should not eat their catch.

While the FDA is charged with randomly testing fresh produce for pesticide residues, their labs are often overwhelmed or just catatonic in their work. A report from the GAO found that turn-around time for pesticides (82,000 samples taken by the FDA from 1983 through 1985) averaged 28 days for the 19 field laboratories, varying from 6.1 days in San Francisco to 164.9 days in New York.[22] At one lab, produce samples sat for an average of seven weeks. At that rate the FDA was doing archeology, not protecting consumers.

Conflict of interest. The European Economic Community, unlike the U.S., has long since banned hormones from their food supply. When the EEC banned the import of hormone-fed U.S. beef, beef lobbyists in the U.S. pressured the government to retaliate with a 100 percent customs tariff, worth $100 million, on European food imports. A treaty was reached, but Europe learned the wrath and influence of the cattle industry. A few large companies and lobbying concerns in America seem to have a disproportionate influence on the safety versus profitability of our food supply.

Inert ingredients? According to the dictionary, "inert" means "having few or no active properties." The EPA must have a different dictionary. Of the 1,200 "inert" ingredients approved for agricultural use by the EPA, 50 cause cancer, birth defects, or neurotoxicity; 50 have chemical structures similar to other proven dangerous chemicals; 800 have no information whatsoever regarding their safety; and 300 are genuinely inert or innocuous.[23]

These "inert" ingredients are used as a carrier system in pesticide spraying. While pesticide guidelines are fraught with loopholes, by listing an ingredient as "inert" a manufacturer does not have to live by any regulations. Inert ingredients have no tolerance standards. While some may be harmful in their own right, other inerts potentiate the action or staying power of pesticides, which increases their overall toxicity. The largest outbreak of farm-worker skin poisoning was caused by the inerts used on a citrus crop. In 1987, the EPA announced a plan to "encourage," but not order, the removal of hazardous inerts from pesticide use.

Circle of poison. Many pesticides that are banned in the U.S. are still produced by U.S. companies who ship these dangerous products to other countries with no pesticide protection, who then use the pesticides on food crops that are often shipped back into the U.S. Enter the Marx Brothers form of federal protection. Although it may have taken decades to ban a pesticide, we eat it anyway. In many cases the FDA does not even test for a banned pesticide, since they naively assume that no one uses it.

Although EDB was banned in the U.S. in 1984, the FDA still allows foreign mangoes to carry EDB residues, saying that a complete ban would harm foreign relationships. Heptachlor, a cousin of the deadly DDT, is also banned in the U.S., but purportedly used on Central American and Philippines fruit. From 1983 through 1985, the FDA did not check any pineapple from the Philippines for any pesticide residues. Over a nine-year period, the FDA did not check any foreign produce for EBDC, a carcinogenic fungicide that is produced in the U.S. and sold to other countries, but banned here.

Aldrin, Dieldrin, DDT, chlordane, and endrin are similar in several respects: they are all proven carcinogens, are all banned in the U.S., and are all used on coffee beans which are shipped into the United States.[24] These green coffee beans are obviously breaking the law, and the FDA knows it, but they do nothing. DBCP is a pesticide that causes cancer and sterility in males and is banned in the U.S. but used extensively worldwide on produce like bananas and pineapples. The FDA does not screen for DBCP on any produce.

At least 25 percent of pesticide exports *from* the U.S. are products that are not approved for American use.[25] Pesticide sales have exploded worldwide, with exports from the U.S. doubling over the past fifteen years. Pesticide use in Africa has increased 500 percent over the past decade.

You might ask the obvious question: "How do these poor struggling nations buy millions of dollars worth of pesticides?" Loans, of course. The World Bank, the Asian and Inter-American Development banks, and the U.S. Agency for International Development often loan money for pesticide purchase. In one year, China was loaned $285 million, which was 19 percent of their pesticide bill; Egypt was loaned $207 million, 83 percent of their bill; and Indonesia, Colombia, Guyana, and other developing nations all borrowed extensively for pesticide purchases.

SOMETIMES IT IS THE PUBLIC'S FAULT

On those rare occasions when all government wheels are synchronized and something is about to be done to remove a harmful agent from the diet, the public may demand a recount of the votes. Such a situation occurred with saccharin. In 1911 the USDA attempted to ban saccharin when scientists declared it to be a food adulterant; by 1951, a rat study had found saccharin to be carcinogenic; and in 1955, the National Academy of Sciences found that "the maximal amount of saccharin likely to be consumed is not hazardous." Three major studies published in 1972, 1973, and 1977 found that saccharin causes bladder cancer. The FDA was about to ban saccharin in 1977, but amid the protests of dieters and diabetics, Congress passed the Saccharin Study and Labeling Act which allows saccharin to exist as long as a warning is on the label. Even when the bureaucrats are willing to override the lobbyists' protests, the public objects to a rational move. Government protectors get understandably confused and return to their lethargic pace.

We also have a tendency to give low priority to food inspection at budget time. As of 1989, the FDA had an annual budget of $48 million and one thousand inspectors to police everything from blood banks and drug companies to all food items. With seriously understaffed offices and low pay, many federal agencies can barely put out fires, much less prevent them. For four years Struktol Co. of Ohio sold a food additive to french-fry and potato-chip manufacturers with the promise, "complies with FDA regulations." Well, the FDA had never heard of their antifoaming agent, which contains several ingredients known to be carcinogenic. No charges have been filed against Struktol officials. In April of 1989 in Los Angeles, state and federal authorities raided a huge operation making cheese and sausage with no licenses or inspections. There were seven plants with hygiene described by the prosecuting district attorney as "so filthy you wouldn't allow your pet to eat the food." Who knows how many other illegal and dangerous food operations continue. Without adequate manpower, the FDA cannot properly police the food industry.

In the very fine print of the EPA's laws was written, "You ban it, you buy it." In other words, if the EPA finds a pesticide or other food agent to be harmful enough to ban, then the EPA must purchase all existing inventories. David Bunn of the consumer action group CALPIRG charges that this law gave pesticide companies a license to kill.[26] The annual budget for the EPA's pesticide control program is $42 million, with the ban-and-buy clause costing them $30 million to purchase three pesticides. Since banning a pesticide literally takes food out of EPA employees mouths, they are extremely reluctant to do it. (This law was changed in October of 1988.)

WHAT ARE ACCEPTABLE RISKS?

Each fall, the new sixth-graders at Harrison Elementary School in Mullica Hill, New Jersey, embark on a nutrition research project. The teacher, Cathy Dilks, and school dietitian, Julie McGrath, like to show the children the importance of proper nutrition by feeding one rat a decent diet and another rat a "junk food" diet. In past years, the experiments have impressed many students with the need for proper nutrition. The 1988 experiment brought a new twist to the story: the health-food rat choked on a cracker and died.[27] Though Mrs. Dilks thought there might be a lesson on death and dying somewhere in this confusion, the real moral to the story is: there are no guarantees in this world.

To a certain extent, we can reduce our risks, then hope for the best. Risks can be ranked based upon statistics. For instance, you have a 1 in 8 billion chance of being hit by a meteor, a 1 in 50 million chance of being bitten by a shark, a 1 in 14 million chance of winning the big lottery, a 1 in 65 chance of dying in a car accident (triple the risk if you drive drunk without a seat belt), a 1 in 3 chance of dying from smoking cigarettes, and a 1 in 2 chance of dying from heart disease simply because you live an American lifestyle. It doesn't pay to worry about pesticide residues while smoking, nor to fret the sharks in the water when driving recklessly to the beach. Keep your risks and fears in perspective.

Similarly, the government tries to assess the risk-to-benefit ratio of using various additives and pesticides in your food supply. By spending X dollars on a project, what will the return on investment be in saved lives or better health? If we double the investment, will we double the return? Or will double the investment only bring another 30 percent added safety? With limited funds, should we spend the extra money for a lower return margin?

Preventive measures tend to peak at a certain level on the graph. New York State spent $43 million one year to outfit all out-dated school buses with seat belts. There had been one death the previous year from lack of seat belts. Is one life worth $43 million? If you are the person or the parent it may be, but could that money have been better spent elsewhere? These are the gut-wrenching questions and objective number-crunching that various branches of the federal government must perform. It is definitely not an enviable position to place a value on human life and calculate the best "return on investment" for preventive measures. But someone has to do it. Otherwise we would spend $8 billion on shark protection, nothing on prenatal care, and end up saving two lives while sacrificing a million others. There has to be a rational, cold, calculating mind somewhere in this emo-

---

Figure 6B THE NUMBERS GAME

A DROP IN THE BUCKET:

One part per million (ppm) = 1 ounce in 32 tons of food
One part per billion (ppb) = 1 drop in 10,000 gallon tank
One part per trillion (ppt) = 1 grain of sugar in Olympic pool

RISKY BUSINESS:

1×10^{-6} = *Cancer risk of one in one million*
1×10^{-5} = *Cancer risk of one in one hundred thousand*
1×10^{-4} = *Cancer risk of one in ten thousand*
1×10^{-3} = *Cancer risk of one in one thousand*

RADIATION CONVERSIONS:

1 Gray (Gy) = 100 rads
1 KiloGray (kGy) = 1,000 gray = 100,000 rads

tionally charged issue. There is no way that we can have a fresh
and plentiful food supply with a zero risk. Some risk is as much a
part of living as oxygen. But we can definitely lower the current
risk without affecting the food supply and without any appreciable increase in costs.

The EPA considers one additional death per million to be
acceptable. Which means that at least 235 Americans each year
die from the use of many different pesticides. According to the
National Academy of Sciences report in 1987, nearly one million
Americans over a seventy-year lifetime (about 14,000 per year)
could get cancer due to pesticide use. However, due to the existence of alternatives, these risks are unnecessary.

We all take risks. Skiing, tanning, eating barbecued burned
food, driving fast on the freeway, standing on ladders, eating
high-fat, low-fiber food, and drinking too much alcohol are all
high-risk lifestyles. The difference is that pesticides are forced
upon us while most other risks are voluntary.

Since the risks of pesticide residues are unnecessarily high, we
need to explore safer alternatives. But I also encourage the reader
to evaluate where your real risks are in life. If you live a healthy
lifestyle, then pesticides could be a high risk that you would like
to eliminate. If you lead an unhealthy lifestyle (i.e., smoking,
obesity, sedentary) then you should take care of these major
risks before worrying about the lesser risks of pesticides.

THE GOVERNMENT CAN DO A BETTER JOB OF SAFEGUARDING THE FOOD SUPPLY

The vast majority of our food is totally uninspected while the
remaining small percentage is marginally inspected. When violations are found, the food has usually been consumed and no
action is taken against the offending party. When you look at
some of the government food inspection practices—using outdated smell and feel tests on beef; allowing "inerts" to be used at
liberty; not testing for known harmful agents that are known to
be there (like salmonella and EDB)—you come away with the

feeling that "government in action" may actually be only two words "government inaction."

The function of the government is to protect the people. With a slight increase in effort and investment, we could have a safe, abundant, and nourishing food supply. Until then, when it comes to food and water, *caveat emptor* (let the buyer beware).

CHAPTER 7
What's in the Food?

*Y*ou picked up this book because you are at least suspicious that your food supply is not as safe as you wish it was. Your suspicions are warranted. The American public, as shown by these examples, now seriously questions the safety of its food: in March of 1989, several grapes from Chile were found to contain cyanide—and that country's $1 billion-per-year fruit industry came crashing down around one industrial saboteur (one worried mother in Oregon even called the state police to track down her ten-year-old daughter and apprehend the grapes in her lunch bucket)[1]; that same week, newspapers carried the story of an Arkansas poultry farm that had to destroy 400,000 chickens due to pesticide contamination, and the chairman of the New York City Produce Association had people calling him all day asking, "What *can* I eat?" Although these stories stunned the nation and made good press, these food hazards are low risk relative to other long term and more serious food safety issues.

America's food industry has come a long way since the colonial era. In the seventeenth and eighteenth centuries, 96 percent of all Americans were farmers; now, only 2 percent of us farm, and they are able to feed the remaining 98 percent of us who do something else for a living. I was raised in farm country and my grandfather farmed in Illinois, so I know that farming is a tough way to make a living. There are occasional slack periods, but basically a farmer works seven days a week and sometimes sixteen hours a day in heat, cold, and mud with the high risk that some capricious storm can devastate the year's income. That unsavory job is avoided by the vast majority of people because of high-tech farming. Some of those techniques are true time savers, including efficient tractors to plow vast acreages, but some of these new farming techniques, such as excessive use of pesticides, hormones, and antibiotics, can lead to problems in the food supply.

Some nutritionists argue that the real "unsafe" food in America is the highly-refined high-fat junk food that many Americans thrive on, not the pesticide residues on broccoli[2]—but there is much more to our twentieth-century foods than just the nutrient categories of carbohydrates, fats, proteins, vitamins, minerals, and water. There is also a mixed stew of questionable added ingredients. Our blessed food cornucopia comes with a warning label.

DRUGS

There are over twenty thousand different animal drugs in wide use today in domestic livestock of which the government can detect only 30 percent in their meat inspection programs. Unfortunately, the FDA has been rather lenient in granting temporary or "emergency" approval to use drugs that have not been tested for safety. It may be years before the FDA ever demands formal safety studies of these "emergency" drugs.

Actually, most of the drugs used in raising beef, pork, and poultry do nothing to safeguard either the animal or the consumer; they are there just to fatten profit margins. Hence, these drugs are optional. The safer alternative would be minimal drug usage. Legally, there is a "drying out" period of days or weeks, depending on the drug, in which the animal is supposed to be drug-free so there will be minimal drug residues in the meat.

Realistically, these guidelines are rarely observed, or enforced by the skeleton crew used by the USDA.

For instance, chloramphenicol is an antibiotic that was banned for use in meat animals in 1968 because it could cause a fatal blood disorder in the consumer. However, it is still in use. A survey in 1984 showed that 95 percent of veterinarians admit to using this drug. Animal drug supply houses sell it without a prescription, so the farmer can bypass the rare vet who will not use it.

HORMONES

In 1979, the FDA proposed to withdraw its approval of hormones (specifically, estradiol benzoate) used to encourage rapid weight gain in animals. Something must have changed their minds: in 1983 they not only withdrew their proposed ban, but also rescinded their order (that had been in effect since 1956) that cattle must be hormone free for sixty days prior to slaughter. Hormones were banned in Europe in 1981 when a rash of early sexual maturation occurred in Italian children; a trend that subsided when meat, chicken, and milk were taken out of their diet. A similar situation happened in Puerto Rico in 1985: over three thousand children were experiencing premature sexual development. Seventeen-month-old infant females started to menstruate; young boys, as well as girls, developed breasts; young girls sexually matured years earlier than would be expected. Once again, the symptoms went away when meat, chicken, and milk were taken out of the diet.

Supposedly, time-release hormone pellets were implanted beneath the skin near the animal's ear or other part not used for human consumption. In 1986, the U.S. Food Safety and Inspection Service found over ninety cattle feedlots that were implanting pellets at illegal points or in double dosages.[3] European health experts have concluded that the risks from hormone use far outweigh the benefits. Lab findings from the National Cattlemen's Association, however, show that hormone levels in beef are only slightly elevated when the hormones have been properly used. For instance, a female child produces 54,000 nanograms (ng) of estrogen (similar to the growth hormone used in cattle rearing) daily, while a pregnant woman produces 20,000,000 ng of estrogen daily. A one-pound steak from a hormone-raised steer will add only 3 ng via the diet. Thus, when properly used, hormones *should* be safe in domestic animals. But according to a more objective journal, veterinarians find about a 25 percent increase in the estrogen levels in a steak from hormone-fed cattle.[4]

In the fall of 1988, Europe rejected American hormone-fed beef. American cattlemen did not want anyone developing the notion that hormone-fed beef was unsafe—such a notion might jeopardize not only U.S. sales, but the $1 billion in beef that Japan buys from the U.S. annually—so, through lobbyist pressure, the U.S. government retaliated with a 100 percent customs duty worth more than $100 million, on European food imports. In a truce, Americans agreed to ship only hormone-free beef to Europe, but under the guise of "high-quality beef."

Most scientists agree that the proper use of hormones in raising animals poses a minimal risk, even to children. Yet many people have the misconception, "If a little is good, then more is better." With that slogan firmly in place, some cattle owners may abuse hormones. Excess hormones in the food supply could cause premature sexual maturation in children, elevate the risk for cancer (especially in women), and induce infertility in some women. Although hormone-fed cattle do grow faster and fatter, most of the added weight is in the form of fat and water, which means that hormone-fed meat is potentially harmful not just from hormones, but from the higher fat content. Also, bulking up cattle like this is a throwback to the earlier part of this century when the beef hucksters would feed salt to their cattle, while en route to market, to encourage water weight gain.

Since many consumers have grown weary of dodging such hazards in their food, nearly four hundred supermarkets nationwide now sell hormone-free beef and chicken. For a listing of stores and producers who handle hormone-free animal products, send $.50 plus a self addressed stamped envelope to CSPI (see Appendix).

ANTIBIOTICS

In the years surrounding World War II, antibiotics were developed to treat previously intractable bacterial infections. The work was hailed as "miraculous." Today, Americans are in danger of squandering the value of miracle antibiotics as we use tons of these wonder drugs merely to encourage rapid weight gain in animals. This category presents a growing problem today, but could be the true apocalyptic sleeper of this entire book. Scientists have presented the distinct possibility that antibiotic-resistant bacteria could cause an epidemic similar in scale to the plagues of medieval Europe. How could such a wonder drug be so misused?

In 1949, Dr. Thomas Jukes, a researcher with American Cyanamid Corporation, found that traces of the antibiotic tetracycline added to the food mash of chickens increased their weight gain by 10 to 20 percent.[5] Piglets did even better. Routine administration of low doses (euphemistically called "subtherapeutic" by the meat industry) of antibiotics were soon added to most animal feed. Not only did the antibiotics encourage faster growth, but they also protected the animals against infection. Without antibiotics, animals had to be kept in clean uncrowded quarters or they would fall prey to the many diseases that crowding fosters.

Farm animals now eat nine million pounds per year of "subtherapeutic" antibiotics, or half of our annual antibiotic production. Antibiotics usually kill the majority of bacteria that come in contact with the drug, but the few bacteria that survive this dousing are able to pass on their drug-resistant abilities to other bacteria in a swapping of genetic material. The creation of "bulletproof" bacteria parallels the creation of "bulletproof" insects, as illustrated in the chapter on pesticides.

Scientists found that the 500 percent increase in salmonella food poisoning over the past three decades may be traced to the use of antibiotics in animal rearing.[6]

Chloramphenicol, the banned antibiotic mentioned previously was linked to an outbreak of food poisoning through hamburger meat. The strain of bacteria involved was found to be resistant to chloramphenicol. If an antibiotic-resistant bacteria in the food supply teams up (exchanges genetic material) with a bacteria that is spread through the air or water supply, then we could create the Black Plague of the twentieth century.

This "subtherapeutic" use of antibiotics poses a frightening scenario, and already may be responsible for 270,000 cases annually of salmonella poisoning, including one hundred to three hundred deaths. There are many well-known scientists, including Dr. Lester Crawford, director of the FDA's Center for Veterinary Medicine, who are strongly opposed to the subtherapeutic use of antibiotics throughout our food supply for various reasons:

> We may start a plague that cannot be stopped with antibiotics
> We are neutralizing the potency of antibiotics to treat other ailments
> By regularly consuming antibiotics, we may kill off the "friendly" bacteria in the intestines. These friendly

Figure 7A: Incidence of Salmonella

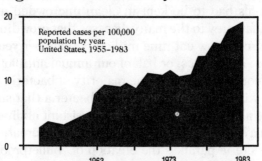

Source: Center for Disease Control

bacteria help to produce vitamins (such as biotin) and compete with unfriendly bacteria (like *Clostridium difficile*) that can cause acute gastrointestinal problems, including diarrhea, pain, and fever
 Pet food contains much higher amounts of antibiotics and has been lethal to human infants.[7] The raw ingredient for pet food is sometimes food that was considered unfit for human consumption

Scientists have known for more than a decade that antibiotics in animal feed are causing widespread mutations in bacteria. The FDA tried to ban nontherapeutic antibiotics in the food supply in 1977, but was blocked by Congress. Each year since 1977, a bill has been introduced in Congress to ban the use of nontherapeutic medication, yet each year the vendors of antibiotics roust enough opposition to defeat these bills. This issue may be more than a time bomb—it could become a nuclear bomb.

IRRADIATION

In 1898 the French scientist Marie Curie left her keys on a photographic plate next to a rock of uranium. When she returned to the lab the next morning, there was an imprint of her keys left on the photographic plate. The world was never the same thereafter. Professor Curie's unprotected fascination with radiation won her two Nobel prizes and an early death from leukemia.
 Until the atomic bomb exploded over the New Mexico desert in 1945, radioactivity was little more than a cheap magician's trick. Radioactive minerals are now a major factor in energy production, medicine, and weapons—and some people would like to see their uses extended to food preservation.
 The technique of food irradiation is actually more than a half century old. USDA scientists found that irradiation destroyed trichinosis worms in pork and were granted a patent on the procedure in 1921. However, until after World War II, radioactive isotopes were rare and expensive, and thus not practical for

widespread food preservation. By 1955, the U.S. Army began a ten-year study on the wholesomeness of preserving food with radioactivity. Some ninety universities were eventually involved in this project.

Although any form of energy (including microwaves and ultra-violet light) can be used to irradiate food, the process usually involves gamma rays from radioactive cobalt-60 or cesium-137, both refuse by-products from nuclear reactors and weapons manufacturing.[8] The basic idea of food irradiation is to blast the food with lethal doses of rays that kill all microbes and enzymes that can deteriorate the food. Irradiation is considered a food additive and is regulated by the 1958 Food Additives Amendment: there are prescribed amounts of radiation to which a food can be exposed, that are measured in "kilorads" or "kiloGrays." Since 1963, the FDA has approved irradiation of food to prevent sprouting, to control insects in harvested wheat, and to eliminate trichina parasites from pork. As of April, 1986, the FDA has approved a much more liberal law allowing irradiation of many food products.

A number of bureaucratic puzzles have presented themselves here. In one case, a food processor was found to be irradiating dried mushrooms. While irradiating dried mushrooms is not approved,you can irradiate vegetable seasonings, which is what the company claimed they were doing. In another case, it is suspected that shrimp from Bangladesh and other Third World countries has been irradiated, although that is illegal. For years, shrimp arriving in the U.S. from these underdeveloped countries would be rejected by USDA inspectors due to filth, insects, or deterioration; but for the past eight years, shrimp arriving from Bangladesh via the Netherlands (a world leader in irradiation) has been astoundingly clean. Inspectors believe that radiation is being used, but can't prove it through any normal test methods.[9]

The radura symbol must be affixed to foods that have been irradiated. Foods that contain only some irradiated ingredients (like TV dinners) need not use the radura. Nutrient loss from irradiated food and traditional food preservation techniques, such as canning and freezing, is about the same.[10]

Proponents of food irradiation downplay the paranoia of radiation by calling their process "cold sterilization," and claim such benefits as:

Replacement of postharvest pesticides, such as the dangerous EDB
Inhibition of the sprouting of potatoes, onions, etc.
Delay of the ripening of fresh fruits and vegetables.
Elimination of many of the bacteria responsible for food poisoning.
Through these benefits, helping to eliminate hunger by bringing more food to undernourished nations.[11]

A mighty impressive list of promises. But there is a dark side, worthy of concern. The FDA reviewed 413 separate studies on the safety of irradiated food and decided that 344 studies told them nothing, 32 showed adverse effects, and 37 supported safety. When food is zapped with radiation, there are substances produced in the food, called unique radiolytic products (URP), which do not exist anywhere else in nature. These URPs give expert scientists throughout the world a queasy feeling about the safety of irradiation. The United Kingdom will not allow irradiated food to be sold in their country; Japan will not accept irradiated fresh produce; and no foreign government will accept

Figure 7B: Radura Symbol

irradiated pork. Syracuse University, a major research center in upstate New York, has banned the use of irradiated foods on campus.[12] In July of 1989, Governor Mario Cuomo of New York signed a bill banning the sale of irradiated food (except spices) in the second most populous state in America. Dr. Richard Piccioni has gathered together many of the studies which show URPs can damage DNA in the cell nucleus.[13] Perhaps irradiation is not as safe as the FDA says.

These URPs are found in trace quantities in irradiated food. The FDA has a policy that trace impurities that are present at less than 50 parts per billion are considered unimportant. However, thirty studies have found that irradiated food in test animals can cause chromosomal damage, anemia, thyroid disease, kidney disease, impaired reproduction, and increased mortality. When malnourished East Indian children were fed wheat that had been recently irradiated, they developed multiple chromosomes in their white blood cells, often considered to be a sign of impending cancer.[14] Rats fed irradiated food over their lifetime developed kidney damage.[15] Animals fed irradiated chicken meat developed testicular tumors.[16] While irradiation seems to be quite lethal to many forms of life, it does not kill botulism bacteria (a deadly form of food poisoning found in improperly canned food)[17] and even enhances the growth of the fungus that produces the lethal aflatoxin.[18]

All of this hoopla of controversy may be for naught. Scientists at the University of California at Davis find that irradiation is inappropriate on most varieties of fresh produce because it makes fruit and vegetables more likely to bruise in transit. Irradiation is also an expensive form of food preservation, thus available only to the larger food conglomerates. To date, little more than spices and incidental food ingredients are irradiated in this country on a large scale, primarily due to high cost and low consumer acceptance.

If irradiation were the only means of avoiding starvation, we would perhaps need to look at it more closely. But as it is, irradiation is nothing more than an expensive high-tech method that is inferior to many alternative food preservation methods and appears to be a marketing ploy to sell radioactive wastes. The recent cataclysmic nuclear-waste dumping by the federal government will cost $100 billion to clean up, and proves that radioactive wastes are not your garden-variety garbage. Transporting, storing, and using radioactive material is dangerous, which would increase if irradiation of food became a common procedure. Using radioactive refuse to preserve our food supply is questionable. Encouraging the widespread handling of radioactive wastes in the wake of the Chernobyl nuclear reactor meltdown in Russia is sheer lunacy.

NATURALLY OCCURING TOXINS

Jackie Gleason, the self-avowed hedonistic entertainer, outlived Euell Gibbons, the famous foraging naturalist. No doubt genetics was Gleason's trump card, but if there was something magical about eating raw natural foods, then Gibbons should have been the longer lived of the two. The popular misconception "if it's natural, then it must be good for you" is far from true. Scorpion venom, botulism, or oleander plant extract are but a few of the very natural and quite lethal substances that nature has produced. The now-banned carcinogenic red dye #2 is made from the flowers of the highly touted health food, the amaranth plant. The list of naturally occurring toxins is extensive and of growing interest to the modern toxicologist.[19]

Essential nutrients. Some nutrients when taken in excessive levels can be toxic, although rarely fatal. The animal form of vitamins A and D, and the mineral selenium, are potentially toxic but also essential nutrients. However, it is extremely rare that nutrient toxicity could develop through food intake. The greatest risk in vitamin supplements is when a child consumes an entire bottle of tasty chewable vitamins loaded with iron for growing children; the iron overload can be dangerous and possibly fatal. Most other nutrient toxicities are rare and reversible. By taking large doses of an isolated mineral, you can create a mineral imbalance which surfaces as a toxicity or deficiency.

While selenium may be a potent force against cancer and pollution, it can also be toxic. Let's compare selenium intake levels:

> average American intake: 30 to 70 micrograms, mcg
>
> recommended intake to protect against pollution: 600 mcg
>
> toxicity: as low as 2,400 mcg according to the NRC[20]

The Chinese people who were experiencing problems with selenium toxicity were consuming about 5,000 mcg per day. In 1988, there was a storm of controversy as certain scientists warned about the risk of too much selenium in our diet.[21] However, researchers at the University of California at Davis found that when high-selenium water is used to irrigate crops, a mere 30 mcg per day of selenium is added to the diet.

Other natural toxins. Many of our naturally occurring toxins are ancient "pesticides" that bring a mixed blessing. In order for humans to obtain nutrients from these mildly poisonous plants, we were forced to develop detoxifying abilities that neutralize the poison's harm. Hence, due to naturally occurring pesticides in plants, humans are better prepared to grapple with the plethora of poisons that we face in twentieth-century America.

A brief list of the more prominent naturally occurring poisons would include:

> *hydrazines* in mushrooms
> *safrole* in black pepper
> *psoralens* in celery, parsnips, and figs
> *solanine* in potatoes
> *quinones* in rhubarb and other plants
> *theobromine* in coffee, tea, and chocolate
> *pyrrolizidine alkaloids* in various herbal teas

isothiocyanate in mustard and horseradish
canavanine in alfalfa sprouts.

As you can see, eating has been a harrowing adventure since
long before the advent of pesticide residues. Some of these "poisons" may also be useful to the body in small amounts: quercetin
and rutin are bioflavonoids that probably enhance the effectiveness of vitamin C, but in high doses may predipitate unhealthy
changes in cells;[22] capsaicin, the active ingredient in hot peppers, can thin out the blood to prevent heart disease, but may
also be weakly carcinogenic. Most of these naturally occurring
poisons will be a minimal problem if you: Eat a wide variety of
foods—not concentrating on any one food in particular will
avoid toxic buildup; and maintain your detox system at optimal
efficiency as described in part 3.

TAINTED BOOZE

In July of 1985 wine lovers around the world were stunned
with the news that some expensive German and Austrian wines
had been sweetened with antifreeze (diethyleneglycol)[23] The
governments of those proud wine producing countries promised
that the strictest laws would be passed to prevent a recurrence.
People are very serious about getting quality alcoholic beverages.
About a decade ago, the Center for Science in the Public Interest
(CSPI) published a report showing the alarming levels of carcinogenic nitrosamines found in alcoholic drinks. The public got concerned. The alcohol industry cleaned up the problem.

It would be nice if alcoholic beverages contained only alcohol;
at least you would know your adversary. Alcohol is a definite risk
factor toward cancer of the mouth and gastro-intestinal tract,
may cause birth defects, and contributes to half of all traffic fatalities. But in moderate use for most adults, alcohol can be a mild
relaxant and can elevate HDL levels that protect against heart
disease.[24] Unfortunately, most alcoholic beverages contain trace

amounts of thousands of different impurities, known as congeners, that can be harmful.[25]

There are seventy different pesticides approved for use on grapes. In 1985, a pesticide (demeton-methyl) was found in wine, although officials considered the amount to be insignificant.[26] This pesticide is an organophosphate with one side effect in humans being neurotoxicity, causing headaches and erratic behavior. Some people could think that they had had too much to drink; the alcohol may not be the culprit, but rather the congeners and pesticide residues.

Most wine and beer manufacturers use sulfites as preservatives. Sulfites can cause serious allergic reactions in about 5 percent of the twenty million asthmatics in this country, which puts one million people at risk. The EPA has ruled that table grapes can have no more than 10 parts per million of sulfite added,[27] but most wines contain 125 to 175 parts per million, or twelve to seventeen times more than the "insignificant" level.

Not until 1985 did scientists have lab equipment that was sensitive enough to detect urethane in trace amounts. Urethane is a known carcinogen and is now found in many different alcoholic beverages as a by-product of the heating or fermentation process.[28] While Canada immediately set enforceable standards regarding allowable urethane levels in liquor, the U.S. has lagged behind in this area, only recently asking the liquor industry to develop its own voluntary standards. While the FDA considers a cancer risk of one in a million to be acceptable, their own scientists find that the cancer risk of urethane in alcohol is ten to one hundred times the "acceptable" level. CSPI scientists think that the problem is much worse, with a cancer risk of five thousand in every one million moderate drinkers. That would put 75,000 people at risk for cancer just from the urethane in liquor. The FDA's chief food toxicologist, Dr. Gary Flamm, has called urethane "a carcinogen that should be feared. Ranking substances by the threat they pose to cause cancer in humans, urethane would be first, second, or third."

The most urethane-contaminated of alcoholic beverages are (worst first): bourbon whiskey, European fruit brandy, cream sherry, port wine, Japanese sake, and Chinese wines; with the safest being gin, vodka, and most beers.

A glass or two of wine for a well-nourished, nonpregnant, non-alcoholic, and active adult probably does no harm and may even be a mild benefit. But the more likely scenario of a marginally nourished American who consumes moderate to high amounts of urethane-tainted booze is a game of Russian roulette with two bullets in the chamber.

FOOD ADDITIVES

Although Columbus missed his destination by about eleven thousand miles, it was the pursuit of food additives that sent his tiny ship out toward the edge of the earth. Food rots quickly with no refrigeration, which makes the flavor and odor become nause-ating. To cover that stench, people in Europe began using the treasured Oriental spices to drown the flavor of rotting food. Roy-alty would pay handsomely for the luxury of ginger, pepper, cin-namon, and vanilla to spice up their food. (The term "salary" is derived from the Latin word for salt, since the Romans used to pay wages with salt, which was a highly prized food preservative and flavor enhancer.)

If every town could produce a varied diet throughout the year for all of its citizens, then there would be no need for additives. But such is not the case.

There are 2,800 additives approved for use by the FDA, with another 10,000 ingredients finding their way into our food system as "incidental" additives via the agriculture and food processing industries.[29] The average American consumes about 1,500 pounds of food per year, of which 150 pounds is additives. (Salt and sugar comprise 93 percent of additives). While one extremist group would like to ban all food additives, the opposing extremists would like to use copious quantities of unsafe addi-tives to make junk food more appealing and have an unlimited shelf life. There should be a rational middle ground.

Most additives are safe, some even beneficial (such as guar

gum and vitamin E), but a few are potential hazards in the diet. In order for an additive to be considered for approval by the FDA it must do one or more of the following to a food:

1. Improve the nutritional value
2. Enhance quality or consumer acceptability
3. Improve the keeping quality
4. Make the food more readily available
5. Facilitate its preparation

Up until about 1980, additives were easily "grandfathered" into FDA approval via the Generally Regarded As Safe (GRAS) list. Today it takes about three to ten years and half a million dollars to perform the studies necessary to get an additive approved by the FDA. Lab animals are given high doses of the additive in question and observed for acute, subchronic, and long term toxicity. The following is a brief description of the main categories of food additives.

Antioxidants help prevent fats from "rusting" (oxidizing), and include such valuable nutrients as vitamins E and C. Although BHA and BHT are probably safe as food additive antioxidants, they should not be taken in pill form as longevity supplements (as was recommended in a best-selling health book).

Preservatives slow down food spoilage by checking the growth of microorganisms. Benzoic acid and sodium nitrate are examples. Nitrates and sulfur preservatives (metabisulfite, sulfur dioxide, etc.) are suspicious members of this group.[30]

Emulsifiers and stabilizers are chemicals that try to keep the mixture of ingredients from separating out of solution. Lecithin from soybean oil and thickening agents like guar gum are examples of nutritious and safe members here. The fiber part of legumes are not only a thickening agent used in food, but also are being tested as a potent cholesterol-lowering drug for use against heart disease. This group is relatively safe.

Dyes are the most questionable of the additives. They are strictly "window dressing" to make unhealthy or aging food look better. The U.S. consumes 6.4 million pounds of food dyes per year. The National Research Council finds the evidence against at least two dyes is overwhelming: they pose a major cancer risk. Four of the seven approved artificial food dyes have been shown to cause cancer in animals. By age twelve, four million U.S. children will have consumed more than one pound (454 grams) of food dyes, with some children taking in up to three pounds of dyes. We do eat with our eyes—that's the problem, because dyes entice us to eat food that is deceivingly pretty. Even FDA employees, who defend junk food in general, are suspicious of food dyes.[31]

You are more likely to be safe with a natural dye, like chlorophyll (green), beta-carotene (yellow), and caramel (brown). Coal tar–based synthetic dyes differ from any chemical found in nature, which provides us with an important clue about the safety of artificial food dyes. There are thirty-five dyes permitted for use on food by the FDA. In an ironic twist, the violet dye formerly used by the USDA to stamp "prime" on beef was found to be carcinogenic.

Norway and Greece do not allow any food dyes. The World Health Organization found only six of the twenty-nine food dyes reviewed to be safe. Red dye #40 is suspected of causing lymph tumors in mice. The yellow dye tartrazine has been suspected of causing behavioral disorders in some sensitive children and probably causes rashes and sniffles in ninety thousand sensitive Americans.

The aggressive food lobbyists, the submissive FDA, and the naive consumer must bear equal blame for the dangerous levels of dyes in American food. Real cherries are not flamboyantly red: only dyes can make them that color. When consumers expect and buy neon-bright foods, the manufacturer is more than willing to supply them. Whenever possible, avoid this category.

Sequestrants prevent mineral ions from reacting with the food by creating a chemical "cage" to keep the mineral inert. EDTA, citric acid, tartaric acid, glycine, and others form this mostly safe category.

Anti-caking agents prevent the clumping that can occur when dry powdered food (like a boxed cake mix) sit in a humid environment. Various forms of aluminum (like sodium silicoaluminate) are used for this purpose in most dry packaged goods in America. Aluminum toxicity has been implicated in Alzheimer's disease, which has become the most common form of senility in this country.[32] Toxic amounts of aluminum are more likely to come from the bulk intake of aluminum-based antacids, although minimizing aluminum from all forms would be a good idea. Other members of this group are relatively safe.

Humectants slow down the drying out of a food by retaining the moisture. These are safe.

Acid-base balancers try to maintain a certain pH for flavor, texture, cooking properties, and shelf life of the food. These are also safe.

Firming and crisping agents attempt to keep fruits and vegetables full of water. Aluminum and sodium salts are often used for this purpose and are questionable but not dangerous additives.

Flavoring agents are there to ensure that eating is a pleasurable experience—nothing wrong with that—but here food manufacturers may know the consumer's palate better than the consumer. Highly refined "junk food" offers increasingly higher levels of fat, salt, sugar, and flavor enhancers (like monosodium glutamate, MSG) to create consumer acceptance. In small amounts, these additives are relatively harmless. In typical American amounts, they may become a significant cause of hypertension, dental caries, obesity, heart disease, cancer, and other common health woes. Sugar is such a prominent additive that it gets its own category.

MSG is a particularly suspicious member here, having been implicated in fetal abnormalities in animals and partial nerve paralysis in humans. Some very intriguing research at the University of Texas has found that vitamin B-6 supplements (50 milligrams daily) prevent and even reverse the problems caused by MSG.[33] It could be that a marginal intake of B-6 makes people less vulnerable to harm from MSG intake.

Sweeteners are the largest category of additives. The average American consumes 132 pounds of sugar yearly. At that massive intake level, sugar has been implicated in dental caries, heart disease, obesity, diabetes, and other diseases that typify America.[34]

Meanwhile, artificial sweeteners have their own long and tainted history, with the banning or near banning of cyclamates and saccharin. Aspartame (or NutraSweet) is an artificial sweetener made from amino acids that may increase the risk of brain tumors, according to an FDA-appointed science panel.[35] Also, Dr. Richard Wurtman at the Massachusetts Institute of Technology has found that large amounts of aspartame can cause nervous-system reactions (everything from headaches to epileptic seizures) in sensitive individuals.[36] Seventy percent of artificial sweeteners are used in soft drinks. Studies show that our increase in the incidence of obesity has continued in spite of the phenomenal consumption of artificial sweeteners in this country. That seems to nullify any reason for the existence of artificial sweeteners.

The FDA has recently approved a new artificial sweetener, acesulfame potassium, to compete in the $1 billion per year artificial sweetener business. Both aspartame and acesulfame are about two hundred times sweeter than sugar. The FDA has proposed lifting the twenty-year-old ban on cyclamates. Sorbitol is a sweetener that does have calories and will not cause cavities, but some people develop gastrointestinal problems from sorbitol. While a little sweetener can make bland but nutritious food more enjoyable, bulking up on sweeteners can do serious harm to your health.

Enzymes speed up or slow down chemical reactions, such as rennin used to curdle milk into cheese. This group is safe.

Flour and bread additives have their own group since bread is a staple food in the Western diet. I would encourage the reader to purchase minimally processed whole grain bread, thus avoiding many suspicious additives that are found in white bread.

Nutritive additives have been directly responsible for preventing death or disease in millions of people. By adding iodine to salt, the government and food industry nearly eradicated goiter in America. (Goiter still affects over 400 million people around the world; there are some inland mountainous regions of the world where the few people who do not have the swollen neck of goiter are chided with the insulting name "bottleneck.")

By adding vitamin D to milk, rickets (soft and deformed bones in children) nearly disappeared in America. By adding thiamin back to white flour, beri-beri has been reduced, although white flour is a sad excuse for the once robust nutritive value of whole wheat. A food is *enriched* when some of the original nutrients that were lost in refining are replaced. A food is *fortified* when nutrients are added that are not normally found in that food.

Finland now adds selenium to its bread to help lower its incredibly high incidence of heart disease from selenium-poor soil. By adding nutrients that are found in low levels in the diet, we could significantly improve the health of the American people for only pennies a day. The minerals chromium, magnesium, calcium, zinc, iron, potassium, and selenium; and the vitamins folic acid, B-6, C beta-carotene, E, and riboflavin could all be safely and cheaply added to food staples to give Americans a quantum leap in health and longevity.

Which ones are safe? So how can you know which of these 2,800 additives are safe? Shop the perimeter of the grocery store: most of the highly processed foods loaded with additives are toward the center of the store. If you eat foods in as close to their natural state as possible, you will minimize your intake of all additives. Otherwise, specific guidelines would be to:

Avoid MSG, nitrates, brominated vegetable oil, artificial food colors, and sulfur agents (for sensitive individuals).

Minimize your intake of saccharin, quinine, and sodium-or aluminum-based anything.

Read your food labels. Take some responsibility for your own health. Do not expect the government to totally protect you. They can't and won't.

BURNED PROTEINS

When proteins are seared at high temperatures they produce benzo-pyrenes, which are known carcinogens. A well-done two-pound steak contains as much cancer-causing substances as you could get from smoking six hundred cigarettes.[37] Unfortunately, Americans are so attached to their barbecues that the average person eats several hundred times more carcinogens from burned food than they breathe from heavily polluted air.[38]

This warning includes fried foods, overheated oils, burned sugars, and so on.[39] Avoid overcooked food of any sort. Although I haven't been able to give up the great American barbecue, I am more cautious in keeping the flames under control and never eating well-done meat. Also, by including the foods and nutrients listed in the "solution" section, you can neutralize much of the potential harm from occasional rational barbecuing.

MICROORGANISMS

In the early 1970s, a jumbo jet took off from Europe bound for America with a real surprise for the entire crew and passengers. The custard filling in their dessert was brimming with a *staphylococcus* bacterial infection, compliments of the acne pustules and poor hygiene of the food preparer. Everyone aboard got severe diarrhea and cramps, including the captain and crew: only through heroics was the plane landed safely. This episode provided the material for the comic movie *Airplane*, but it wasn't so funny for the people on this transatlantic flight. Since then, the Federal Aviation Administration has required that half the crew eat one food and the other half eat a different food, just to avoid another potential disaster.

There are strangers in our food supply. Just as much as you need food, so do the tiny trespassers that include bacteria, molds, fungus, worms, and others. Most food has at least some traces of microorganisms, but when allowed to proliferate through ideal conditions, germs can become a serious health risk. FDA microbiologists estimate that 69 million to 275 million episodes of diarrhea per year occur in the United States, compliments of food microorganisms.[40] The U.S. Center for Disease Control estimates that nine thousand Americans each year die from food-borne infections. Most of these deaths are older adults, children, infants, and sick people who are unable to defend themselves against infection and severe dehydration.

Medical services, lost wages, and recalled food cost America $1 billion to $10 billion per year from food-borne infections.[41] Of all the things you could worry about in your food supply, this category outweighs the rest in sheer dollars and fatalities, yet is more prosaic than the exotic categories like DDT residues on carrots. Make no mistake about it, food-borne infections are a very serious health issue.

The main culprits here include:[42]

Salmonella. About one out of every thousand cases is fatal. By USDA admission, 37 percent of all poultry, 10 percent of all pork, and 5 percent of red meat is contaminated with salmonella when it is sold. Also, salmonella can exist in dairy products, especially unpasteurized milk. A 1985 outbreak of salmonella from poor hygiene in a dairy processing plant led to 197,000 people getting ill and fourteen deaths.[43]

Staphylococcus. Found in the skin, nose, and throat of most adults, it can be easily transmitted through poor food handling. Accounts for about one-third of all food-borne infections.

Campylobacter. A recently discovered but increasingly prominent infection that is often antibiotic resistant. In a five-year period from 1981 to 1986, campylobacter incidence increased by 523 percent in California.[44] Found on meat, poultry, and unpasteurized dairy products, it is spread through fecal to meat contact, which occurs continuously in slaughter houses.

Listeria. Just identified in the 1980s and found

Figure 7C: Cycle of Contamination

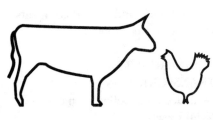

CATTLE RANCHES AND CHICKEN FARMS
—Animals surrounded by own excrement, which harbors bacteria
—Cramped animals spread bacteria to one another
—Feces contaminate feed, and animals ingest bacteria
—Rodents and insects help spread bacteria
—Drugs to enhance animal growth breed resistant bacteria

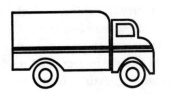

PRESLAUGHTER TRANSPORTATION
—Storage areas contaminated from previous cargo
—Animals ingest contaminated feed
—Animals surrounded by own excrement

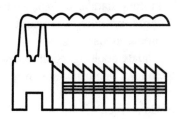

SLAUGHTERHOUSE
—Unsanitary environment spreads bacteria
—Unsanitary workers cross-contaminate products
—Unsanitary equipment spreads bacteria

POULTRY SLAUGHTER
—Defeathering equipment spreads dirt and feces
—Eviscerating machines spread feces on birds
—Birds mingle in chill bath, allowing cross-contamination

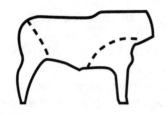

PROCESSED MEAT PRODUCTION
—Human and mechanical handling (boning, grinding, slicing) spreads bacteria
—Combined and reworked meats increase bacterial levels

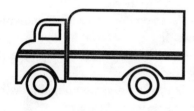

POSTSLAUGHTER TRANSPORTATION
—Inadequate cooling promotes bacterial growth
—Inadequate temperature maintenance in truck/train cars promotes bacterial growth

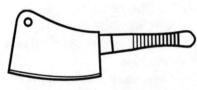

WHOLESALE/RETAIL HANDLING
—Unsanitary machinery, workers and utensils spread bacteria
—Inadequate temperature maintenance in storage freezers and retail cases causes growth of bacteria

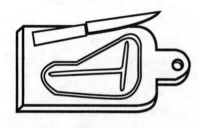

CONSUMER/KITCHEN
—Unsanitary hands, utensils, cutting boards, sponges, and counters contaminate foods
—Inadequate cooking, cooling, and storage allows bacterial growth

(Source: New York City Department of Consumer Affairs)

mostly in contaminated dairy products and red meat. From 20 to 50 percent of all diagnosed cases are fatal. In 1985, a factory in Los Angeles producing Mexican-style cheese, Jalisco, caused 47 deaths and stillbirths and 147 illnesses.[45] Listeria exists throughout nature, but is most likely to occur in unpasteurized dairy products. A very lethal and new member of this group.

Clostridium botulinum. A bacteria that grows in anaerobic conditions, such as improperly canned products, and creates one of the most lethal natural substances known to humans. If equally distributed, one ounce of botulism extract (or less than a whiskey glass), could kill everyone in America. Due to quality control in canning factories, this condition is relatively rare, but 20 percent of cases are fatal. Neurotoxic symptoms include double vision and paralysis of respiratory tract. Seek medical help immediately.

Clostridium perfringens. Found throughout nature, but most likely to infest food that is left out of the refrigerator. Rarely fatal, but quite uncomfortable.

E. coli. Spread by fecal to food contact, from poor hygiene in slaughtering plants and restaurants. Rarely fatal, but growing in incidence.

Shigella. Spread through poor hygiene of fecal to food contact. More common in poor nations where overcrowding, flies, and raw sewage create ideal breeding grounds.

Yersinia. Present throughout nature, but most likely to cause food-borne infections when foods are eaten uncooked. Victims have appendicitis-like symptoms.

Giardia. A protozoa that exists in the intestines of many mammals. Can be spread through contaminated water, food washed with contaminated water, and contaminated workers. Can become a long term chronic infection in the intestines. Now found in the drinking water in high mountain streams, due to sheep and bear fecal contamination.

Vibrio (including cholera). Found throughout warm coastal waters. Most likely to infect people through shellfish that are held at room temperature. Rare but deadly.

Bacillus cereus.[46] Found widely throughout vegetation and soil. Spread by allowing starchy foods (like corn, potato, vegetables, puddings, soups, and rice) to stay at the ideal breeding temperature.

Hepatitis A. This is a virus that attacks the consumer with flu-like symptoms and can be spread by fecal contact. Nationwide, 27,869 cases of hepatitis A were reported to the Center for Disease Control during the year 1987. That represented a 23 percent increase over the previous year.[47] It is usually spread by an infected food handler who does not practice good hygiene.

High-speed processing machines in slaughterhouses allow fecal contact to the meat, which means much of our meat and poultry has been innoculated with one or more of these villains. One of the real worries here is that widespread use of subtherapeutic antibiotics will produce an epidemic of food-borne infections that are resistant to antibiotic treatment. Also, don't look to the government for protection here: the USDA does not inspect meat for bacteria nor does it reject meat because of bacterial infestation, taking the position that bacterial contamination is inevitable.[48] There are a number of consumer action groups who constantly petition and badger the USDA to change this bizarre stance.

Aflatoxins are basically a mold, or fungus, that grows on grains (like corn, wheat, and rye), legumes (like pinto beans and peanuts), and nuts (like sunflower seeds and walnuts). Aflatoxins are about twenty-one times more lethal than DDT and are one of the more potent carcinogens ever tested. Around the world, the incidence of liver cancer follows immediately behind aflatoxins in food. The most likely source of aflatoxins are peanuts and peanut butter that are poorly stored in a warm humid region. Even trace amounts in the diet of pregnant women can cause mental retardation in their offspring.[49] A rural region of Georgia, where the people eat a diet high in homegrown peanuts, has twice the national incidence of mental retardation in infants. Aflatoxins are more prevalent on a growing plant that is stressed, such as during a drought or poor soil conditions.[50]

Although the FDA has set a tolerance of 20 parts per billion of aflatoxin as allowable, test animals die of liver cancer when fed a diet that contains only 5 parts per billion. In order to minimize your intake of aflatoxins, buy only peanuts and peanut butter from quality high volume interstate vendors. Obviously, avoid eating any moldy looking nuts, grains, or legumes.

Ergot is another poison that is produced by the mold *Claviceps purpurea* that grows on rye grains during cool rainy summers. Such a condition probably brought about the Salem witch trials in eighteenth-century New England, since ergot is a substance similar to the hallucinogenic drug, LSD, and can cause people to act demonically possessed.[51]

Raw milk is another item worthy of concern. Although there are vague unproven health claims associated with consuming unpasteurized milk, more than one thousand Americans have become ill and at least twenty have died since 1980 from foodborne infections transmitted through unpasteurized milk.[52]

How to defend yourself? Minimize the ideal requirements that allow microorganisms to thrive:

Time. Under ideal conditions, one bacteria could multiply into a thriving colony of two million within only seven hours.[53] Since all food is infected with at least one bacteria, you can't give them the ideal conditions to duplicate.

Temperature. From 60 to 120 degrees F. (15.5 to 48.8 C.) most microorganisms reproduce rapidly. Avoid this temperature range by keeping food either hot on the stove or cold in the refrigerator—never left out at room temperature.

High fluid content. Dried foods, like brown rice and pinto beans, do not have enough fluid to support bacterial growth. Moist foods are easier targets for microorganisms.

High protein content. Meat, eggs, dairy, fish, pork, and poultry are all ideal breeding grounds with the protein supply providing for rapid growth of microorganisms.

Surface area. When food is ground up (like hamburger or potato salad) you increase the growth rate for microorganisms.

Hygiene. Though bacteria are everywhere, you can reduce the innoculation of food through good hygiene: wash hands after using the bathroom or blowing the nose, keep food surface areas clean, make sure there are no insects to transmit diseases, and keep infected workers away from food.

PESTICIDE RESIDUES

The U.S. now uses about 1.2 billion pounds of pesticides and herbicides per year in 50,000 different products with 600 active ingredients. Ten pounds of pesticides and herbicides are used annually for every man, woman, and child in this country. Experts estimate that only 2 percent of the pesticides hit the bugs with the remaining 98 percent going into the air, soil, water, or food supply. Either we breathe it, eat it, drink it, or let it lie in the soil to possibly seep into next year's crop.

Only twenty-eight of the six hundred available active pesticide ingredients are of major concern to the National Research Council, which finds that 80 percent of our health risk is due to using thirteen pesticides on fifteen food crops. Listed in order, with the items of greatest concern first: tomatoes, beef, potatoes, oranges, lettuce, apples, peaches, pork, wheat, soybeans, beans, carrots, chicken, corn, and grapes.[54] The thirteen pesticides include one herbicide (linuron), two insecticides (permethrin, chlordimeform), and ten fungicides. One herbicide (linuron) represents 98 percent of the total cancer risk from all herbicides. With our incredible brain pool of scientists and Nobel laureates in this country, we should find substitutes for these few chemicals that pose such a disproportionate risk to our food supply.

Pesticides can make a fabulously nutritious food more of a question mark. For instance, broccoli is high in vitamin C, calcium, folacin, vitamin A, and the cancer-fighting indoles. All well and good. But there are fifty different pesticides used on broccoli. Since you cannot peel broccoli and many pesticides are systemic (become part of the plant and cannot be washed off), much of that pesticide residue is consumed. Hence, there is a risk versus benefit to broccoli that has nutritionists wondering, "Do I recommend that people eat this?" Buy organic broccoli or soak your commercial broccoli in warm water and Ivory soap (no additives) for fifteen minutes, then scrub and rinse. Other produce has a similar shower of pesticides throughout its growing season. Apples can have 110 different pesticides used on the crop, 70 on bell peppers, 100 on tomatoes, and so on.

According to the EPA, excessive pesticide residues are found on about 3 percent of all domestic produce and 6 percent of all foreign produce. However, the Natural Resources Defense Council conducted a yearlong study that had more disturbing findings: 63 percent of all strawberries, 55 percent of all peaches, and 52 percent of all cherries tested had detectable levels of pesticide residues.[55] There were thirty different pesticides detected on carrots, with 17 percent of the carrots containing detectable levels of DDT, which has been banned for fifteen years but persists in the soil.

The National Research Council has calculated that if all produce had the maximum allowable pesticide residue (ADI) of all pesticides approved for that crop, in other words a worst-case scenario that would not violate any laws, the cancer risk increases 3,000-fold, from the EPA's acceptable 1 in 1 million to a dismal 3000 in 1 million. If such is true, then 10,000 Americans die each year from cancer caused by pesticide misuse.

With consumer action groups to disclose this information and intelligent consumers to heed the advice, only 52 percent of Americans have confidence that the government adequately protects our food supply, while 73 percent feel that we should use fewer pesticides to insure a safer food supply, even it that change brings higher prices with it.[56]

The residues in food may not always be pesticides, but rather could include chemicals used to process the food. For instance, methylene chloride was the primary solvent used to extract caffeine from coffee for many years. The National Toxicology Program found that methylene chloride causes liver and lung cancer in lab animals.[57] Since 1967, the FDA has allowed methylene chloride residue levels of up to 10 parts per million in decaffeinated coffee. According to many experts, including the FDA, that is one thousand times higher than a safe level that could easily be obtained with modern equipment. Some companies now decaffeinate their coffee with steam extraction methods, which are safe. Check your label.

Fresh fruits and vegetables are about 70 to 90 percent water. In order to keep the produce from shriveling, looking bad, and losing weight and value, produce merchants (both packers and grocery chains) often apply waxes to seal in the produce. This "shrink wrap" embalming approach may be cost effective to the vendor, cutting moisture loss by 30 to 40 percent, but it is quite unhealthy to the consumer. The FDA has approved six different waxes for use on eighteen different produce items. Approved waxes include shellac, paraffin, palm oil derivatives, and synthetic resins—all items that are also used to wax your kitchen floor, car, or fine wood furniture. Waxes cannot be washed off with normal warm water soaking. Fungicides, like orthophenylphenol (also used to deworm sheep), are applied along with the wax to keep fungus from growing on the plant. Not only does this permanently bond the fungicide to the produce, but 90 percent of all fungicides are known to cause cancer.

According to FDA law, the grocery store must display a sign noting that waxes or postharvest pesticides have been applied to the produce. In reality, no one complies with this law and the FDA admits that it does not have the manpower to enforce it. Waxes are a mild risk, yet waxes with fungicides are a major risk that cannot be scrubbed off even by the wary consumer.

Produce items that are approved by the FDA for waxing include: apples, avocados, bell peppers, cantaloupes, cucumbers, eggplants, grapefruits, lemons, limes, melons, oranges, parsnips, passion fruits, peaches, pineapples, pumpkins, rutabagas, squashes, sweet potatoes, tomatoes, and turnips. In a consumer poll, 96 percent of the people were concerned about the coatings used to enhance the appearance of fresh produce. Next time you can see your reflection in that bright shiny apple, think about it.

A main reason that waxes and fungicides must be used is the lengthy period from harvest to the grocery store shelves. The average produce today travels 1200 miles to the consumer. It costs New York City residents an extra $2,000 per truckload to get broccoli from California out of season. Generally speaking, for every $2 spent growing a food, another $1 is spent moving it. Many people in Florida may wonder why they buy California oranges (and vice versa), or why New Yorkers buy apples grown in Washington: the problem is that large grocery-store chains make produce contracts with mega-produce farms, regardless of their location. If grocery chains bought more local produce, it would be fresher, require less chemicals to keep it looking decent, use less energy, and made customers happier about patronizing local produce.

DESIGNER FOODS

Nearly 8,000 new food products were introduced to American grocery shelves in 1987. Most of them boasted some type of nutritional modification, including 400 with "reduced calories," 159 lower in fat, 120 with lower sugar content, and 55 with added fiber.[58] Efforts to make good food better are to be commended; but we should not tamper heavily with foods.

Some people claim that sedentary Americans need low-calorie food to be able to continue to enjoy eating—Yet low-calorie options don't seem to improve our health picture at all. The Institute of Food Technologists finds that in 1974 there were 28.8 million obese Americans, of which 8.4 million were severely obese. By 1980, after the introduction of hundreds of low-calorie designer foods, there were 34 million obese Americans, of which 13 million were severely obese.

Designer foods include those breakfast pastries that can be toasted. The fat that is used in these pastries must stay solid at toasting temperatures of 180 degrees F. No one know what such a chemically altered fat does in the body. We now have a fat substitute that is a sucrose polyester. The body doesn't know what to do with it, since it is a totally foreign molecule.

While scientists have improved foods with greater insect resistance or higher protein content, the further we deviate from the time-tested molecules found in natural foods, the greater the risk of creating a substance that is toxic to the body. I highly encourage people to eat real foods in moderation and exercise off the extra calories to maintain a decent figure. Saccharin, cyclamates, synthetic food dyes, and others are all grim reminders of nonnutrients that can be harmful in the body.

CONTAINER RESIDUES

You eat more than the food in front of you. Depending on your kitchen utensils, you may also be eating trace amounts of plastic, metal, and lead. Glass, stainless steel, enameled steel, and hard food-grade plastics are all reasonably safe. But soft plastics have various ingredients that can migrate into the food and create a problem.

Acrylonitrile is found in soft plastics and the foods that are housed in them, such as tub margarine and olive oil.[59] Upon ingesting acrylonitrile, lab animals get cancer and bacteria has mutagenic changes. Humans working in the acrylonitrile factory and inhaling vapors showed an increased risk for cancer in all sites, especially the lungs.

Canned foods contain trace amounts of tin, cadmium, and lead (if the seam is leaded). Wax milk cartons contain trace amounts of dioxin, which is used to formulate the wax paper. Quart plastic bottles of soft drinks are particularly suspicious since the carbonated water will accelerate the migration of plastic chemicals from the container.

Though there is some concern that excess aluminum in the diet can precipitate Alzheimer's disease, aluminum pots and soft drink cans will not contribute large amounts of aluminum to the diet unless there is considerable acid food in the container to dissolve greater amounts of the aluminum.

Nearly all ceramics have a glaze to protect the finish. Most of these are lead based, and some glazes are applied at lower kiln temperatures, so that the glaze is not inert and can have lead migrate into the food or beverage. Lead is a vicious food and water pollutant that should be seriously avoided, if you have lead-glazed ceramic kitchenware or cups from Third World countries, you may wish to have them tested or relegate them to show pieces. Although the FDA has a standard of only allowing 7 parts of lead per million to leach from a plate in 24 hours (new recommended level: 0.1ppm), they cannot/do not check the 500 million pieces of ceramics that are imported into this country each year. Please use safe ceramics that are fired at properly high temperatures. This area can be the downfall of many otherwise healthy families. If you have a favorite set of ceramic dishes you would like to have tested, write to the U.S. Potter's Association, 518 Market St., East Liverpool, OH 43920 for a list of fifteen laboratories that can test your dinnerware for its safety, or write to Frandon Enterprises, 511 N. 46 St., Seattle, WA 96103.

Just exactly what are the implications of having trace amounts of harmful agents migrating into the food from food containers? No one has thoroughly researched this area, but I would highly encourage the reader to buy milk in gallon plastic containers, minimize the use of quart soft drink containers, avoid any suspicious ceramic ware, and stick to the reliable safety of glass and stainless steel whenever possible.

FISH

Fish is supposed to be healthy food. However, from the Great Lakes to the Gulf of Mexico to the Pacific and Atlantic coasts and many rivers and lakes in between, we have shamelessly polluted our water and fish. Safe eating of fish is an unusual topic for several reasons.

There is no mandatory inspection of fish or shellfish. In 1986, the FDA examined six pounds of fish for every one million pounds that were eaten. In Los Angeles harbor alone, 57 million pounds of fish were landed in 1985 with only thirty fish inspected by the FDA. Of the hundreds of known contaminants in fish, "action" levels have been assigned to only a dozen pollutants. If you eat more than two and half pounds of certain kinds of fish per year, then you are exceeding ADI limits set by the FDA.

A study by the U.S. General Accounting Office mysteriously concluded that there is no need for a mandatory federal fish inspection program, like the one used for meat and poultry.[60] While Dr. Frank Young, commissioner of the FDA, defends American seafood as safe, that same report shows the disproportionate number of food-borne illnesses that are linked to eating fish.[61] Although the FDA has known for fifteen years about the rampant

figure 7d: Fish creates a disproportionate amount of food-borne disease
outbreak = two or more cases of food-borne illness linked to a common food source

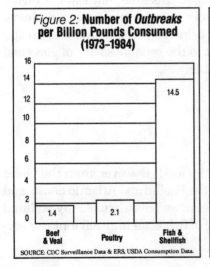

Figure 2: **Number of *Outbreaks* per Billion Pounds Consumed (1973–1984)**

SOURCE: CDC Surveillance Data & ERS, USDA Consumption Data.

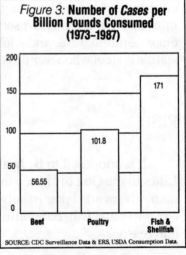

Figure 3: **Number of *Cases* per Billion Pounds Consumed (1973–1987)**

SOURCE: CDC Surveillance Data & ERS, USDA Consumption Data.

problems in the safety of our seafood supply, they proposed some changes in 1975 which were quickly shot down by the fish industry and state governments.[62] While there is minimal voluntary inspection of domestic fish, 64 percent of our fish is imported with virtually no inspection at all.

Fish is supposed to be healthy food. Due to frequent endorsements from many health experts, Americans now eat 11 percent more fish than in 1980. Fish is high in a special type of fat (EPA), protein, vitamin B-6, selenium, and other valuable nutrients; but in some fish, the risks outweigh the benefits. Although average seafood consumption in America is 15 pounds per person annually, real seafood lovers eat up to 180 pounds per year.[63] Even 15 pounds per year could be a health risk if consuming the wrong kind of fish. With the increased consumption of fish, the National Marine Fisheries Service has been overwhelmed and now inspects less and less of the total fish catch.

Fish rots quickly. This is due to high levels of polyunsaturated fatty acids. Many commercial fishing vessels catch fish and do not process it until they return to harbor. This makes shopping for fresh fish a real treasure hunt.

The sushi craze A longstanding tradition in some ethnic groups and a recent craze in upscale American restaurants is eating raw fish (sushi). There are parasites, like tapeworms, roundworms, and various bacteria, that can only be neutralized by cooking the fish.[64] In one outbreak, 1,017 raw-clam lovers developed intestinal cramps, diarrhea, and vomiting from gastro-enteritis via the bacteria in raw shellfish.[65] Anyone with cancer, diabetes, or other immune-impairing disease should avoid raw fish completely.[66]

Repositories of pollution. Most of our indiscriminate pollution ends up in some body of water and becomes more concentrated higher up the food chain—ending with large predatory fish being the most lethal. There is about a 10,000-fold increase in the concentration of a pollutant from water to larger fish. The U.S. spews 32 billion gallons of toxic chemicals and sewage into the sea *every day.* The results have been devastating as one-third of American shellfish are illegal to eat due to contamination from bacteria, viruses and toxic chemicals.[67]

According to Larry Skinner, an ecologist with the New York Department of Environmental Conservation, a person eating an eight-ounce serving of trout from Lake Ontario once a week would have a cancer risk of 1 in 200.[68] That is 5000 times the "acceptable risk" level of one cancer in one million people used by the EPA! Fortunately, commercial fishing is banned in Lake Ontario. Researchers found that pregnant women eating two to three meals per week of contaminated fish (PCB is often the problem) gave birth to infants with weak reflexes, sluggish movement, and behavioral problems.[69]

In some polluted lakes and streams, researchers have found that two out of three fish have cancer themselves!

PCB is now a ubiquitous pollutant that is particularly concentrated in freshwater fish in northeastern America and near big city bays. Pregnant and lactating women should avoid fish from these regions. Ironically, studies around the world show that the consumption of *clean, healthy* fish is a major protective factor in the prevention of breast cancer.[70] There will be many victims and martyrs before this pollution scandal is cleared up. (See the "PCB" section in chapter 5.)

In 1983, the FDA found DDT in 334 of 386 samples of domestic fish tested, even though DDT was banned eleven years prior to that time. In 1984, the National Oceanic and Atmospheric Administration studied the water quality and fish samples around the nation. Worst offenders were Los Angeles, Boston, Salem (Massachusetts), and New York harbors. All had water and fish laced with DDT, PCB, heavy metals, and sundry pollutants. Things haven't improved much since then. A group of scientists find that government "action" levels for DDT and dieldrin in Great Lakes sport fish are providing no protection to the consumer.[71]

Much of the 1.2 billion pounds of pesticides and herbicides

and 90 billion pounds of pollutants produced annually in America end up being washed into streams, rivers, lakes, underground aquifers, and oceans. Missouri state health officials have advised against eating fish from the Mississippi and Missouri rivers due to lethal levels of the insecticide chlordane.

Some toxins in fish are naturally occurring. Ciguatera is a toxin found in warm-water fish, like groupers, snapper, barracuda, tuna, amberjack, mackerel, and eels. The ciguatera poison in the fish comes from concentrating the poison found in tiny sea creatures (dinoflagellates) that are consumed. The large fish store ciguatera harmlessly in their fatty tissue; but ciguatera poisons the central nervous system in human consumers with such bizarre symptoms as "sensory reversal"—that is, the patient perceives hot objects as cold, and vice versa. While a new testing kit from the University of Hawaii can detect ciguatera, no cooking process will detoxify the poison. The Center for Disease Control estimates that up to 150,000 cases of ciguatera poisoning occur each year around the world; however, if you eat a variety of fish and avoid concentrations of fatty tissue by broiling the fish over a fire, then it is unlikely that ciguatera will be your nemesis. Puffer fish are a delicacy in Japan, but with an 80 percent fatality rate in those eating the wrong part of the fish, only licensed chefs can prepare this food.

Heavy toxic metals have a tendency to concentrate in fish, especially shellfish which eat by "vacuuming" the bottom of a bay and digesting the organic matter therein. Shellfish caught in big-city bays and harbors are quite suspect. Excess chromium (from metal-plating industries) can cause kidney damage; lead can cause impaired mental development; and arsenic can cause cancer. In March of 1989 the Florida Department of Health and Rehabilitative Services issued a warning against eating certain fish caught in the Everglades area: various species of game fish contained four times the amount of mercury considered "acceptable" by federal standards.

The upshot of all this information is summed up nicely by Dr. Les Kaufman, a research scientist at the New England Aquarium in Boston. "The environmental prophecies of the late '60s and

'70s are unfortunately coming to pass. People have to look at the environment as an organism. That's not hippie talk. It's reality."[72] Our irresponsible dumping into waterways has lessened our valuable seafood populations, and made unsafe many other kinds of fish.

Some guidelines that can help make fish an enjoyable, nutritious, and relatively harmless food:

-Small is beautiful. While larger predatory fish have higher concentrations of pollutants, smaller fish are safer.

-Avoid the organ meats of most fish, especially shellfish. That includes foods where the entire fish is thrown into a soup or casserole.

-Trim away the fat in fish. Most pollutants are fat soluble and concentrate in fatty tissue. Do not use the drippings of fish. Best cooking methods are to broil, bake on a rack, or boil in water.

-Pregnant and lactating women need to be particularly cautious of suspicious fish, since the contaminants can cause fetal abnormalities. Minimize or avoid bluefish, striped bass, swordfish, shark, and limit tuna consumption (from high mercury content) to less than a half pound per week.

-Eat a varied diet. Don't make fish your only entree item and don't eat too much of any one type of fish. Avoid fish caught near major industrial areas. Safest are ocean fish caught offshore: cod, haddock, pollock, yellowfin tuna, flounder, and ocean perch. Salmon has remained surprisingly uncontaminated. If you eat shellfish, make it a snack, not a meal. Eat only cooked shellfish. Catfish and swordfish win the booby prize for most tainted. Even catfish raised on pond farms is usually exposed to the pesticide runoff from nearby farms.

-We need mandatory fish inspection. Although fish poses unique problems to a food inspection program, we need some protection in this healthy food commodity. A fish inspection program would safeguard our food and return the public's sense of confidence in fish.

SUMMARY

As you can see, you have every reason to be concerned about the safety of your food supply. However, the "solution" section of this book shows you how to reduce your intake of toxins while increasing your tolerance of unavoidable toxins. It may seem to be an odd ending to this chapter, but try to enjoy your food while using judicious caution.

CHAPTER 8
What's in the Water?

Anne Anderson had known only one person in her whole life with leukemia, so it seemed like uncommonly bad luck when her own three-year-old son, Jimmy, was diagnosed with this lethal form of cancer of the bone marrow.[1] Then she found out that two other children in her neighborhood had leukemia, and began asking if something in their area could be causing this unique cluster of rare childhood cancer. No one would answer Anne's questions back in 1976, nor would anyone even listen to them. After twelve children in the area developed leukemia, Anne enlisted the help of a Harvard statistician who calculated that Anne's neighborhood in Woburn, Massachusetts, had 7.5 times the national incidence of leukemia. People began listening. Eventually, several major industrial polluters were caught, sued, and settled out of court for contaminating the municipal water well with toxic chemicals, like trichloroethylene.

Woburn is hardly a rare case. In 1978, Love Canal in upstate New York became a disaster area as Hooker Chemical plant dumped inconceivable amounts of pollutants, which dramatically affected the health of locals. In 1983 Times Beach, Missouri, had to be evacuated because their ground water was thoroughly polluted with PCB. The EPA has identified over 28,000 potential hazardous waste sites around the country that are probably leaking into drinking water sources. Departing from their normally staid and reserved language, the EPA has called toxic contamination of our water supply "a ticking time bomb, ready to go off."[2]

WATER: THE ULTIMATE NUTRIENT

Most Americans could live weeks if not months without food, but we would die within a day or two without water. Two-thirds of an adult body is water. Water's functions are many. It:

- lubricates, as in mucus and sweat
- provides structure and cushioning, as in the muscles and skin
- becomes a solvent, dissolving most water soluble substances
- is the medium of the blood
- is a reactant in millions of chemical reactions; by an enzyme inserting one molecule of water in between two beads on a "necklace," molecules can be broken down into smaller usable parts through hydrolysis
- dilutes waste matter
- regulates body temperature
- provides traction (on the fingertips)
- protects exposed areas of the body (like the eyes and nose)
- keeps the body at a neutral pH.[3] And much, much more.

Optimal amounts of water will reduce the incidence of infections, constipation, kidney stones, and other common maladies. The average person drinks about one liter of water daily, while the wiser and more active person drinks two to four liters of clean fluids daily. Water is truly the ultimate nutrient.

When astronauts look down on this emerald green planet, they see mostly sea. Two-thirds of the earth's surface is covered with water, yet 99 percent of all water on earth is unavailable for human consumption because it is salt water, or locked in polar ice caps, found in remote regions, or in sandy aquifers under the earth's surface. Americans have had a tendency to think of our water supply as unlimited and cheap. It isn't. Many scientists predict that the next great resource crisis will be over water, not oil. Israel is reluctant to give up the West Bank land acquired during the Six Day War because underneath that bleak landscape is one of the largest aquifers in the Middle East. Throughout the planet Earth, and especially in America, we have polluted an alarmingly high percentage of our precious drinking water. The purpose of this chapter is to show you how to protect yourself from our increasingly dangerous water supply.

WATER POLLUTION USA

Each year American dumps 71 billion gallons of hazardous wastes into landfills and waterways: no doubt many of these contaminants are causing varied health problems. A study by the California Department of Health Services found that pregnant women who drank bottled water had a lower incidence of miscarriages and birth defects than women drinking tap water. Stomach cancer has also been related to the quality of drinking water.[4]

According to the Congressional Office of Technology Assessment, America has more than 600,000 open and closed solid waste facilities, with 35,000 of these dump sites threatening the ground water supply. We have 2.5 million underground gasoline tanks and another one million tanks storing industrial chemicals.[5] According to the EPA, at least 25 percent of these tanks leak. A leak of one gallon of gasoline per day can render unsafe the drinking-water supply for 50,000 people. We also have an additional 180,000 pits and ponds for holding liquid wastes from industrial and mining operations; of the 26,000 ponds that contain toxic waste, 70 percent have no barrier to prevent them from leaking into underground water supplies.

The Department of Defense produces 500,000 tons of hazardous waste annually at 333 sites around the country. Half of these federal sites are in violation of federal pollution laws. Another five hundred different federal nuclear sites are violating pollution laws by illegally dumping radioactive waste under the guise of "national security." For over thirty years, the Army dumped nerve gas and other toxic wastes at the Aberdeen Proving Ground, which led to pollution of nearby drinking sources and a creek flowing into the Chesapeake Bay.

The results of this widespread pollution has been devastating to our precious water supplies. In a 1984 study by the National Cancer Institute, there were 1,565 chemical contaminants found in American drinking water, of which 117 are known or suspected carcinogens. A 1985 study by the EPA found 1,338 different contaminants. A consumer action group, the Center for Responsive Law, conducted its own study, finding 2,110 compounds in drinking water, of which 190 are known or suspected to be harmful to health. Ninety percent of the chemical contaminants in our water supply have not even been identified.[6]

The pesticide EDB has been found in more than seven hundred wells in Florida. Over 2,450 wells in California are tainted with the pesticide DBCP.[7] By 1980, the EPA found that 350 hazardous-waste sites had caused the closure of five hundred wells in thirty-two states. As of 1989, all major aquifers in New Jersey have been affected and over one thousand wells have been closed in that state since 1971 due to its dubious distinction as the "toxic waste capital" of America, with ten of the fifty worst toxic waste sites in America. An EPA survey of 945 public water supplies found that nearly 30 percent were contaminated with organic chemicals. As reality continues to surface through fact gathering, the problem worsens.

Richard Arlington of Fort Edward, New York, found out how precarious our water supply really is. In the middle of the night he was called by a state health official who told him not to use the water and to evacuate his home immediately—his home water well had been contaminated with industrial wastes from a nearby factory, and the carcinogenic chemical TCE was found at two hundred times the allowable level.

At first, it looks like a big-city problem: 41 percent of the contaminated wells in California are in Los Angeles County. However, farm areas are at risk because pesticide and herbicide runoff ends up in the water system. More than 1,700 wells in the farming region of Fresno County, California, have been tainted with DBCP. Nebraska, Iowa, Minnesota, and Wisconsin have all instigated their own water protection laws due to polluted water supplies from farming. Strip-mining in the West, uranium mining in the Southwest, acid mine drainage and industry in the East, and oil and gas drilling in the South have made water pollution an equal-opportunity villain.

You can run but you cannot hide from this water pollution mess. Nine of every ten rural residents rely on groundwater, serving nearly forty million people.[8] Researchers at Cornell University find that nearly two-thirds of rural households in America use drinking water that fails to comply with EPA standards. In sparsely populated Idaho, radioactive and chemical contamination from a U.S. nuclear weapons facility has polluted fifty square miles of the underground water tables.

Laws are getting more strict and businesses do not intentionally set out to poison the landscape and residents; but money is the engine of our economic system. Right now, dumping toxic wastes in land disposal facilities costs only 25 to 50 percent the price of proper disposal in a toxic waste site or incineration. Many responsible industries have shown efforts to improve the situation: the 3M corporation has cut hazardous waste generation by 50 percent, saving themselves (by recycling) $292 million since 1975.

GOVERNMENTAL PROTECTION

Unfortunately, governmental protection of our precious water resources has been dismally absent. Until 1986 only twenty-two of the seven hundred widespread contaminants in drinking water were regulated. Of the thousands of contaminants found in American drinking water, the EPA has established a Maximum Contaminant Level (MCL) for only eighteen chemicals. Even though laws are purposefully vague and lenient, there have been tens of thousands of violations of the water pollution laws each year—yet in the ten years following the Safe Drinking Water Act of 1974, the EPA referred only twenty-one cases to the Justice Department for prosecution.

Legally, small businesses who produce less than 2,640 pounds of hazardous waste each year can dump their wastes anywhere. Although asbestos is a known carcinogen when inhaled, there is no EPA guideline for asbestos in the water supply. Legally, a community using groundwater is required to test for inorganic contamination (lead, arsenic, and nitrates) only once every three years. Legally, more than 11.5 billion gallons of liquid waste is injected deep into the earth each year. While proponents of deep injection claim it is a safer alternative, over the course of two years the nation's largest waste disposal firm leaked 45 million gallons of hazardous waste that was destined for deep injection into nearby aquifers before the EPA shut down the system. Although bottled water is under the jurisdiction of the FDA, there are no guidelines regarding the quality of bottled water, nor does the manufacturer have to list the source of their water supply. It need only comply with EPA guidelines, which, as you can see, are not very reassuring.

When chlorine is used to disinfect municipal water supplies, it can react with decaying organic matter (like leaves) to create a known carcinogen, trihalomethanes (THM). The European Economic Community has set a safety standard for THM of 1 part per billion (ppb); Germany and Switzerland use 25 ppb for their guideline; but the EPA uses 100 ppb as an "action" level. Water systems that serve fewer than 10,000 people, which accounts for 46 million Americans, do not have to comply with any standard for THM.

After decades of data collection, in May of 1989 the EPA proposed Maximum Contaminant Levels (MCL) for thirty-eight known carcinogens in the American drinking water supply. However, local water officials will have eighteen months to comply, with longer phase-in periods allowed if economic hardship can be proved.

Anne Anderson, the mother whose son died of leukemia, was criticized by others with the comment, "The city wouldn't let us drink bad water!" With flimsy laws, minimal enforcement personnel, and guidelines written more for economic conveniences than public protection . . . don't look to the government to insure the safety of your water supply.

CONTAMINANT STEW: WHAT'S IN THE WATER?

Chlorine. In 1908, Jersey City, New Jersey, was the first town in the U.S. to disinfect their municipal drinking water with chlorine. A new era of health was ushered in as outbreaks of cholera, dysentery, and typhoid were seriously reduced. However, due to excessive use of chlorine, it is now more of a hazard than a help. In 1974, the EPA found that chlorinated water increases the risk for cancer in lab animals, and since then many other scientists have found similar conclusions. Researchers now find that the risk of bladder cancer triples for people who consume chlorinated water for forty years.[9] The incidence of bladder, colon, and rectal cancer also increases with long-term exposure to chlorinated tap water.

When you think about it, chlorine is bleach—a deadly poison. Chlorinated hydrocarbons (like DDT) are among the most deadly chemicals created. Chlorine by-products, like chloroform, are also known carcinogens. Chlorine, if used, should be cautiously applied to our drinking water.

The safer alternatives to chlorine include ozone, chlorine dioxide, chloramines, and ultraviolet light. Ozone, a safer but slightly more costly water treatment method, is being successfully used in Europe and in twenty-six plants in the U.S.

Bacteria and viruses. Although the poisonous nature of chlorine does a decent job of subduing plagues through our water supply, over a twelve-year period there were 106,000 cases of water-borne infections in the U.S., including hepatitis A and giardia.

Asbestos is found in certain rock formations, particularly in the western U.S., that come in contact with drinking water. Although it is a known carcinogen in the air, ingestion of asbestos is not as well understood. The National Research Council has calculated that one million fibers of asbestos per liter of water could cause cancer beyond the acceptable one in one million people, as set by the EPA. Eleven percent of the 365 urban water systems surveyed by the EPA had concentrations of asbestos greater than ten million fibers per liter. Although San Franciscans are blessed with otherwise healthy water from their high mountain Hetch Hetchy reservoir, bay area drinking water contains around 100 million fibers of asbestos per liter.

Synthetic organic chemicals (SOC). These chemicals are by-products of industry—everything from solvents used to degrease jet engines to cleaning solvents for computer microchips. Trichloroethylene and benzene are commonly found in water supplies and are carcinogenic. These chemicals can be absorbed in the intestinal tract, inhaled while you enjoy your hot shower (due to their volatile nature), or absorbed into the skin while you lounge in your tub.

Some households in high-risk areas have had to install water filtration systems to remove these chemicals from all household water, not just tap water, to be able to bathe in reasonable safety. Many of these solvents are known carcinogens, and most can also cross the placental barrier and have been known to cause liver problems in newborns who got poisoned through mother's milk.[10]

One large industrial site in the Silicon Valley of San Jose, California, leaked 50,000 gallons of a solvent into the nearby water supply. Residents became alarmed when there was a three-fold increase in the norm for birth defects and a two-fold increase for spontaneous abortions. Major cardiac defects were 2.5 times the county average for newborns. Unfortunately, but not surprisingly, another bay area hospital has recently experienced a fifteen-fold increase in rare heart defects in infants.[11]

The symptoms of mild SOC toxicity in adults could easily be confused with the flu: nausea, headache, dizziness, fatigue, stomachaches, and diarrhea. Those most at risk for serious problems are pregnant women, infants, and young children.

Over two hundred industrial facilities dot the shores of West Virginia's Kanawha River. The EPA says that the health of the 220,000 residents in this valley is in jeopardy due to water and air pollution.[12]

Pesticides. One category of SOC, pesticides, has accounted for a major share of water pollution in this country. The California Assembly Office of Research found fifty-seven different pesticides in three thousands wells statewide. Farm use was blamed for twenty-two of these pesticides, while the others were from industrial dumping and household use.

Chlordane, used for termite control, is found in many freshwater streams, lakes, and drinking supplies throughout this country; it is not only carcinogenic but is toxic to the central nervous system. The fumigant EDB is such a potent carcinogen that health officials consider the "action" level to be the detectable level of 20 parts per *trillion*.

Over 2,500 wells in California and hundreds of others across the nation have been contaminated with the fumigant DBCP. Health officials estimate that in California alone over 16,000 people will contract cancer due to DBCP in drinking water. Stomach cancer and lymphoid leukemia are much more common in areas with DBCP-laced drinking water. DBCP persists in the soil and water with a half-life of 141 years.[13] Once DBCP was banned, the fumigants that replaced it have done similar damage to drinking water supplies.

Nitrates. If you stop for a drink at a public rest area along Highway 99, the central artery in California, you will see a sign that reads "Pregnant women and children should not drink this water." Farmers fertilize their fields with forms of nitrogen, nitrates. Rain rinses some of this fertilizer into the waterways and eventually into the drinking water supplies. The nitrates from fertilizer can be broken down in the intestinal tract to nitrites, which are absorbed, oxidize blood cells, and leave the infant with "blue baby" disease, or methemoglobinemia. This can result in death or brain damage. Nitrates and nitrites are also carcinogenic and have been linked to stomach cancer in humans. Recognizing this threat to health, Nebraska has adopted a management program to regulate the use of fertilizers so that water supplies are not tainted, as occurs in many agricultural regions. Nitrates are particularly dangerous to pregnant and lactating women and young children.

Radon. When underground water is naturally exposed to decaying uranium, radon is the by-product. Radon affects up to half the drinking water systems in this country and is particularly dangerous when the water is heated or agitated, such as in a shower, because it can then be inhaled as a gas. Although the EPA recognizes the hazard posed by radon in water, there is an even greater and more unmanageable threat from radon in the air, which is probably the number-two cause of lung cancer in this country.

Fluoride. In small amounts, fluoride in the water helps to harden calcium salts in the teeth and bones. Prudently added to municipal drinking water, fluoride drastically reduces the incidence of dental caries and osteoporosis; but when excessive levels of fluoride are naturally present in the water, fluorosis (mottling of teeth) can occur. The Surgeon General of the U.S. considers fluorosis to be a "cosmetic problem." New studies show that excess fluoride in the drinking water may increase the risk for certain types of cancer.

Lead. Thousands of years ago, lead was originally mined as a by-product of silver mining. Soon, people found its usefulness: it doesn't rust, is soft and pliable yet hard. However, over 2,400 years ago Hippocrates warned about the adverse health effects from the use of lead.[14] In the nineteenth century, scientists had unequivocal findings showing lead toxicity in humans. Yet we continued to mine it: lead can stop bullets and X rays, makes a nice paint base, and is useful in batteries.

Water from lead pipes, lead solder to join pipes, lead contaminated water supplies, and lead lined water coolers accounts for 15 to 40 percent of the lead that Americans ingest. A million drinking fountains in schools across this country are lead-lined and contain forty times the upper limit of acceptable lead levels in water.[15] The EPA plans to lower allowable lead levels in water from the current 50 parts per billion to a safer 10 ppb. At the new safer level, forty million Americans are drinking water with toxic amounts of lead.[16]

Soft water, which is low in magnesium or calcium; high-acid water, which is mostly from acid rain in the eastern U.S.; and warm water will carry the most lead. Some states have mysteriously high levels of lead in the tap water. Illinois water, for instance, has four times the acceptable levels of lead in it, or 200 ppb.

What to do? Your city may be willing to test your tap water for lead. If not, contact one of the following companies who provide testing services to the public for a fee: WaterTest (1-800-426-8378); Suburban Water Testing (1-800-433-6595).

Bottled water and home filtration systems are viable alternatives to the mysterious toxic stew that spews forth from many water taps. This subject is thoroughly discussed in chapter 9.

WASTING OF WATER

How can we expect our cities to provide us with healthy purified water when 40 to 90 percent of our water supply is used to irrigate crops, cool turbines, and flush toilets? One reason for our water pollution dilemma is waste. In addition to jealously guarding the purity of our precious water reserves, we need to either conserve water or have dual water systems, with one pipeline for drinking and another water pipe for non-consumption uses.

Americans consume two to four times more water than our European counterparts. Forty percent of all water used daily in the U.S. is for agriculture, much of this for farms in the arid West. The federal government spends $4 billion annually subsidizing water for farms, which encourages profligate waste: farmers pay one half cent for water that would cost a city dweller in California one dollar. At this price, some farmers choose to flood fields and cast conservation to the wind.

Farmers aren't the only ones wasting water. Many cities are desperately trying to prop up their ailing water delivery systems. About half of the municipal water supply in Boston leaks into the ground due to corroded pipes. New York has an equally disastrous system.

You and I are also at fault. Toilets use up to five gallons (nineteen liters) per flush, although more efficient toilets use less than one-third the water. Trying to maintain plush golf greens in the Southwest desert, excessive watering of lawns, and frequent washing of cars are other wasteful habits of Americans. When apartments convert from "help yourself" general water use to everyone paying for their own (metered), consumption is cut in half.

St. Petersburg, Florida, and Denver, Colorado, have initiated a dual water system which promises to safeguard drinking water while cutting the cost of water for industrial and farming purposes.

WATER, WATER, EVERYWHERE, AND NOT A DROP TO DRINK

This famous line, the original of which was recited by the Ancient Mariners (in Coleridge's poem about a becalmed ship), soon begin to apply to Americans. Although some of our pollutants, pesticides, herbicides, and fertilizers end up tainting the food supply; much of these contaminants end up in the water. Our health suffers accordingly.

Until government, industry, and agriculture can be coerced into a more responsible approach to our water supply, I would encourage you to buy bottled water or a quality home filtration system.

PART THREE
The Solution: A Four-Point Program

CHAPTER 9

How to Reduce Your Intake of Toxins

Y ou may have waded through the previous chapters with a heavy heart, constantly thinking, "Then what can I do?" The answers is, "You can do plenty to protect yourself." This entire section is a four-point program to lower your risk from food and water pollutants. Step one, this chapter, is to minimize your intake of toxins. The next three chapters aim to increase your tolerance of unavoidable toxins.

The following safe-eating precepts are listed in order, with most important first.

Eat less fat. Most pollutants are fat soluble and hence hide themselves in fatty tissue. By eating less fat (especially animal fat), you not only lower your risk for heart disease, cancer, and other common ailments, but you also substantially reduce your intake of pollutants. Since pollutants bioaccumulate further up the food chain, it is extremely important to minimize your intake of animal fats. Many pastries, french fries, and other deep-fried items are cooked in animal lard that is a reservoir of pollutants.

The average American consumes about 45 percent of his or her calories from fat. If we could cut this number down to 30 percent or less, we would find ourselves in better health and with less risk from pollutants. This means eating less:

167

fatty meats and the marbling of meats (as in hamburger, prime rib, bologna, sausage, etc.)
gravy, lard, meat drippings
high-fat dairy products (ice cream, butter, sour
cream, cheese, etc.)
deep-fried foods

Eat a wide variety Do not focus on any one food, since that
food may be a source of unknown pollutants. If you eat small
amounts of various different poisons, you probably will not
become a statistic. If you rely heavily on just a few foods for your
grocery list, then you run a gamble that these foods may not be
safe.

I have met many vegetarians who eat considerable quantities
of cheese or nuts in order to get the protein they miss from not
eating animal food. High-fat cheese contains some of the herbicides and pesticides that were sprayed on the pasture land which
fed the dairy cattle. Nearly all nuts contain some aflatoxins, and
some nuts have concentrated amounts of this deadly toxin.

I don't mean to discourage vegetarians, because this can be a
potentially healthy lifestyle. Just don't "jump out of the frying
pan and into the fire" by trading one risk for another. I don't
think we should stop eating dairy and nut products, but don't
make them the epicenter of your diet. By eating a varied diet,
you have at least evenly distributed your intake of toxins, which
is actually a major victory on your part.

Eat more fiber. Fiber is indigestible food matter, which acts as
a sponge to soak up toxins in the intestinal tract. When scientists
fed a variety of pollutants and questionable food additives to rats,
the rats got sick and died. The same experiments were repeated,
this time in conjunction with a high-fiber diet. The rats survived
unscathed.[1]

Prior to 1960, many scientists considered fiber to be useless
since it is indigestible. Today, fiber is recognized as one of our
true allies in protecting us from food pollutants: we are only
beginning to understand its importance on health. For instance,

the cabbage family (cabbage, broccoli, cauliflower, brussel sprouts) contain a potent anticancer agent called indoles. There has been a steady rise in the incidence of and death from colon cancer in the U.S. Experts have speculated that our many commonly occurring food toxins, such as pesticide residues, are causing this problem. Fiber binds poisons, including toxic heavy metals, in the intestinal tract and carries them out with the feces, where they belong.

Buy organic. This is not always a viable option for some people, due to the cost and availability of organic produce. Some produce items, like apples, broccoli, carrots, celery, peaches, pears, and spinach are highly recommended as organic purchases, since the commercial varieties are often heavily laced with risky pesticides. (More in this chapter.)

Grow your own. A home garden can produce cheap, tasty, clean, and nutritious foods. You don't need much space, time, or money for such a project. (More in this chapter.)

A kitchen sprout garden. You can have your own cheap, clean, tasty fresh greens year-round in any climate with only two minutes of effort per day. (More in this chapter.)

Peel it. Fruits, vegetables, grains, legumes, nuts, and any other foods that have a disposable "wrapper" are much safer food items, since the outer coating carries much of the pesticides with it. Even though bananas, corn, grapefruit, melons, oranges, and similar produce may be heavily sprayed, you eat little of this poison because you throw away the "wrapper." However, there are some systemic poisons, like Alar, that are not lost with the peeling.

Peel all root crops, like carrots, potatoes, beets, and onions, unless they are organic. Worms (nematodes) near these root crops are killed by gassing the soil with potent nematocides, which sit in direct contact with the root crop throughout its life.

Waxes and fungicides that are mixed in to coat shiny-looking produce (like green peppers, cucumbers, and apples) are unhealthy. Although you cannot wash or peel these off in green peppers, you can broil the pepper near a flame to loosen the outer skin. Remove the outer leaves of produce like cabbage, lettuce, kale, endive, and spinach. Many grains, legumes, nuts, and seeds also fall into this category, so avoid sucking on the outer shell of whole sunflower seeds and pistachio nuts.

Eat lower on the food chain. Toxins concentrate with each successive predator. If the water has a little pollution, then the algae that grows in the water will have even more toxins, and the small fish that eat the algae have even higher concentrations of pollution. And on it goes. In mercury-polluted water, the worst thing to eat is the last creature on the biological chain, i.e., the "top dog": swordfish and tuna.

Unfortunately, this means that some of the wild game, like bear and wildcat, that would normally be pristine clean, may now be unfit for consumption, depending on the region that the creature lives in. "Lower on the food chain" means a semivegetarian lifestyle: have some lean ground beef with your tacos or spaghetti, or have some fish or chicken with your vegetables and rice. But try to avoid the John Wayne pizza-size steaks that have traditionally been the focal point of many American meals.

Eat natural. The issue of food additives can become a complex one: "Which additives are safe? How will I remember all of this?" We can simplify matters considerably by eating foods as close to their natural state as possible. Hence, a fresh peeled orange is a healthier choice than frozen orange juice, which is better than a powdered orange drink. A potato (peeled) is better than instant mashed potatoes, which are better than barbecue-flavored potato chips.

Shop the perimeter of the grocery store and eat natural foods. These two rules will cut your food-additive intake by 90 percent. When you buy processed foods, choose the ones with a minimal list of ingredients.

Avoid nuts and grains that may be moldy. Aflatoxins are an unforgiving carcinogen that hides on moldy nuts, grains, and seeds. Be cautious of local peanuts and peanut butter, which do not have to comply with federal standards on aflatoxins. Former president Jimmy Carter's mother, father, and brother all died from pancreatic cancer, and one of his sisters was just diagnosed with this usually fatal disease. The Carters ran a large family peanut farm for many years in Georgia. Something, which could be aflatoxins from moldy peanuts, has caused a rare form of cancer in four family members.

Cook it. Do not eat raw animal food. Everything from raw fish to poorly cooked pork to raw unpasteurized milk can be hazardous. Up to 275 million cases of diarrhea each year in America could be avoided by following good hygienic standards, like cooking your food. Most fruits and some vegetables can be safely eaten raw, but make sure even these foods have been thoroughly washed or peeled, whichever is appropriate.

Cool it. Do not let food stand at room temperature (60 to 120 degrees F., 15 to 49 degrees C.) for more than an hour. All food has some bacteria in it and bacteria multiply rapidly at room temperature. You can stunt bacterial growth by keeping food in the refrigerator or freezer.

Wash it. If you cannot peel it and it is not organic, then use warm water or a mild soapy solution to clean and rinse your fresh produce. Ivory soap shavings provide a cheap no-additive soap for washing produce.

The "Dirty 15." The National Academy of Sciences found that 78 percent of our pesticide risk comes from only fifteen foods, due to the potency or frequency of spraying on these food items. The worst are listed first: tomatoes; beef; potatoes; oranges; lettuce; apples; peaches; pork; wheat; soybeans; beans; carrots; chicken; corn; and grapes.

The pesticide risk is escalated substantially when these food items are processed and concentrated, such as in catsup, grape jelly, beef jerky, etc. Minimize your intake of high-risk food items, buy organic, or grow your own.

The FDA has found that certain food items contain more chemical residues than others. Again, the worst are listed first:[2]

> baked potato (with peel)
> spinach (fresh or frozen)
> raisins
> sweet pepper, green and raw
> collards
> strawberries
> squash
> frankfurters
> peanuts, dry roasted
> pumpkin pie
> candy, plain milk chocolate

Once again, minimize intake of these items; peel, wash, or buy organic if available.

Avoid very hot foods and beverages. Worldwide studies find a major increase in the incidence of cancer in regions that commonly eat very hot food or beverages.[3] It could be that the frequent burning and healing of mouth and esophagus tissues brings about changes in the DNA, which leads to cancer.

Buy local. Produce shipped from distant lands and shores must be picked green, or sealed in wax, or gassed with preservatives.

Buy in season. Fresh produce that is available out of season either has been shipped from a foreign grower, which makes it suspect, or was gassed and stored months previously.

Avoid burned foods especially overcooked proteins. Burning changes the chemical structure of food into benzopyrenes, a.k.a. polycyclic aromatic hydrocarbons, or just PAHs.

Minimize naturally occurring toxins. Since these are usually present in small quantities and humans have evolved an ability to neutralize small amounts of these poisons, eating a varied diet cuts the risk substantially (see chapter 7 for more information). Also, keep your intake of mushrooms to less than a cup per week and do not regularly eat potato skins or parsnips.

Realistic standards. Be suspicious of "perfect"-looking produce. Up to 60 percent of pesticides used in America are for cosmetic purposes only. Often, that perfect-looking piece of fruit has been heavily sprayed to prevent harmless blemishes that lower consumer acceptance. We all know that real oranges are not fluorescent orange and that real peaches have some minor skin blemishes. Unrealistically pretty produce has often been chemically protected, to the detriment of your health.

Safe fish. Since we have used our waterways as open sewers for many decades, fish is no longer the blatantly healthy food that it once was. Smaller fish are safer than larger fish, since the concentration of pollutants increases as you move up the food chain. Avoid fish organ meats and soups which include fish organs. Trim away the fat in fish. Do not use fish fat drippings for sauces. Do not eat raw fish. Minimize your intake of shellfish, since shellfish are bottom filter feeders, where pollutants settle. Seriously restrict your intake of freshwater fish in the Great Lakes, upstate New York, bays near big cities, and various suspect farming and agriculture communities. Fish categories to limit: bluefish, striped bass, swordfish, and shark. Limit tuna consumption to less than a half pound per week, due to mercury content. Ocean salmon has remained surprisingly clean amid this pollution issue.

Buy American. Minimize your intake of imported produce, which may contain banned pesticides and unacceptably high levels of approved pesticides.

Substitute oats. Oats are a hardy grass plant that grows well in the arid northern plains. Because of this characteristic, oats rarely need much pesticide application.[4] If you prepare your own cakes, breads, and cookies, start substituting one-quarter to one-half whole grain oat flour with your whole wheat flour and use more oat-based bread and cereal products.

No peelings. Although some recipes will call for orange or lemon peeling, beware of the hazards in commercial citrus peels. Although by adding the peeling of an orange to a blender you will triple your vitamin C intake, the hazards outweigh the risks. Use only organic citrus when you need some peeling shavings for a recipe.

The same nasty chemicals in these peelings are often found in fresh-squeezed orange juice, frozen orange juice concentrate, and even orange herb tea, since intense mechanical squeezing of the orange will extract much of the poisons that coat the skin.

Buy from the west. Produce grown in the humid southeast often needs more pesticide and fungicide applications than produce grown in drier regions of the country. If you have a choice, buy produce from the drier western regions of the U.S.

Minimum booze. If you drink alcohol, do so in moderation. Pregnant women, people who are driving or operating machinery, alcoholics, and certain ethnic groups (such as American Indians and Asians) should avoid alcohol. Best alcoholic selections from an impurity standpoint: gin, vodka, beer, and white wine. Worst: bourbon, whiskey, European fruit brandy, cream sherry, port wine and oriental wines.

Less liver. Eating less liver for some people may be as easy as standing in fewer forest fires—they are equally unpleasant. However, if you are a liver lover, beware. Liver is normally one of the most nutrient-dense foods in all of nature—a repository of vitamins, (like lipoic acid and choline), minerals, and protein—but the liver is also the detoxifying organ in all animals. Hence it collects pollutants in far greater concentration than any other region of the body, except perhaps fatty tissue.

Tread cautiously in "ethnic" foods Americans use the same adventuresome spirit dining as they do in sports and vacations. We now pride ourselves on savoring ethnic foods from around the world through restaurants and ethnic grocery stores. But be careful: An FDA task force investigated ninety-two ethnic food stores in 1986 and 1987. Almost all stores featured food products from southeast Asia. Federal agents found that 75 to 80 percent of the stores have products in cans and jars which are obviously unfit for consumption.[5] Some products had been on the shelves for over seven years.

Many of these developing countries have an entirely different set of rules for hygiene, food additives, and pesticide residues—or no rules at all. If you favor ethnic foods, be very cautious.

Food containers. *Avoid* foreign ceramics, like plates and coffee cups, unless you are certain that the leaded glaze is safe. Keep your intake of canned food to a minimum, due to trace amounts of cadmium and lead that leach from the can into the food. Minimize use of soft plastics to hold food. Soft plastics, including soft drink quart bottles and small sandwich bags, have petroleum-based chemicals that can migrate into the food. Buy milk in plastic containers rather than wax cartons, since a small amount of dioxin leaches out of the wax cartons. Do not store food in open cans, like leaving orange juice in an open can in the refrigerator.

ORGANIC

In the beginning, there were insects. In the end, there will be even more insects—regardless of what humans do. Biologists tell us that if humanity meets with some untimely apocalyptic finale, like a thermonuclear war or greenhouse effect, insects will survive anyway. The 1.2 billion pounds of pesticides applied annually to American fields have been no more than a minor inconvenience for crop insects—a chemical puzzle to detoxify and then move on to dinner. Survival depends on an organism's ability to adapt to an ever-changing environment, we should recognize the vast superiority of insects in this adaptation skill, due to their teeming numbers of offspring and short generation time.

We cannot purge the world of insects; but we can learn to use biological principles to create safer food without wreaking havoc on the environment. In addition to the immediate health risks posed by pesticide residues, the major source of groundwater pollution in America is from chemicals used in conventional farming. Our current commercial farming methods are destined for extinction—or we are. A new report by the National Academy of Sciences finds that LISA farmers can get equal or better crop yields without the arsenal of poisons employed in commercial farming.[6] LISA farming is a profitable and realistic way to farm.

Commercial farmers once felt that they could eradicate their archrivals in the fields. Yet, with the tenfold increase in pesticide use over the past four decades, crop loss to insects has doubled. There are over 450 species of insects that have developed a resistance to pesticides. It is now the farmer, not the insect, who is more likely to experience cancer or birth defects by using chemical farming techniques.

What is "organic"? "Organic," according to the dictionary, means "involving carbon," which would technically include all sorts of pesticides. "Organic" as popularized by J. I. Rodale, founder of the *Prevention* magazine empire, means "raised without pesticides, synthetic fertilizers, or other related chemicals." There is an implication that organic food is unadulterated, clean, pure, pristine, natural, and healthier—but "organic" has no legal meaning in federal law. "Natural" can be applied to nearly any food loaded with sugar, salt, hydrogenated fat, pesticide residues, and white flour.

The USDA recognizes the label "naturally grown" for poultry and meat, indicating that the animals were raised without growth stimulants, hormones, and other drugs. "Natural" meat and poultry merely means that no chemicals were added *after* slaughter. The ruckus raised in 1988 over European rejection of American hormone-fed beef led to the term "high quality beef," meaning no hormones used in rearing.

Semantics have become an issue. In a government poll, 63 percent of Americans believed that "natural" foods were more nutritious and 47 percent of the people were willing to pay a 10 percent premium on these foods. Now there is a temptation by unscrupulous food processors to call their food "natural" or "organic," because of the profit motive. Thus far, the federal government has declined a role in regulating organic foods. There needs to be clear-cut legal definitions for these words so that the consumer knows what he or she is getting.

As of 1989, sixteen states had laws governing "organic" meat and produce.[7] In those states, there is a maximum $1000 fine for the illegal use of the word "organic." Consumers in the other thirty-four states are unprotected from deceiving business practices. Five states will provide information to farmers interested in LISA methods.[8] (According to most state organic laws, organic produce may contain up to 10 percent of the FDA allowable levels of pesticides, since neighbors spraying their crops could slightly contaminate the LISA farm.)

How does LISA farming work? By creating healthy soil, rotating crops, and employing friendly natural predators, the LISA farmer is able to get equal or superior crops without blasting the fields with poison. Scientists have found that a plant's own natural insect resistance can be enhanced by providing a healthy soil environment. The soil is a living organism, composed of bacteria, worms, and other creatures who collectively decompose organic matter into fertilizer and keep the soil loosely packed. Many forms of life weave a tapestry that creates "healthy soil." When we douse these life-forms with poisonous chemicals, we take away the natural fertility process in the soil. LISA farming encourages soil fertility through the use of compost, manure, sea kelp, fish emulsion, pH (acid/base) balancing, and more.

Friendly bugs? After a bitter and expensive twenty-seven-year war against the alfalfa weevil, victory may be near for American farmers. A tiny harmless wasp has saved farmers in the northeast about $8 million per year in pesticide costs and provides near 100 percent control of the alfalfa weevil, a success level that its chemical counterpart could not even approach.[9] Friendly insects do not eat the food crop, but dine heavily on the crop-destroying insects.

For example, the insects *Cryptolaemus* (mealybug destroyer) will gorge on mealybugs, aphids, and other scaly insect. *Encarsia formosa* feeds on white fly. Green lacewings eat most soft-bodied insects. Ladybugs will dine sumptuously on aphids, small worms, and other soft bodied insects. You can buy 32,000 cooperative and hungry ladybugs for about $25. My wife and I once used ladybugs to quickly rid her parent's citrus trees of a serious aphid blight.

We had a heavy infestation of aphids in our orange trees last year. The aphids were being protected and "milked" for their nectar by an endless stream of ants who were living in their nest in the ground and commuting up the tree trunk to their aphid farm. We applied a sticky substance (called "Tanglefoot") around the tree trunk, which shut down the ant's commute: they could no longer defend their aphid colonies, and soon the natural predators ate the aphids. The trees got better quickly. Normally, aphids require heavy and frequent pesticide application. For $4 worth of sticky stuff and fifteen minutes of effort, the problem was solved without poisons being applied to our precious orange crops.

Bugs aren't the only helpers available to the LISA farmer. Ducks and geese are voracious predators of snails and slugs. Bats eat up to three hundred insects daily with no harm to crops or humans. There is preliminary evidence that a bacteria (*Bacillus Laterosporus*) living on fresh produce in the fields help to contain yeast growth. This same *Laterosporus* also protects us from systemic yeast infections like *Candida*. Pesticides kill *Laterosporus*, which may explain the alarming rate of Candida infections in Americans. LISA farming allows the friendly

Laterosporus to live. LISA farmers also employ gigantic vacuum cleaners to suck the bugs off the plants. There are also crop sprays, like Safer Insecticidal Soap (containing potassium salts of fatty acids), that kill bugs effectively without harming the environment, the nearby water supply, or the consumer.

Goats can be incredibly effective at clearing weeds and brush. Range-management specialists in Canada had tried everything from fire to herbicides to bulldozing with no success in keeping weeds off of a 15,000-acre grazing reserve. Goats happily ate the weeds, left the grassland for cattle, and later provided meat after their job was done.[10] This is an example of the wise use of natural resources: converting useless plants into high-quality protein, rather than poisoning the landscape.

Crop rotation. For thousands of years, humans have rotated crops to keep down weed and pest numbers. Only with the advent of chemical farming since World War II have farmers abandoned crop rotation. University of California scientist Phil Roberts finds that one of the most effective methods of reducing chemical dependency while combatting insects and plant diseases is crop rotation. This sounds mundane amid our high-tech world of satellite communications and lap-top portable computers, but it works.

Get the lead out. Lead pollution may be the most crucial issue of this whole book, yet it gets little publicity. LISA farming drastically cuts the amount of lead taken in by plants. Nina Bassuk, a plant physiologist at Cornell University, found that in soils with a balanced pH (6.5–7) and high amounts of organic compost (40 to 50 percent of volume), lead uptake was near zero, even in soil that was heavily saturated with lead (3,000 parts per million). LISA farming may be more than just the *wiser* alternative, it may be the *only* way to protect ourselves from our serious lead pollution.

Bad attitude. The farming community has been through a rough decade. Bank foreclosures, falling commodity prices, and the falling value of farm real estate all spelled trouble for our productive American farmers. They are just beginning to come out of that slump. The annual harvest in America yields about $57 billion for the farmers, of which $14 billion comes from government subsidies.[11]

Here is the problem. Many commercial farmers would like to break away from the dangerous and expensive chemical dependency they have developed, yet government subsidies encourage chemical farming and penalize anyone for rotating crops. There is a serious attitude adjustment necessary by the federal government before we can make any headway into LISA farming. In 1989, the USDA began its long-awaited program to encourage LISA farming—with a trivial allowance of $4.5 million for the year.

Perhaps the pendulum is beginning to swing toward LISA farming. In 1980, less than 1 percent of our 2.2 million farmers employed LISA methods. Today, over 2 percent are organic farmers, with a total of 5 percent of American farmers making a concerted effort to use less poisons on the crops. That's not much, but it is a start.

Money. Although a small but energetic band of environmentalists have been telling us for decades that chemical farming is unwise, change is finally coming; but because of money, not because of health issues. Costs of developing and testing a new pesticide have risen from $6 million in 1976 to over $30 million today. Also, in recent years twenty-six pesticides have been banned or closely regulated.

The increased cost to the pesticide manufacturer is passed onto the farmer, who then finds chemical farming to be prohibitively expensive. Organic farmers now save about $90 to $100 per acre in corn and $45 per acre in soybeans by employing LISA methods. Also, demand for organic produce now outstrips supply. From 1987 to 1989, demand for organic produce doubled, with a current $3 billion in annual income.[12] For the past five years, the organic farming industry has had an annual growth rate of 30 percent, an enviable track record for any business.

Yet even that stratospheric growth was dwarfed in 1989 with the Alar incident. Organic apple prices jumped by 30 percent in two weeks, and even at that price you couldn't find any. In 1988, Lucky Food Stores introduced organic produce in a few test markets, and the program was so profitable that two hundred other Lucky stores followed suit. Organic produce is expected to grow from its current 2-percent share of the market to 9 percent within the coming decade.

When Dale Cochran, the Secretary of Agriculture in Iowa, returned from a fact-finding tour of Europe, he was enthusiastic about the prospects of selling organic meat and produce to West Germany, where demand also exceeds supply.[13] Money, the true engine of our society, appears to be driving us toward LISA farming.

And big farms, too? A main criticism levied against organic farming is that it is not practical for anything more than a small farm operation of less than two hundred acres. Not so: Just ask Delmar Akerlund, who operates an extremely profitable and non-subsidized LISA grain and cattle farm on 760 acres near Valley, Nebraska;[14] or ask Cliff and Naioma Benson, who farm 3,000 acres of organic wheat in northeast Colorado—although their harvest is two-thirds that of their neighbors, and requires a more intense level of management, the Bensons also get a premium for their crop that makes it quite profitable; or ask Stephen Garnett, who profitably raises natural beef on his 520-acre Virginia farm, seventy-five miles from Washington, D.C.[15]—he uses no growth hormones (since he does not castrate the males, hence they make their own hormones), needs no antibiotics (since the cattle are allowed to roam), and without the cramped quarters of commercial stockyards there is little risk of infections—Garnett sells everything he can produce, and at a premium price; or ask the Spray brothers, who have run a 650-acre LISA farm in central Ohio for the past ten years—their crop yields are from 13 to 41 percent *above* the county average;[16] or ask Paul Keene, who has profitably worked his 500-acre LISA farm, known widely as Walnut Acres, in Pennsylvania since 1946.

Not long ago, organic farmers were a scattered lot of eccentrically dedicated people who could barely pay their own rent. There was a certain altruistic romance that kept them in the business. Today, there are about 40,000 organic farmers with some political clout and much science background who earn an increasingly enviable profit. For more information in LISA/organic farming, see the appendix for relevant organizations, or contact: IPM Practitioner, Box 7414, Berkeley, CA 94707, for newsletters and various books on the subject.

GROW YOUR OWN

Years ago, my wife and I were driving through the gorgeous citrus valley north of Los Angeles, and we stopped to buy a large box of fresh oranges. That night the box of oranges was near our bed in the hotel room, and we both awoke with merciless headaches from the stench of the pesticide residues on the oranges. Years later, we moved into a house with four orange trees: we have never sprayed the trees, yet they produce the most flavorful and healthy crop of oranges imaginable. Fresh unsprayed oranges have a pleasant aroma, not the pungent stench that was coming from the heavily sprayed oranges that we purchased. The best way to control the quality of your fresh produce is to grow some of your own food.

Most Americans spend considerable time and money cultivating ornamental plants, trees, and an entirely useless lawn. Lawns were initiated during the decadently wasteful monarch era in Europe. It was a flagrant insult to the peasant to say: "See, I have so much money that I waste my vast acreage on useless plants, while you have to grow your own food." Lawns became a symbol of affluence.

Outside of America, most other people put their precious land to work to raise fresh, tasty, cheap, and clean produce. Why not spend the same time and money nurturing plants that you can eat? Instead of ornamental bushes around your house, put in dwarf fruit trees. Instead of a lawn, put in a low-maintenance herb and vegetable garden. Instead of those shade trees, put in nut and fruit trees that also provide shade.

You don't need much yard space. You can grow cherry tomatoes in a hanging basket or fruit trees in a small, flat, trained shape (called "espaliering") against a sunny wall. Bean poles magnify your yard space ten-fold by growing upward. A typical quarter-acre city lot, if planned wisely, can feed a family of four with fresh produce for most of the year. You not only feed your family with clean healthy food, but by planting trees, you reduce the greenhouse effect. Children who are reluctant vegetable eaters often will eat something from their own yard. Rosalind Creasy has written a complete guide to "edible landscaping" for the homeowner that is a favorite of mine.[17]

There are some hints you may need before you get started on your home garden. If your property was once heavily sprayed with chemicals, then you may want to plant an interim crop, like annual rye grass, clover, or alfalfa. The dense fibrous root systems of these crops will take up lingering pesticides and herbicides. Discard this crop, do not even mulch it. Another way to break down poisons in the soil is to expose them to the ultraviolet radiation of sunshine. Borrow your neighbor's powered rototiller and till up the soil twice a month during sunny weather. This action will chemically degrade much of the residue poisons.

Once you begin your crop, realize the cardinal rules of successful gardening: healthy soil, prevention of bug problems, and crop rotation. Healthy soil needs plenty of compost or manure and a balanced pH of 6.5 to 7. Once the initial work of nourishing the soil has begun, your work load in the garden will diminish considerably. Be cautious of free fertilizer, such as sludge from the nearby sewage plant. Sludge can contain toxic heavy metals like lead and cadmium.

Prevention is another key issue. By monitoring your crops early in the season, you can deal with bug problems before they become uncontrollable. By laying down plastic sheets or hay between the garden rows, you can keep weed problems to a minimum.

Rotate your crops annually and plant alternating rows of crops in your garden. This keeps down insects. Find out what grows well in your climate. Purchase seed and plant varieties that are disease-resistant and hardy for your climate. Become familiar with Integrated Pest Management principles. There are more resources in the appendix.

Ruth Stout was a lovable lady in upstate New York who decided that gardening should not be such a chore, and who wrote several good books on minimum-effort gardening. She devised her own low-maintenance gardening system and continued gardening for the next forty-five years until her death at age ninety-six. Although her garden was small, she boasted that she never had to buy store produce in all those years. She obviously canned some of her vegetables and fruits to get her through the winters.

Get a good gardening book. Be willing to spend some time and a little money in the beginning. After the first year, the time and money required are much less, especially when you plant fruit or nut trees. Gardening can be a cheap, enjoyable, low-maintenance, nutritious project that also brings an indescribable spiritual joy in eating your own food.

SPROUT YOUR OWN GARDEN

Sprouts are the ultimate no-work, year-round, no-dirt, pesticide-free, absolutely fresh garden. Kids love the fascinating process of seed sprouting and are more likely to eat these vegetables than store-bought produce. Sprouting improves the quality of the protein, increases vitamin levels,[18] reduces the digestion-interfering agents called phytates and much of the naturally occurring toxins,[19] and adds considerable water and fiber to the diet.[20]

Lettuce salads have somehow become synonymous with a healthy lifestyle; yet leafy produce, like cabbage, kale, spinach,and lettuce absorb more pesticides than other crops due to their extensive exposed surface area. Also, lettuce is a weak plant that often gets heavy spraying to avoid the cosmetic damage from pests that would make it unsellable; and it has precious few nutrients to offer. Sprouts make a vastly superior alternative to lettuce.

The essence of sprouting is to keep the seeds wet enough that they sprout, but not so damp that mold grows on them. Most grain, legume, and vegetable seeds will sprout. Favorite sprouting seeds include: alfalfa; peas, like dwarf gray, early Alaska, Laxton progress, and others; and beans, like executive bunch, top crop bunch, Burpee stringless, and so on.

Not every plant sprout should be considered edible, since some plants (like potatoes) provide their new shoots with a toxic substance to protect the plant through its early growth phase.

Sprouting method: You will need a glass jar (quart size or larger), a screen for the top, and a rubber band to hold the screen in place. There are also commercial sprouting kits available in most health-food stores. Place one or two tablespoons of seeds in your glass container with the screen secured on the top. The seeds will expand about tenfold as they sprout, so allow enough room for their expansion. Fill the container half full of water and let stand overnight. Next morning drain and rinse the seeds. Let stand inverted over the sink for proper drainage. Rinse and drain twice each day for the next four or five days. Keep the jar in a dimly lit area.

Larger seeds, like peas and beans, should not be allowed to grow more than a half inch long, since they will develop a bitter flavor. Mung bean sprouts can get up to two inches in length without bitter flavor. Wheat, barley, oats, and other grass plants make terrific sprouts. Smaller seeds, like alfalfa, can grow to an inch in length without any bitter flavor. For some extra vitamin A, let the alfalfa sprouts sit in a sunny window for the last day before eating. The green color indicates beta-carotene, the plant version of vitamin A, which is an accessory pigment in photosynthesis.

In excess quantities, sprouts can blunt the immune system in humans. Do not eat more than two cups of sprouts daily. In the most remote small town, in the depths of winter, with little effort or money and no risks, you can enjoy a fresh healthy green garden through sprouting. We have been avid sprouters for the past eight years and rarely purchase expensive, nutrient-poor, heavily sprayed lettuce for our salads.

IN SEARCH OF CLEAN WATER

Water pollution is a front-page issue in America. There is plenty of scientific and government evidence that the abundant and clean tap water supply we took for granted is no longer readily available to many Americans. If you live in a community that uses rivers or wells for municipal water and has nearby farming and/or industry, then you should be suspicious of your water quality. Once you accept the grim reality of drinking water pollution, you are then faced with a choice: purify your water at home, or have someone else do it (bottled water).

Home purifiers. [21] There are three basic types of home filtration units:

Figure 9A: YOUR KITCHEN SPROUT GARDEN

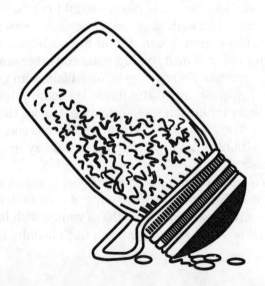

Carbon filters from activated charcoal that is compressed into a solid block
Reverse osmosis (RO) membranes
Distillation

Solid block carbon filters are quite effective at removing chlorine (and the derivative trihalomethanes), bacteria, asbestos particles, and petroleum distillates like pesticides and gasoline. Carbon filters also leave most dissolved minerals in the water, which is good if you want to derive the nutritional benefits of the calcium, magnesium, and fluoride in your drinking water, but is bad if you have heavy metal contamination (like mercury, lead, and arsenic) in your municipal water or household plumbing. Carbon filters should be solid core (not granular), should come with a prefiltration device to screen out sediment, and should be replaced about every six months to avoid bacterial buildup on the filter.

Reverse osmosis (RO) uses water pressure to force water through a semipermeable membrane which screens out impurities. RO has the advantage of eliminating nearly all contaminants. Since RO removes all minerals, you will be protected from lead poisoning, but will lose the essential minerals of calcium, magnesium, and fluoride from your drinking water. Fluoride is critical for the proper hardening of bones and teeth. Pregnant women and growing children should take fluoride supplements if RO is chosen. Also, some hard waters contribute up to 350 milligrams of calcium and 150 milligrams of magnesium daily to the diet. Losing that significant mineral intake should alert the RO user to food choices or a mineral supplement to compensate for the loss.

The disadvantages of RO include:

High initial cost
Low volume of water output (not practical for commercial applications)

Figure 9B. Effectiveness of Various Water Filtration Methods
(√ = removes most of this category)

WATER IMPURITIES	WATER FILTRATION METHODS		
	quality high density carbon filter	reverse osmosis	distillation
toxic heavy metals —arsenic —lead —mercury —cadmium		√	√
trihalomethanes —chlorine —chloroform	√	√?	√
microbes —Giardia —E. Coli —most bacteria, worms	√	√	√
synthetic organic chemicals —benzene —pesticide/herbicide —PCB, DDT —petroleum distillates	√	√	√
asbestos	√	√	√
nitrates	√?	√	√
useful minerals —calcium —magnesium —fluoride	leaves them in	√	√
flavor	good	better	strange
cost (purchase & maintain)	reasonable	high	high

Lower efficiency at removing chlorine and related trihalomethanes

Water waste. RO loses seven gallons of water for every one gallon of drinking water obtained since the unit must continuously rinse the membrane of the removed impurities.

Distillation is how nature uses the energy of the sun to convert salty ocean water into pure rain water. If you apply enough heat to a body of water, then the water molecules will vaporize, leaving behind most of the impurities. The water vapors are then recaptured through cooling tubes.

Distillation is extremely effective at removing most impurities, except perhaps some volatile pollutants that vaporize along with the water molecules; but it is very expensive to buy and maintain, since it uses considerable electricity and the unit must often be cleaned of impurities. Distilled water also tastes strange, since it lacks the usual "body" that you become accustomed to with the assortment of dissolved minerals in drinking water.

I suggest that you find out what the prevailing water problems are in your community. You can test for lead in your tap water by sending a sample of your water to a number of different testing labs. (See chapter 8 for names and phone numbers.) If lead is a key problem, then a carbon filter will not work for you. If your municipal water supply is relatively clean and cost is a concern of yours, then you should be able to buy a good multistage carbon filtration unit for under $200 that will economically serve your family for many years to come.

Bottled water. Then there is the argument: "Why bother with home filtration? Let the experts handle that." Some bottled water is obtained from deep wells or mountain streams. Of all these, the cleanest and least suspicious water sources would be high mountain reservoirs in the western U.S., since the prevailing jet stream over America blows pollutants in an easterly direction and dumps them in the eastern mountains as acid rain.

Up to 25 percent of water bottlers take the local water supply and purify it. Some have very sophisticated equipment; some don't. Some are very scrupulous business people; and some aren't. By virtue of the reigning law on the subject, the Safe Drinking Water Act of 1974, the federal government has basically stayed out of regulating the bottled-water industry. Government regulation of bottled water is based on the premise that these products should meet only the same set of health quality standards as tap water—which is like saying that the only requirement for getting into Congress is that you not be a convicted felon.

In 1975, when bottled water was a dusty esoteric grocery shelf item, federal apathy was okay. But by 1985, the industry had grown by 300 percent.[22] Today, the bottled water industry is a more than $2 billion per year business. There needs to be a "referee" in this melee of free enterprise.

A 1982 study conducted by the New York State Department of Health found dangerous organic chemical contaminants (like tetrachloroethene, benzene, and toluene) in 68 percent of the bottled water products tested. That same year, the Suffolk County Health Service in New York conducted a similar study of bottled water and found it to be comparably contaminated as the region's tap water, where two-thousand wells were found to be polluted. The club sodas and seltzers tested were different. They were *worse* than the region's questionable tap water, containing more chloroform.

The California Assembly Office of Research also published its own study, in 1985, which analyzed bottled water, again finding horrific tales of contamination from gasoline, flies, roaches, mercury, and many carcinogenic chemicals. Since 85 percent of the bottled-water business is concentrated in California, New York, Illinois, Florida, and Texas; it is not surprising that those states have made the greatest advances in regulating bottled water. Even more prominent have been the peer review efforts of the International Bottled Water Association (IBWA), to which 85 percent of the bottled water manufacturers belong. The IBWA recommends that its members monitor their water for 129 different contaminants and requires yearly plant inspections.

Bottled water can be convenient, tasty, and a healthy substitute for tap water; but it is also expensive—at least one-thousand times the price of tap water. Avoid using "mineral waters" as your main drinking water, since the government standards on mineral waters are much more lenient than for tap water. Most importantly, patronize a reputable water dealer who can give you a detailed chemical analysis of their bottled water, the origin of their source water, and their filtration methods. Your county health department may be able to tell you of what, if any, water contamination problems you need to be aware.

There have been numerous instances of "bottled-water" distributors who merely added sugar or some other flavoring agent to the municipal tap water and sold it for a steep markup. Near many supermarkets you will find drinking water vending machines that boast of "EPA approved" drinking water. As you have seen in the chapter on water contamination, "EPA approved" means they are using your local tap water, and should provide little comfort to the customer. There are advantages and disadvantages to each method of clean water. Choose the method that is right for your budget and local water problems.

For centuries Europeans have respected the difference between washing water (tap) and drinking water (potable). For centuries, we didn't have to worry about that issue. Due to our gross negligence in agricultural and industrial pollution, we no longer have that privilege.

CHAPTER 10
Foods that Increase Your Tolerance of Toxins

*L*ife would be grim indeed if we munched away at mealtime knowing that our food was laced with both man-made and naturally occurring toxins. But take heart! Nature has not set us adrift on a raft going over Yosemite Falls. While there is a frightening array of poisons in many foods, there is an equally impressive list of protective agents in others. If you choose your foods wisely, you can cancel the harm done by unavoidable toxins. That's what this book is all about: making the right choices. Because people who select their food primarily for taste, cost, and convenience (which is what the average American does) are assuming that lucky guessing will carry them safely through life. That may be an unwise gamble.

Historically, groups of humans survived or perished based upon a somewhat random selection of their diet. Lead poisoning helped to speed the downfall of the Roman civilization: the Romans made a mistake in selecting lead for their base metal to make wine goblets and water pipes. The Aztecs of Mexico got lucky by combining beans with corn in their diet. They didn't do this because their nutritional biochemists told them about the need for complementary proteins—they were just fortunate enough to choose a nutritious diet. Hence, the secret to surviving was to blindly grope your way through the indigenous food supply to include enough nutrients and exclude most of the toxins.

This is the first generation in human history to have enough knowledge about our diet that we can consciously include what we need and exclude what is harmful. That selection process may be somewhat like hopscotching through a mine field, given our rampant pollution, but it is still better than the "luck of the draw" that our ancestors faced. We know what to do—they had to guess. We could wait a couple centuries and find out if our current diet allows us to pass the acid test of Darwin's "survival of the fittest"; or we can arm ourselves with nutrients and protective foods to survive the gauntlet of eating in the 1990s. This chapter introduces you to foods that have been scientifically proven to reduce the harm done by pollutants.

"Balance" is a key word here. We have all heard the trite expression, "Eat a balanced diet," meaning to include a wide variety of foods. This sounds like theoretical pablum until one really investigates the dazzling array of pharmacological agents in our diet.

> If you regularly eat a small amount of cabbage, it may protect you from cancer. If you eat too much raw cabbage without enough iodide in the diet, you could get goiter.
>
> Regular intake of onions could protect you from cancer. But too much onion will not only keep friends at arm's length, but will send your blood sugar levels into a skydive.
>
> Regular intake of soybeans may protect you from chemical carcinogens and viruses. An excess of soybeans could cause infertility problems, due to the estrogenlike activity of some substances found in soybeans and peas.
>
> Regular intake of yogurt will provide you with protection against carcinogens, microbes, and other harmful agents in the diet. Too much yogurt could spark a milk protein allergy.

Regular intake of small amounts of rice, barley, and other grains will provide you with major protection against carcinogens through the phytic acid in grains. Too much grains in the diet may cause a deficiency due to phytic acid binding to essential minerals.

Eating may sound like a complex and dangerous pastime, but it isn't. Just keep the aphorism, "Eat a balanced diet," in mind and select more often from the "superfoods" outlined in this chapter than you do from the dangerous foods mentioned in the previous chapters.

Disease is rarely the product of one catastrophic event in the body. More often, disease is the cumulative effect of unhealthy forces overwhelming healthy forces. In small quantities, many food poisons may be fairly innocuous. But in normal American quantities these poisons probably wreak havoc on the health of millions of people. Without food, we die—but with the typical poor food selections that Americans make, we also die. If your food "friends" can overwhelm your food "enemies" in number and potency, then you may be rewarded with a long and vigorous life.

FOODS AS PROTECTORS AND HEALERS?

Penicillin was discovered rather by accident in the 1920s when Sir Alexander Fleming found that bread mold killed bacteria in petri dishes; which explains why an age-old remedy for wounds was a "mold poultice." Birth control pills were also stumbled upon haphazardly when some bright mind noticed the contraceptive effect of cactus plants, which contain estrogen-like compounds. From cactus, birth control pills—pardon the pun—were born. Curare was introduced to medicine thousands of years after natives in South America had been using this paralyzing plant extract to stun their prey. The potent heart medicine, digitalis, is from the common plant foxglove. Over two thousand years ago, healers recommended willow extract for goutlike symptoms. Today, we call willow extract aspirin. Potent chemicals are not restricted to plants with scientific names found only in steamy distant jungles; there are also pharmacological agents in some of the foods at your local grocery store.

Prior to World War I, physicians were restricted to mostly herbs and foods for medicines. Witness an excerpt from a 1927 article in the professional journal for doctors, *American Medicine:* "Apple is therapeutically effective in all conditions of acidosis, gout, rheumatism, jaundice, all liver and gall bladder troubles, and nervous and skin diseases caused by sluggish liver, hyperacidity, and states of autointoxication." Then came the explosion of chemical knowledge that followed World War II. Physicians became understandably distracted with new potent synthetic drugs and dropped nature's healing agents of foods and herbs from the medicine bag.

BACK TO NATURE?

Why has there been a recent resurgence of interest in natural healers?

Questionable wonder drugs. Many of the new wonder drugs have proven to be less wonderful than anticipated. Many are expensive, dangerous, laden with side effects, and none offer protection against food pollutants. While most modern drugs are relatively new and untested, the natural substances discussed in this chapter have been "field tested" for several million years. The long-term effects of many drugs are unknown. Clofibrate, a drug commonly prescribed to lower serum cholesterol, has a cancer risk 85,000 times higher than normal exposure to PCB.[1] Phenobarbitol, a commonly prescribed sedative, has a similar cancer risk.

The foods that are discussed in this chapter have virtually no toxicity, no side effects, are very inexpensive, and are available without a prescription. Irwin Ziment, M.D., professor of medicine at the University of California Los Angeles School of Medicine, notes: "The use of food as a drug had always been important until the modern drug industry arose in the nineteenth century." Dr. Ziment considers foods to be potent drugs and sees a return to the concept of foods as medicines.

New sensitive lab equipment. It wasn't until the last decade that sensitive enough lab equipment was available to separate and identify the thousands of trace components in foods. New lab equipment is so sensitive that if you dropped a sugar cube into a large reservoir of water, the scientists could take a sample of water at the other end of the reservoir and tell you exactly what molecules were in the sugar cube in parts per trillion. Although herbal folklore claimed cures for certain ailments, it wasn't until the modern scientist could extract, purify, and test these food ingredients that he or she became convinced of their value.

Need for pollution protection. Our pollution problem is taking a staggering toll on our health. We need something to protect us from the many poisons in the food, water, and air supply. While cancer is relatively rare in most underdeveloped nations around the world, in America cancer is the number-two cause of death for adults *and children*.[2] While the EPA considers a cancer risk of one per million to be "acceptable," 130 of every one million American children get cancer each year, with a third of those coming from leukemia. Cancer has escalated its plague upon society by growing from 4 percent of all deaths in 1900 to 21 percent of all American deaths in 1981. Our food, air, and water pollution is the major reason for such a drastic increase in cancer incidence.[3] After several decades of intense and expensive medical research, a Harvard physician has provided statistics to show that we have lost the war against cancer.[4] Even allowing for the aging population, cancer incidence and death rate have both increased since 1962. Two-thirds of cancer patients cannot be cured.

Many of the brightest minds in cancer research are now examining the only realistic alternative: prevention of cancer through nutrition. Because even if we begin major environmental cleanup efforts now, it will be decades before we have a clean food and water supply, due to the time necessary for pollutants to chemically decay. Rather than feel helpless or wait for our phlegmatic Congress to act, you can protect yourself with the many natural components that are available.

Gifts from Nature. We are beginning to realize our limitations at understanding health problems and creating chemical solutions. It is easy to get an agog feeling about modern science: we have laptop portable computers; we have split the atom, been to the moon, and sent robot spaceships to both Mars and Venus. We communicate by satellites, perform surgery with lasers, and tinker with the cell's DNA like a mechanic fixing a car. In spite of these impressive accomplishments, scientists still cannot make an apple or a baby . . . or weave a spiderweb . . . or create an antibody for immune protection. Many items in nature seem mundane next to the wizardry of science, yet it is these "mundane" substances that can offer us protection from both manmade and naturally occurring poisons in the food and water supply. This doesn't mean we should stop trying to understand nature and to fix problems when we can; but in our enthusiasm for modern science, we have erroneously categorized natural remedies as inferior to man-made solutions.

Science thought it had the upper hand on nature with genetic engineering. Scientists had isolated one of the immune factors (interferon) that zaps cancer cells and, through genetic engineering, had created some interferon in the lab. They had hoped for a "magic bullet" against cancer, but interferon was a serious disappointment. Apparently, the human immune system that successfully battles cancer cells does so with a multitude of weapons that work with the enviable coordination of a well trained army—an army that we are only beginning to understand.

My purpose in this little discussion is not to discourage us from making advances in science, but rather to admit our limitations and accept the many chemical gifts that nature offers us. The $46-billion-per-year American pharmaceutical industry knows of the largesse of nature—one-fourth of all prescription drugs are from plants. Mega-billion-dollar multinational drug companies, prestigious research universities, and well-funded government scientists have all been chasing the elusive "protection against cancer." Nature has already given us powerful chemo-preventive agents in the form of:

> *minerals,* like selenium
> *vitamins*, like beta-carotene, vitamin C, vitamin E
> *foods*, like garlic and yogurt
> *food components*, like indoles from cruciferous vegetables.

The evidence has finally reached critical mass for some organizations. Dr. Peter Greenwald, director of the National Cancer Institute, has approved funding for over thirty different studies that look at foods and nutrients to prevent cancer.[5] For instance, twenty-two thousand Harvard physicians are participating in a study to see if supplements of beta-carotene can prevent cancer. Thirty thousand farmers in China are being given a combination of minerals and vitamins to slow the deterioration of their precancerous esophagus condition.

Why do the majority of scientists, physicians, and politicians still ignore these chemo-protective gifts from nature and try to build better chemicals in the lab? One reason is that these natural chemicals cannot be patented, and hence are not profitable to research or market. In nature, there are chemo-protective agents that boggle the minds of our brightest scientists. We cannot duplicate these chemicals; we do not even fully understand how they work; but we know that they do work—and we can use them to protect us from the staggering collection of poisons in our food, water, and air supply.

Take charge of your own life. Don't expect your doctor to care for your body. He or she may be able to help during occasional health emergencies, but it is you who must bear 99 percent of the responsibility for your health. If you consume typical American quantities of food and water poisons, your health may well deteriorate beyond the point at which medicine can help you. Do something now before it is too late.

SYNERGISTIC FORCES IN FOODS

Foods provide a delicately balanced combination of known and unknown factors that have synergistic action—one plus one equals four. Although 1000 milligrams of vitamin C daily has been shown to reduce the risk for stomach cancer, a small glass of orange juice containing only 37 milligrams of vitamin C is *twice* as likely to lower the chances for stomach cancer! *Something* in oranges is even more chemo-protective than vitamin C. Calcium in milk is better absorbed than calcium from supplement pills. Chromium from yeast is two to ten times more effective than elemental chromium found in pills. When researchers isolated a potent antibiotic from yogurt, they worked with Merck Drug Company to patent and produce the antibiotic—but they were disappointed when this yogurt antibiotic did not turn out to be the "magic bullet" against intestinal infections. Since then (1963), researchers have found at least seven distinct natural antibiotics in yogurt that are capable of killing a variety of microorganisms. Yogurt also contains other microbe killers, including lactic acid, acetic acid, benzoic acid, and hydrogen peroxide. The net effect of yogurt is more than one could expect from the individual components that have been isolated. So it goes for many foods.

THE TYPICAL AMERICAN DIET

Worrying about pesticide residues in an otherwise horrendous diet is like a kamikaze pilot making sure his seat belt is fastened. Though Americans seem to be more health conscious, we are also eating more pizza, cookies, ice cream, and doughnuts.[6] These high-fat, high-sugar foods take the place of more protective foods, and the net effect is double jeopardy: danger from what you eat, and danger from what you are not eating enough of.

Many extensive scientific surveys find the American diet wanting in a long list of essential nutrients, including vitamins A, D, E, and C, beta-carotene, riboflavin, pyridoxine (B-6), folacin, pantothenic acid, the minerals, calcium, magnesium, potassium, zinc, iron, copper, chromium, selenium, the major food components of protein, complex carbohydrates, fiber, special fatty acids, and even water. Data from over 11,000 Americans showed that on the particular day surveyed:[7]

41 percent did not eat fruit

82 percent did not eat cruciferous vegetables

72 percent did not eat vitamin C–rich fruits or vegetables

80 percent did not eat vitamin A–rich fruits or vegetables

84 percent did not eat high-fiber grain food, like bread or cereal

The American diet becomes a double-edged sword: we eat too much poison and not enough protective foods and nutrients. The catastrophic results are obvious in our health woes. While many Americans are aware of the risks in pesticide residues, few are aware of the protective value of a well-planned diet. Safe eating means more than just avoiding dietary poisons, it also means fortifying the body with essential nutrients and fantastically protective food factors.

HOW DO FOODS PROTECT US FROM FOOD TOXINS?

-By spurring on the body to produce more toxin scavengers, like GSH

-By bolstering the immune system

-By wrapping the virus or bacteria in a "strait-jacket" to prevent it from parasitically attaching to a healthy host cell

-By stimulating certain detoxifying enzyme systems, like the liver's cytochrome P450[8]

-By shutting down the oncogene in your human cells that acts like a traitor to participate in cancer growth

-By directly killing tumor cells

-By directly killing bacteria and viruses that may cause cancer or food poisoning

-By binding up substances, like bile acids, that can decay into a carcinogenic substance

-By caging toxic heavy metals and carrying them out of the body

-By attaching to fats, to stop the carcinogenic fat "rusting" process

-By providing essential nutrients that allow the body to better defend itself against pollutants and invading microbes

-And more

There are several stages necessary in order for cancer to turn into full-blown metastasis, which is the stage at which cancer spreads its evilness to other parts of the body. First, there is the "initiation" phase, in which something (radiation, pesticide residues, smoking, natural toxins,etc.) attacks the DNA in the cell nucleus, leaving the cell staggering with the blow: most cells recover; some don't. On to phase two, called "promotion." Something must then help accelerate the rate at which the battered cell reproduces its nonkosher DNA. At that point, a tumor may exist. What causes the tumor to worsen from benign to malignant to metastasis throughout the body is a subject of great interest in labs around the world.

Various nutrition factors can interrupt this deadly cancer progression at each point along the way. Indoles from the cabbage family rev up the detoxification system of the body to produce more glutathione peroxidase (GSH), which is a "Rambo" enzyme that destroys assailants intent on disrupting the cell's precious DNA. Beta-carotene is a food nutrient that boosts the body's immune system while also being directly toxic to tumor cells. Other carotenoids from plants are potent antioxidants, meaning that they can neutralize chemical saboteurs within the body. Garlic and yogurt produce substances which can kill viruses, some of which can trigger a cancer cascade.

Perhaps you thought food was just for dining pleasure, but there is an ingenious array of protective chemicals in certain foods. Choose the right foods and the chemical war within you shifts in your favor.

SUPERFOODS

Of the foods that help protect your body from damage through food pollution, there is a small and elite band of superstars. Some are so chock-full of protective factors that you would need a prescription for these foods if they came only in pill form. Eat these foods often.

Yogurt. Thousands of years ago, some careless chef left out his or her warm milk on a hot summer's day. Fortunately, a favorable bacteria (*Lactobacillus*) landed in the milk and began fermenting the lactose (milk sugar) into lactic acid. The end result was a thick creamy food. Not wanting to waste food, the chef tasted the product, declared it acceptable, and lived to tell about it. Yogurt was born.

If *Lactobacillus* bacteria is the mother of yogurt, then Dr. Elias Metchnikoff was the father. Dr. Metchnikoff was a Nobel laureate (in 1908 for work in immunology), friend to Louis Pasteur, and one of the more preeminent researchers of his era. He was convinced that poisons in the intestinal tract were the cause of disease and death, and that these poisons could be arrested by the action of microbes from fermented milk. In 1900, Dr. Metchnikoff was able to isolate one of the fermenting bacteria in yogurt (no small task in those days of primitive lab equipment), prove the efficacy of the bacteria in animal studies, and even provide the *Lactobacillus* culture to a food company who began selling yogurt and fermented milk in a commercial venture. Both brilliant and altruistic, Dr. Metchnikoff refused his share of the profits in the yogurt industry that he spawned.

Since then, wild undocumented reports of superhuman longevity through yogurt have poured in from around the world. Groups in Russia, Bulgaria, Africa, France, and elsewhere have proclaimed yogurt as their elixir of life and propagator of vigorous health. Scientists had considered the yogurt legend as "rubbish" or "too good to be true"—until they started researching yogurt. Now there is abundant evidence to show that yogurt may prevent a host of ailments, including heart disease, cancer, and intestinal problems, and may prolong life by bolstering the immune system.[9] Yogurt is an all-star in protecting you from food pollutants.

Diarrhea from bacterial infection is *the* most common problem from our tainted food supply. In a study using infants who had to be hospitalized for severe diarrhea, one cup of yogurt fed three times daily provided quicker recovery than the standard medical treatment of Kaopectate and neomycin. Children given the yogurt recovered in an average of less than three days, while children on the more traditional medical protocol took five days to recover.[10] In another study, five hundred Japanese servicemen who drank a cup of yakult (fermented milk drink) daily for six months remained healthy, while over 10 percent of the group not drinking yakult got dysentery.

E. coli is a common bacteria found in tainted food. Italian researchers found that yogurt significantly reduced the number of *E. coli* bacteria in adult intestines.[11] Yogurt bacteria (*Lactobacillus bulgaricus*) also improved the growth and survival rate of lab animals who were deliberately infested with *E. coli*.[12] *Salmonella* is a bacteria that causes one of the most common and dangerous types of food infections. Rats fed yogurt and then *Salmonella* survived much better than rats given milk and then *Salmonella*.[13]

Virtually nothing in the medicine bag of modern drugs works

against viral infections. Yogurt does. Mice injected with lethal doses of influenza virus had a 100 percent *mortality* rate, while mice fed yogurt and then injected with flu virus had a 100 percent *survival* rate.[14] Rats kept on a diet that included a continuous supply of yogurt were better able to survive a host of infectious microorganisms.[15] In test tube studies (in vitro), yogurt was effective at killing bacteria strains that even modern antibiotics can't kill.[16]

Because of the unrestrained use of subtherapeutic antibiotics in rearing domestic animals, we have bred a new generation of antibiotic-resistant food infections that could also mutate into a plague of major proportions. It is comforting to know that yogurt may provide substantial protection against these new and exotic bacteria. Although several antibiotics have been isolated from yogurt cultures,[17] it becomes increasingly obvious that yogurt is a complexly woven tapestry of antimicrobial factors which add up to more than the sum of the parts. Many of us have been victimized by the "trots" of diarrhea from tainted food: if you dine out frequently or travel to foreign countries, yogurt can be your valuable ally against deadly microbes in the food and water supply.

One of the leading experts on yogurt, Dr. Khem Shahani from the University of Nebraska, considers the antibiotics in yogurt to be more potent than the prescription variety, a common side effect of which is to kill the friendly bacterial colonies in the gut, which then leads to diarrhea. Yogurt is able to control the diarrhea that frequently results from taking oral antibiotics.[18] Essentially, yogurt is more effective against many bacterial and viral intestinal infections that the best drugs on the market, and without the usual side effects.

Food pollution blunts the immune system and introduces infections that are considered "opportunistic," meaning that they can only become a problem when the host's immune defenses are down. But yogurt can stimulate a poisoned and lethargic immune system to work better. Yogurt not only contains its own antibiotics that function like a heat-seeking missile to directly kill hostile bacteria, but yogurt also has other weapons against microbes. It can simultaneously bolster the body's own immune system, like military aid to a friendly nation to allow them to better fight their own war. Yogurt added to the diet of mice greatly increased antibody production and increased the spleen reservoir of various immune factors.[19] In both mice and humans, yogurt tripled the production of interferon (a natural weapon against infections and cancer) and raised the levels of natural killer cells more effectively than the side-effect-laden prescription drug, Levaelsole. In another experiment, trace amounts of yogurt added to human blood in vitro caused a major increase in the output of interferon.[20] Within fifteen days, yogurt-fed mice showed measurable improvements in immune function, both in the digestive tract and bloodstream.

I am suspicious that pollution-bludgeoned immune systems are at least partly responsible for the epidemic of new and exotic infections in America: *Candida,* Epstein-Barr virus (chronic fatigue syndrome), toxic shock syndrome (supposedly due to tampons), AIDS, nonspecific urinary tract infections (NSU), and others. Yogurt helps to offset the harm done by pollutants. Yogurt bacteria is even clinically effective at treating vaginal tract infections.[21]

Cancer may be the end result of years of exposure to food toxins. Yogurt helps to prevent cancer, slow down the growth of tumor cells in the gastrointestinal tract, and even bolster the immune system to destroy active tumor cells.[22] Researchers find that certain enzymes that occur naturally in human intestines can change harmless substances in the colon into potent carcinogenic agents;[23] yogurt was able to reduce these dangerous enzyme levels in the intestines by 40 to 60 percent.[24] Yogurt seems to swing the tide of intestinal bacteria away from hostile and toward friendly, greatly reducing the risk for colon cancer.[25] Although Finnish people eat a high-risk cancer diet (high in fat and animal protein, and low in fiber), they have a very low incidence of colon cancer, probably due to their regular consumption of yogurt.

And yogurt may be able to lower the risk of cancer beyond the intestinal tract where it is directly exposed. When scientists looked at the diet of 1010 women with breast cancer and a comparable group without breast cancer, they found that there was a "dose dependent" relationship between yogurt intake and risk for breast cancer—the more yogurt consumed, the lower the risk.[26] A similar study in the Netherlands showed comparable results:[27] Rats fed yogurt and then exposed to a list of carcinogens were less likely to develop cancer.[28]

A shocking report from Bulgaria in 1962 found that 59 percent of 258 mice implanted with a highly malignant type of cancer cells (sarcoma) were *cured* by yogurt. More recent trials found less astounding but still promising results—yogurt did squelch tumor growth in 30 percent of mice with implanted sarcomas.[29] Yogurt bacteria creates a substance (blastolysin) that works like a chemotherapy agent against certain malignant tumor cells (sarcoma S180).[30] Yogurt as adjunct therapy to help cure cancer patients? Maybe.

At least thirty million Americans are lactose (milk sugar) intolerant,[31] meaning that they cannot derive the major nutritional benefits from milk without experiencing considerable intestinal discomfort. Yogurt assists in milk sugar digestion to make milk more tolerable,[32] the end result being that people who cannot drink milk can consume yogurt without digestive problems.[33] (People with milk allergies, however, must avoid yogurt, since their problem is due to a protein intolerance.)

After a five thousand-year track record as a legendary therapeutic agent, yogurt is finally taking its rightful place in science as a potent protective food that should be in your diet often. As an additional side benefit, yogurt bacteria compete with the bacteria that make intestinal gas, lowering the "wind" output of all people. Yogurt helps to make a high-fiber diet less socially offensive. How much more friendly can a food get? Dr. Metchnikoff would swell with pride if he could see the data on yogurt now.

How to use it. Try to buy active cultured yogurt in low-fat or non-fat form. Kefir and acidophilus milk also contain active yogurt cultures. *Lactobacillus acidophilus, thermophilus,* and *bulgaricus* are the friendly bacteria strains that are hopefully listed on the container label. Use yogurt in cooking in lieu of cream, to thicken mashed potatoes or as part of cake frosting. We eat a bowl of yogurt nearly every morning with some wheat germ and fruit preserves mixed in. We also make yogurt cream cheese, by gently spooning the yogurt into a clean nylon stocking, then letting it hang over a bowl for two days. Yogurt cream cheese is lower in fat and calories than cream cheese, with all the benefits of yogurt and the same smooth rich texture of cream cheese. We add yogurt cream cheese with some jam to whole wheat tortillas or crepes, roll them up, and warm them in the microwave for a tasty entree.

If you eat enough yogurt, store-bought yogurt can become expensive: an alternative is to purchase your own yogurt maker. There are numerous nifty yogurt makers on the market, but if you cannot find one in your local stores, Walnut Acre Farms (listed in the Appendix) has them by mail order. An even cheaper alternative (as we do) is to create your own yogurt maker. The basic idea in yogurt production is to:

-Boil the milk in order to kill off the competitive bacteria that would hinder the growth of the *Lactobacillus.*

-Simmer the milk to steam off water for a thicker yogurt mixture.

-Once the milk has cooled, innoculate the milk with a spoonful of fresh active yogurt culture (the starter).

-Let the concoction ferment at a warm temperature.

Yogurt probably originated in the Middle East where the primordial batch of yogurt sat out in summer desert heat most of the daylight hours. Duplicate the environment of a summer's day in Baghdad and you will have delicious thick yogurt.

Recipe for yogurt:

-Scald 8 cups of milk with one cup of added powdered milk. This means that the milk is starting to foam, but not yet at a rolling boil.

-Turn heat down and simmer for at least 5 minutes; the longer you simmer (up to 45 minutes) the thicker your yogurt will be.

-While the milk is simmering, place 2 tablespoons of live cultured good-tasting yogurt in each of two quart-glass peanut butter jars and stir briefly with a plastic spoon until creamy.

-After simmering milk, let the temperature drop to 49 degrees C. (112 F.). You don't want to kill the yogurt bacteria with milk that is too hot.

-Add about a cup of the warm milk to the yogurt starter in each of two jars and stir gently but thoroughly. Then add the rest of the milk to the glass jars.

-Place the jars (uncovered) in a picnic thermos (the size that holds a six pack of beer). Close the thermos lid and leave for 6–10 hours. The longer it sits, the thicker it gets. (Do not open container and peek while the fermentation is occurring.)

You have just cut the cost of yogurt from $14.40 per gallon to $2.10 per gallon (cost of milk).

Garlic. If there were a heavyweight match for champion among the superfoods, surely garlic and yogurt would be wrestling for the title. Allicin is both the potent antibiotic in garlic and also the pungent smell factor. Its odor is infamous: gophers, insects, vampires, and squeamish humans shrink from its presence. An ancient critic long ago spawned the legend that when Satan crawled out of Hell, in his first two footsteps on earth, garlic and onions grew. The ancient Egyptians worshipped garlic. Pliny, a famous Roman naturalist living in the first century A.D., recommended garlic for sixty-one different ailments. Louis Pasteur noted that garlic killed all the bacteria on his petri dish. Circa 1900, a large tuberculosis ward in Dublin, Ireland, reported remarkable cure rates by eating, inhaling, and smearing garlic on the chest as an ointment. And garlic can become your personal bodyguard against food pollutants.

Eating garlic often is like dropping an atom bomb on the various disease-causing microbes in your body and diet. Garlic is more effective against bacteria than tetracycline, one of the more potent prescription antibiotics used in modern medicine.[34] Garlic was able to kill the food infection microbes of *Salmonella* and *E. coli* bacteria in test-tube experiments.[35]

Cryptococcus neoformans is a formidable yeast/bacteria that attacks the central nervous system of humans and is spreading worldwide: even dilute garlic kills *Cryptococcus*.[36] Some very intriguing research shows that garlic rubbed on fungal skin lesions had a near 100 percent cure rate.[37] Garlic is a unique selective toxin to at least seventeen different strains of fungi and even more potent than the drug of choice (nystatin) against yeast infections.[38] Garlic was effective at eliminating *Candida* yeast infections in experimental chickens.[39] Since fungal infections on food is one of the more potent toxins in the food supply, garlic may even provide some protection against the dreaded aflatoxins; and it seems to be equally effective in killing viruses.[40]

Doctors in a poor and remote province of China had no antibiotics and an epidemic of meningitis—an infection of the spinal fluid that can cause brain damage or death—on their hands. The doctors looked into their herb medical books and found references to garlic as an antibacterial agent, so they fed and injected garlic to their meningitis patients and produced a 68 percent cure rate, which is impressive even by modern hospital standards.[41] Garlic apparently was able to cross the sieve (blood-brain barrier) that protects the brain form foreign compounds (many modern antibiotics will not cross the blood-brain barrier). American researchers at Georgetown University also found that garlic obliterated colonies of mycobacteria in petri dishes.[42]

And garlic seems to be lethal on tumor cells. The American Cancer Institute is so impressed with the chemo-protective effects of garlic and onions that they have approved several grants for major universities to study how these modest, stinky, little vegetables can do what wonder drugs cannot.[43] Dr. Tariq Abdullah of Florida found that killer white blood cells from garlic-fed people were able to kill 139 percent more tumor cells than killer white cells from non–garlic eaters.[44] Garlic and onion oils fed to lab animals were able to decrease the number and incidence of skin tumors.[45] Raw garlic fed to mice with a genetic weakness toward cancer was able to substantially decrease the number of expected tumors.[46]Chinese researchers find that a high intake of garlic and onions cuts the risk for stomach cancer, the most common type worldwide, in half.[47]

Garlic may even be able to protect the lungs: it apparently has antioxidant properties that quench free radical destruction of lung tissue, such as occurs in bronchitis, emphysema, and lung cancer.[48] And garlic protects against carcinogenic agents: when Japanese scientists pretreated cells with garlic extract and then exposed them to carcinogenic agents, there was bolstered immunity and a lower cancer rate in the garlic-treated cells.[49] Garlic even provides some liver protection against carcinogenic chemicals.[50]

Garlic has the unusual properties of being able to protect the body against both cancer or microbial invasion. Garlic is deadly to abnormal cells, but nontoxic to human cells—the ultimate selective toxin that pharmaceutical companies have been seeking; the ultimate cheap, nontoxic, over-the-counter wonder drug.[51]

How to use it. Garlic's unique flavor and odor make it lots of friends in gourmet cooking. However, some people do not care for the taste. There are a number of deodorized versions of garlic, none of which have any therapeutic value except Kyolic. In removing the smell component, allicin, most companies have also removed the health benefits of garlic.

We keep fresh garlic bulbs in bulk and use them whole in various dishes, including soups, stews, casseroles, baked beans, etc. Add a whole clove or two to your steamed or microwaved vegetables—cooking removes some of the pungent flavor, bringing out a more subtle gourmet experience. Chop up the garlic bulbs initially, so that no one gets a large mouthful of this pungent herb. As your family grows accustomed to the flavor, you can add it more often to various dishes and in greater quantity.

Fresh pressed garlic is now available in glass jars in most grocery stores, to avoid the messy pressing activity that keeps many people from using this valuable vegetable. Chopped or pressed garlic could accompany fried, boiled, or braised meats, chicken, and fish. There are a number of good cookbooks to provide you with a palatable introduction to garlic uses in the kitchen.[52] One

Figure 10A:

Apple Chutney

4 cups peeled, cored, and chopped tart apples (about 16)
½ cup chopped onions
3 cloves garlic, fresh crushed
½ cup chopped green peppers
1 pound raisins
2 cups brown sugar, packed

2 cups vinegar
2 small hot red chiles
3 tablespoons mustard seeds
1 tablespoon minced gingerroot
1 teaspoon salt
½ teaspoon ground allspice
pinch ground cloves

COMBINE apples, onions, garlic, green peppers, raisins, brown sugar, vinegar, red chiles, mustard seeds, gingerroot, salt, allspice, and cloves in large saucepan. Simmer 2 hours or until thick, stirring occasionally to prevent sticking. Pour, boiling hot, into hot sterilized jars, leaving ¼-inch head space. Adjust lids. Process 10 minutes in boiling water bath.

Makes about 2½ quarts.

of our favorite condiments that we use on various foods is chutney, which employs garlic, onions, ginger, and hot peppers—all foods that merit your regular consumption. It also has a spicy zingy flavor that has become a favorite of mine.

Carotenoids. Next time you find yourself awestruck by the kaleidoscopic beauty of a wooded hillside in the autumn, give thanks for carotenoids. They are more than just another pretty face. They are among the more potent antioxidants ever found and may be the major factor that prevents food pollutants from exploding into cancer in your body. Carotenoids, including the famous beta-carotene, are a group of at least five hundred different pigments that assist chlorophyll in photosynthesis, the process "patented" by green plants that harnesses the energy of the sun to combine carbon dioxide and water into 16 billion tons of sugar each year worldwide. When the autumn angles of the sun mysteriously trigger the tree to go into hibernation, the green chlorophyll recedes, leaving behind the reds, yellows, oranges, and purples of carotenoids to dazzle the spectator.

Most scientists now accept the theory that aging and cancer occur due to the destructive effect of free radicals, which also contribute to much of the harm from food and water pollutants. Dr. Roy Walford, a leading researcher at the UCLA School of Medicine, calls free radicals "the great white sharks in the chemical sea of life."[53] By feeding these "hungry sharks" some expendable meat (antioxidants), you can lessen the cellular damage done by free radicals.

Imagine the biochemistry of the cell as a dance. Free radicals are the bullies who move in to molest the fine ladies. Antioxidants are the suicidial security crew who have a "take-no-prisoners" approach to law enforcement. Decades into the great chase for some chemo-protective agent against cancer, researchers now dub beta-carotene "the most efficient quencher of singlet oxygen thus far discovered."[54] Which means that beta-carotene is the toughest security crew ever found to prevent damage to the dancers.

People who eat more beta-carotene have much less cancer of the:

-pancreas, a particularly fatal variety of cancer.[55]
-larynx, bladder, breast, cervix, and prostate.[56]
-bladder.[57]
-lung and stomach.[58]
-colon.[59]
-prostate.[60]

There are many more studies showing the amazing protective role of beta-carotene against cancer. Of Italian women studied, those who consumed less than 3,300 international units (i.u.) daily of beta-carotene had eight times more cervical cancer than women consuming at least the Recommended Dietary Allowance (RDA) of 5,000 i.u.[61] The new preferred unit of measurement for vitamin A and beta-carotene is retinol equivalents (RE). 5,000 i.u. equals 1,000 RE.

Researchers find that beta-carotene is quite effective at preventing chemically and virally induced cancer. All totaled, an Oxford physician conservatively estimates that adequate intake of beta-carotene alone could cut cancer incidence by one-third.[62] Anyone who is eating less than a rational amount of beta-carotene is walking into a barrage of enemy gunfire (ingested pollutants) with no protection.

Not only can carotenoids help prevent cancer, but beta-carotene may be able to change tumorous cells back into normal cells, a feat which until now was considered impossible.[63] In human patients with lung cancer, large doses of vitamin A were both directly toxic to tumor cells and also elevated the patients' immune levels to begin evicting cancer cells.[64]

One of the ways that beta-carotene may be so effective against cancer is because it can elevate the levels of several key players in the immune system: T4 lymphocytes, T-helper cells, and natural killer cells.[65] Mice fed carrot juice *after* exposure to various carcinogenic chemicals had fewer tumors, yet mice fed some carrot juice *before* exposure to the nasty chemicals had even fewer.[66]

Fortunately, only dehydration destroys large quantities of beta-carotene, so cooked and microwaved vegetables are still decent sources of this free-radical shield.[67]

How much beta-carotene is enough? In many of these studies, an extra 5,000 i.u. of beta-carotene (found in one small carrot) could drastically lower cancer risks. The evidence has so impressed the experts in power that the National Cancer Institute and the Harvard School of Public Health both have large-scale studies under way using beta-carotene to reduce cancer risks.

So far, all we have talked about is beta-carotene. What about the other five hundred or so related carotenoid compounds? Do they also have anticancer and antipollution capabilities? Probably. Even though less than 10 percent of the five hundred or more carotenoids have some vitamin A activity, many of them have the ability to:

- stimulate the immune system
- quench destructive free radicals
- reverse damage to the DNA molecule
- prevent mutations in the cell
- protect against cell damage from ultra-violet sunlight.[68]

One of the carotenoids is canthaxanthin, which is most often seen commercially as a "tanning" pill to give people a quasi-tan look by saturating the skin with orangish pigments. Dr. Norman Krinsky, noted expert on antioxidants and professor at the Tufts University School of Medicine in Boston, has found that canthaxanthin blocks tumor growth in animals. Yet canthaxanthin has no vitamin A activity, which beta-carotene does.

One USDA researcher, Dr. Frederick Khachik, found that foods high in carotenoids were even more effective than beta-carotene at lowering the risk for cancer. One carotenoid, called lutein, found in broccoli, brussel sprouts, and cabbage, also seems to have a cancer-protective ability. Which is just another reason for emphasizing nutritional protection from foods, since our understanding of natural chemopreventive agents is far from clear. Dr.

Hans Stich, a cancer expert in British Columbia, considers the carotenoid experience to show scientists of the "cocktail effect" of synergistic action—many antioxidants working together in concert to create a formidable anticancer effect which is greater than the sum of the parts.

People who are exposed to the typical high doses of pollutants from food, water, and air should increase their intake of beta-carotene and the carotenoid family. Carotenoids have been found to be amazingly safe: no toxicity has been found in carotenoids and beta-carotene (plant version of vitamin A), while toxicity of performed vitamin A (from liver) can easily be reached and can cause birth defects when taken during pregnancy. You are eating enough beta-carotene when your palms turn a mild orange color—that is the saturation point for any health benefits. (If the whites of your eyes are orangish, then you are beyond saturation and should subtract beta-carotene from your program.) Be cautious with supplements of preformed vitamin A from fish liver oil. This can easily become toxic, especially when eating a diet high in beta-carotene.

How to use. Dark green leafy vegetables (like kale and spinach), green vegetables (like broccoli and peas), orange fruits (like apricots and cantaloupe), and orange vegetables (like carrots, sweet potatoes, and pumpkins) are all rich sources of beta-carotene along with undetermined amounts of other carotenoids. One slice of pumpkin pie contains 3,700 i.u. of beta-carotene, while a large carrot has 11,000 i.u. In all but the northern regions of the U.S., some fresh green leafy vegetable will grow even in fall and winter. Collards are a favorite cold-weather green along the Atlantic seaboard and in the deep south. Green leaves from mustard, dandelion, collard, beets, kale, turnips, and other crops all provide valuable mixed carotenoids to the diet. It is relatively easy to get a rich and protective intake of carotenoids when eating lots of fruits and vegetables.

One of our favorite recipes uses equal amounts of grated carrots and grated cabbage, with a sprinkling of sunflower seeds, raisins, and Italian salad dressing for a fabulous cold vegetable salad.

Cruciferous vegetables. Until 1982, the idea that foods may help prevent cancer was heresy, except among isolated pockets of "food faddists." A group of researchers in 1950 fed either beets or cabbage to two sets of guinea pigs, then exposed the animals to harmful levels of X-radiation. The cabbage-fed rodents had a lower incidence of both hemorrhage and death.[69] Rather than speculate that cabbage protected the animals from X-ray harm, the scientists concluded in their article that something in beets became highly toxic when exposed to radiation. Since then, studies have shown that cabbage cuts the death rate in half among animals exposed to radiation:[70] beets don't cause cancer, but cabbage might prevent it. Actually, the ancient Romans reportedly ran their doctors out of town and for a period of years maintained good health by eating their cabbages. A small regular intake of cabbages is probably good medicine against food pollution.

Cabbage belongs to the cruciferous family of vegetables, which also includes broccoli, brussels sprouts, cauliflower, cress, horse-radish, kale, kohlrabi, mustard, radish rutabaga, and turnips. These plants, officially called *brassica*, were coined "cruciferous" because botanists in the Middle Ages thought that the four-petaled flowers of these vegetables resembled a crucifix.

By the mid 1970s the link between nutrition and cancer was still considered "fringe thinking." However, the true pioneers of science don't mind being nonconformists, because they only add to their knowledge base by trying something that hasn't yet been done. Lee Wattenberg, M.D., of the University of Minnesota Medical School, had been feeding small amounts of cruciferous vegetables to lab animals, then injecting them with proven carcinogens. Many of the animals did not get cancer. Dr. Wattenberg eventually isolated an active compound from cabbage (indoles) that alone was able to protect animals from potent carcinogens.[71] With typical scientific understatement, Dr. Wattenberg named these striking anticarcinogens "minor dietary constituents" (MDC). Other protective MDCs found in cruciferous vegetables have more strenuous names: dithiolthiones, isothiocyanates, and lutein.

Indoles seemed to be a mighty shield against the dreaded foe, cancer. Some rats were given indole protection and then injected with with low-dose long-term carcinogens, such as would occur in the typical American lifestyle. All of the unprotected rats died of tumors, while 54 percent of the indole-protected rats survived. This landmark work produced little more than a yawn in those days. Yet in our heavily polluted times, these MDCs may be just as important as eating enough protein and vitamin C.

Later, Dr. Saxon Graham, of the State University of New York, conducted a study that looked at the diets of 256 white male patients with colon cancer and a control group of 783 patients of identical ages who did not have colon cancer. The men who reported eating the most vegetables had the lowest risk for cancer—and of the vegetables, the one food that stood out above the crowd was cabbage. One serving of cabbage per week cut the risk for colon cancer by 66 percent![72] The diet-cancer link had reached critical mass: before the ink was dry on Dr. Graham's article, labs all over the country were gearing up for studies on the nutrition-cancer link. By 1982, the prestigious National Academy of Sciences issued its technical report, *Diet, Nutrition, and Cancer,* which explored the hundreds of ways in which diet can cause or prevent cancer.[73] This report estimated that at least 30 percent of all cancer was nutritionally related. Departing from the normal dry language of the scientist, they proclaimed: "Spread the message that cancer is not as inevitable as death and taxes." We had emerged from the Dark Ages of nutritional science. Since then, other scientists have estimated that nutrition (not enough protective nutrients and/or too many harmful dietary factors) is responsible for up to 90 percent of all cancers.

In 1978, the Japanese National Cancer Center provided their people with a twelve-point program to help prevent cancer, of which eight points involved nutritional recommendations. One of their points was to encourage the intake of rational levels of supplements.[74] All of this hoopla surrounding nutrition as chemopreventive agents against cancer started with the lowly cabbage.

Further evidence for the protective abilities of cruciferous vegetables came out of Dr. Geir Hoff's lab in Norway. Dr. Hoff and associates examined the colons of 155 people in their fifties who had no signs of colon cancer. Half of these people had polyps growing in the colon (polyps are abnormal tissue that can be a prelude to cancer); the other half of the group, with no polyps, ate more cruciferous vegetables than the polyp-infested group. Most impressive for the scientists was the blatant dose-dependent relationship; that is, the more you give of a substance, the greater the effect. The more cruciferous foods consumed, the lower the chance for polyps; while the less cruciferous vegetables consumed, the greater the risk for polyps, and the larger and more abnormal the polyps.[75]

Cruciferous vegetables were then found to extend their cancer protection outside of the gastrointestinal tract, into the bladder.[76] As the evidence continues to gather, six out of seven major epidemiological studies show that cruciferous vegetables protect against cancer of the colon, stomach, lung, esophagus, larynx, rectum, prostate, and bladder. While the weight of the evidence endorses cruciferous vegetables, there are also trace amounts of naturally occurring toxins in these precious foods. Clearly, though, people who eat more broccoli (which also contains beta-carotene and vitamin C) have a lower incidence of cancer.[77]

Cruciferous vegetables may be your primary ally against the *extremely* carcinogenic effects of aflatoxin mold found on grains, nuts, and legumes. Scientists at Johns Hopkins University found that lab animals protected with cruciferous vegetables had about 10 percent the incidence of liver cancer from aflatoxin molds as compared to unprotected animals.[78] A follow-up study also found that an MDC substance isolated form cruciferous vegetables, dithiolthiones, reduced cancer from aflatoxins by 40 to 80 percent, depending on the amount of dithiolthiones used.[79] Brussels sprouts provided comparable protection from other liver carcinogens.[80] (Peanut butter is a cheap and tasty source of protein, calories, and niacin; yet may also contain the dreaded aflatoxins. If you send your kids to school with a peanut butter sandwich, include a small wedge of cabbage for their protection.)

The MDCs in cruciferous vegetables are also able to put your body's detoxification system in overdrive to produce more GSH (glutathione), which is one of the "heavyweight bouncers" that acts as an antioxidant and detoxification substance. Dithiolthiones were also able to increase a protective enzyme system in the body (glutathione transferase).

Lab animals fed cauliflower juice had less intestinal damage from nitroso compounds, which result from nitrates in the water and food supply. While indoles help prevent cancer when fed *before* exposure to a toxin, indoles seem useless if fed after the carcinogen. However, another MDC in cruciferous vegetables, iso-thiocyanates, do provide some "morning-after" protection against carcinogens. Cruciferous vegetables seem to have an army, air force, and navy of MDCs against pollutants and cancer. If one of the MDCs doesn't get the job done, another will.

Heavily salted cruciferous vegetables, such as sauerkraut or the Japanese version, hakusai, may do more harm than good.[81] Keep your intake under one half pound per day of raw cabbage, turnips, and kale, since these cruciferous vegetables contain substances, goitrin and thiocyanate, which can create goiter, a mental and physical growth-stunting in children. As I have been advocating throughout this book, eat a wide variety of foods, with emphasis on including the protective foods of this chapter and minimizing the harmful foods of the previous chapter. The message that stands out in neon letters from this research is: "Eat small amounts of cruciferous vegetables regularly."

How to use. It is best to purchase organic broccoli and cauliflower, since these plants are directly exposed to some potent pesticides. Barring the possibility of buying organic, make sure that you soak your commercial broccoli in warm water for five minutes and then scrub it clean while rinsing. Cabbage is safer since you can peel off the outer layer of leaves. It is preferable to eat most cruciferous vegetables cooked, to neutralize the goiter factors.

Several times a week, we make a soup out of leftover vegetables. Using garlic, onion, ginger, turmeric, rosemary, thyme, and other herb flavorings with a pinch of soy sauce or salt, you can make some mighty tasty soups and casseroles out of leftover cruciferous vegetables along with some grains (like barley or rice) and poultry or fish. Fresh or frozen cruciferous vegetables best retain their nutritive value when steamed or microwaved. Avoid the high fat sauces, like blue cheese dressing, that can nullify the extraordinary benefits of cruciferous vegetables. We often use a delicious buttermilk salad dressing, available in most grocery stores, on our steamy hot cruciferous vegetables.

Legumes. While studying for my Master's degree, I took a course in the biology of ecology. On one memorable field trip to the local sewage treatment plant, the plant manager explained the process of sewage treatment in minute detail. He noted that the end product of sewage sludge can be obtained free and is rich in organic compost, which nearly always yields a healthy crop of tomatoes. Yes, after passing through the chemical torture chamber of the human intestines, and then the multiple stages of fermentation in a big city sewage plant, the tomato seeds could still sprout. That is nature's plan.

Seeds are miniature spaceships, sent out by plants with the fervent hope that their offspring will be able to sprout new life elsewhere. In order to fulfill that plan, many seeds come in "hard shell cases," or wrapped in poison (as apricot seeds contain the cyanide compound laetrile), or with a protective coating of chemicals to escape normal digestion. These seed-protective "antinutrients" were once considered useless at best, and potentially very harmful. Yet new research finds these "antinutrients" to be more like a genie in a bottle to help us in our quest to prevent cancer and viral infections.

The MDCs in legumes include lectins, saponins, phytates, tannins, and protease inhibitors. These MDCs may be able to help us contain cancer in ways that new wonder drugs have failed to. Legumes include most beans (soy, garbanzo, kidney, lima, pinto, etc.), peas, lentils, and even peanuts. Leguminous plants are a balm on the earth since they can fix nitrogen from the air into the soil, hence adding fertility to the earth rather than needing to be fertilized. The merits of legumes read like curriculum vitae for a Nobel laureate.

Legumes are rich in a special type of fiber, pectin, that is water soluble and can neutralize carcinogens and fats in the intestinal tract; they are as rich in pectin as apples. Legumes also attract less bile acid in the intestinal tract. Bile acids are produced internally and are essential for proper fat digestion, but the breakdown products of bile acids can become dangerously carcinogenic, so a minimum of bile acids is best. On oat bran diets, human bile acid production *rose* by 65 percent, while bean diets *lowered* bile acid production by 30 percent.[82] Though oat fiber does help lower fats in the blood, bean fiber is equally effective at that important role.

Of those MDCs in legumes, phytic acid turns out to be a champion antioxidant, smothering the destructive free radical compounds in a suicidal venture and preventing damage to the fatty portion of cell membranes.[83] Another MDC, lignan, found in beans may help ward off breast and colon cancer. Lignan is converted by bacteria into a hormonelike compound that protects the entire body from cancer cells.

Another MDC in legumes, protease inhibitors (PIs), have risen from the lowly ranks of "antinutrient" to "chemopreventive agent" in just the past few years. Protein foods, like meat and milk, must be hacked up into smaller pieces, called amino acids, in the intestinal tract by protease enzymes, which act like an "axe" to cut up the protein into smaller bits. Proteases are necessary for you to derive any nutritional benefit from protein in the diet; yet excess protease enzymes can be commandeered by tumor cells and used to axe their way through tough connective protein and cell membranes to reach the vulnerable DNA molecule within. PIs from legumes put a thick "sheath" around the excess "axes" of proteases to prevent their destructive use by tumor cells. PIs seemed to have been originally designed by nature to protect a plant seed from digestion in the long, dark, scary ride through an animal's intestinal tract. The protected seed would then be excreted unscathed, amid rich compost, for a comfortable and safe beginning to life.

PIs also act as antioxidants to quell the wrecking balls of free radicals that can instigate cancer.[84] In another new discovery, at New York University School of Medicine, Dr. Walter Troll has found that PIs also prevent your body's cells from joining in the wildly eratic growth of tumor cells. Oncogenes (short for oncology genes) are "switches" buried in all human DNA that can be activated to encourage participation in the suicidal building process of cancer cells.[85] PIs cover the oncogene "switch" to prevent cancer cells from enlisting the aid of your own cells.

And if these tricks aren't impressive enough, Dr. Ann Kennedy at the University of Pennsylvania has found that PIs also act like a "heat seeking missile," with a selective toxicity only for cancer cells.[86] Pharmaceutical companies have spent billions of dollars in research trying to find some chemical that will kill cancer cells but leave normal healthy cells untouched. Nature gave that gift to us long ago in the form of PIs. Dr. Kennedy also finds that PIs can perform what was considered the impossible: reverse the DNA damage that can lead to cancer.[87] DNA damage is like having someone spray graffiti all over the architect's blueprints to your home: the damage seems irreparable. Somehow, PIs help the DNA blueprints to "remember" the original healthy drawings and return to that form.

PIs are also effective against viruses. The few drugs available that claim to work against viruses act on the patient's cellular DNA in a dangerous meddling that could lead to cancer as a long-term side effect. Viruses travel in a dormant state, wrapped in a protective protein overcoat, like a lion traveling in a circus cage. In order for a virus to become entrenched in a host, several steps are necessary:

-That protein overcoat must be dissolved by a protease; letting the "lion" out of the cage.
-The virus must be able to penetrate the cell membrane by stealing a protease; using spare "axes" to hack their way into the DNA compartment.
-The virus must then commandeer the host cell DNA (perhaps by switching on the oncogene) to man-

ufacture more viruses; like a terrorist taking over a factory and demanding new products to further the terrorist's cause.

PIs are able to interfere with each phase of the virus's trai-
torous operation. Some studies have shown that high concentrations of soybean compounds shut down 100 percent of
viral activity. Among the viruses that can be squelched by
PIs: myxoviruses (flu, mumps), retroviruses (AIDS, leukemia),
poxviruses (smallpox), and coronaviruses (respiratory infections). After finding all of the impressive data on PIs, I can
only quote the venerable Butch Cassidy and the Sundance
Kid as they were being relentlessly tracked by a determined
posse: "Who *are* those guys?"
    PIs are found in higher levels in legumes (especially soy and
garbanzo beans), with smaller quantities in all seed foods: walnuts, pecans, sunflower seeds, cereal grains (wheat, rice, corn,
oats, barley, and amaranth), sweet potatoes, and bananas. Egg-
plant contains appreciable amounts of PIs while half of the protein in green tomatoes is in the form of PIs. For the most part,
PIs survive cooking and processing, the exception to this rule
being cooked potatoes.
    Although some researchers have protested that legume
antinutrients like PIs may not be as magical and as safe as they
appear, the bulk of the research says that these MDCs in legumes
might be able to inhibit all types of cancer (except stomach cancer), and with no apparent side effects.[88] However, peas and, to
a lesser extent, soybeans have been found to contain substances
that are natural contraceptives.[89] Certain substances in these
plants will imitate estrogen in your body, to discourage a healthy
implantation of a fertilized egg, just the way birth control pills
work. Although I wouldn't consider peas and soybeans to be a
reliable birth control method, if you are trying to get pregnant
then minimize your intake of peas and soybeans. Also, to avoid
other estrogenic activity in foods and nutrients, avoid taking
more than 100 i.u. per day of vitamin E or 100 mg per day of
bioflavonoids, or consuming excessive ginger.

Although the Japanese have a high rate of stomach cancer, probably due to their high intake of salted foods, they have one of the lowest overall cancer rates among the world's advanced nations. Ironically, nearly all soybeans grown in the U.S. are consumed in Japan or by our livestock; but the U.S. has one of the highest cancer rates in the world. I often find it puzzling why we Americans sell our best foods, like wheat germ and soybeans to other nations or feedlots, but don't eat them ourselves. The various MDCs in legumes have become a bona fide scientific phenomenon in the war against tainted foods and cancer.[90]

How to use. The notorious drawback for legumes is their legendary "wind making" ability; flatulence or farting. Although this is a subject that only a proctologist could discuss with a straight face, it bears elaboration since it is an embarrassing problem caused by an otherwise very healthy food group. Flatulence in beans is brought on when intestinal bacteria ferment a type of carbohydrate (oligosaccharides) that is heavily concentrated in beans. The result is methane gas. However, as you continue to eat beans, your body will start to generate more digestive enzymes for these oligosaccharides so that flatulence diminishes the more frequently you have beans in your diet. A steady intake of yogurt also cuts down on the flatulence from beans, because *Lactobacillus* competes with methane-making intestinal bacteria. Adding onions, garlic, mustard, and ginger to beans will further reduce flatulence. You can also reduce flatulence in legumes by sprouting them. But the most effective way of making "low wind" beans is as follows:

-Rinse beans.
-Cover with water in a pan, with an extra 2 inches
of water to allow for expansion of beans as they swell.
-Bring water to a boil for two minutes.
-Turn off heat. Cover the pan. Let stand for one hour.
-Drain this water. Rinse beans again.
-Cover beans with water again.
-Add your favorite seasonings. Ours include hefty

portions of onions and garlic with smaller portions of hot peppers, butter, and salt.
    -Pressure cook for 25 minutes.

At that point, you have great cooked beans for hot soup, like black bean and barley soup, or cold three bean salad (see below). Or you can chop up the beans with an electric mixer to make refried beans for a taco filling (if you used pinto beans) or hummus (if you used garbanzo beans). Garbanzo beans not only offer the least amount of flatulence problem, but also are one of the highest-protein plant foods available.

Noreen Quillin's Blue Ribbon No-Work Three-Bean Salad:

    -Add equal amounts of 3 (or 4 or 5) different cooked beans (use pressure cooker) to a mixing bowl. Soy, garbanzo, kidney, lima, green, string, pinto, and other beans are all viable candidates. Make the color combination pleasing.
    -Add a healthy amount of fresh cut, sweet red onion bits, with a lesser amount of fried garlic
    -Thoroughly mix in a small amount of Italian dressing, just enough for flavor and moisture.
    Makes a terrific hot weather entree, or salad, or starch, or stand-alone snack.

Seaweed. Vegetables of the sea, or seaweeds, have become the Rodney Dangerfield of healthy foods—they don't get no respect. Admittedly, it took us a while to develop an appreciation for their unique flavor. However, seaweed has a five thousand-year history of praise from healers. The source book for the Bible's account of the great flood (*The Epic of Gilgamesh*) mentioned a plant from the sea that would bestow eternal youth and immortality on the eater. Five thousand years ago, the Father of Chinese medicine advocated plants of the sea for those wanting long life. In A.D. 500 Confucius extolled the virtues of seaweed.[91] In the Andes Mountains of South America, groups of natives carry pouches filled with dried seaweed and protect it like the family treasure. They follow this tradition because seaweed contains enough iodine to prevent goiter, which is extremely common in the inland regions of the world. Seaweeds could help solve the world's deteriorating-food crisis. Seaweeds provide special types of soluble fiber, like carageenan and guar gum, that are considered some of the most effective at lowering the risk for cancer and heart disease; and seaweed provides a shield to protect you against virus, fungi, toxic heavy metals, chemical toxins, and can lower the risk for cancer in a number of truly ingenious ways.

Dr. Jane Teas, of the Harvard University School of Public Health, found that low breast-cancer rates in Japan may be due to their consumption of seaweed; since the coastal areas, where more seaweed is eaten, have an even lower incidence of breast cancer.[92] Dr. Teas followed up her epidemiological work with seaweed tests on lab animals, which also showed a decrease in the rate of breast cancer.[93] Premenopausal women in Japan have one-third the breast cancer incidence, while postmenopausal Japanese women have one-ninth of the breast cancer incidence when compared to their American counterparts.[94]

In other studies, intake of seaweed was found to significantly protect animals from breast cancer, leukemia, and other forms of cancer.[95] Dr. Yamamoto was able to isolate the MDC, fucoidan, from seaweeds. Fucoidan is a substance that apparently stimulates the immune system of animals to become wildly predatory on tumor cells. Researchers at the University of Hawaii even found that seaweed extract (Viva-Natural) helped to contain and even reduce lung cancer in experimental mice by stimulating the natural immune defense system.[96] Seaweed extract may someday become a "kinder, gentler" therapy for cancer patients.

There is an army of MDCs in seaweed that act in various ways to lower cancer risk. One MDC, alginic acid, is known to dilute carcinogens in the intestines and to neutralize bile acids that can also elevate cancer risk.[97] Another MDC, beta-sitosterol, has been credited with anticancer properties in the colon.[98] There are also a number of MDCs in seaweed which have antibiotic activity against a range of different bacteria, such as those in the intestines which can produce carcinogenic agents.[99] Also, seaweed provides antioxidants to protect against free-radical cancer risks.[100]

Seaweed's potent antibiotic abilities are legendary. An American marine biologist, J. M. Sieburth, noticed the lack of bacteria in penguin intestines, and later found that seaweed was responsible.[101] Since then, scientists have noted that various MDCs in seaweed are potently effective against many strains of bacteria, fungus, and virus. Test-tube studies find that seaweed extract is as effective as prescription antibiotics against common food-poisoning bacteria (*Staphylococcus aureus, Streptococcus pyogenes,* and *E. coli*); the ubiquitous human fungus (*Candida albicans*); and one of the bacteria responsible for pneumonia.[102]

Cows fed seaweed over a seven-year period had only one incidence of mastitis (an udder infection dreaded by dairy farmers), while a similar group of cows without seaweed in the diet had nine cases of mastitis. The seaweed-fed cows also produced more milk. Interestingly enough, farmers along the sea coasts in Europe have followed the centuries-old folklore of feeding seaweed to their cattle. Seaweed also has proven abilities to destroy intestinal parasites, which can become a problem if you eat poorly cooked foods.[103]

Meanwhile, seaweed has MDCs that work effectively against many viruses. Remember that man-made drugs are relatively dangerous and ineffective against viruses. One MDC in seaweed, sulfated saccharides, seems to rampantly destroy flu, polio, herpes, and other viruses.

One of the most serious hazards in our food and water supply is toxic trace minerals, like lead, cadmium, and strontium. The richly absorbant properties of seaweed have been shown to bind toxic metals in the intestines and move them out with the feces. Even more startling news is that long term continuous dietary intake of seaweed can reduce radioactive strontium that is deposited in bone tissue.[104] Radioactive strontium, which is in the atmosphere from nuclear accidents like Chernobyl and from nuclear weapons testing, ends up in the food and water supply and can induce leukemia.

Figure 10B: THE THERAPEUTIC PROTECTIVE VALUE
OF SUPERFOODS

MINOR DIETARY CONSTITUENT	FOUND IN THIS FOOD	PROTECTS AGAINST
acidophilin, bulgarican, lactic acid, acetic acid, benzoic acid, hydrogen peroxide, blastolysin	yogurt	viruses, E. coli, salmonella, bacteria, cancer cells, lactose intolerance
antibiotics, antivirals, allicin, antioxidants	garlic	bacteria, viruses, yeasts, molds, tumor cells, toxic chemicals
beta-carotene, chlorophyll, antioxidants, lutein carotenoids, canthaxanthin	dark green and dark orange fruits & vegetables	virus, toxic chemicals, tumor cells, lowered immune system, air pollution, smoke, sunlight
indoles, dithiolthiones, isothiocyanates, lutein immune stimulants	cruciferous vegetables	Xrays, toxic chemicals, cancer throughout body, aflatoxins, nitrates

Figure 10B: THE THERAPEUTIC PROTECTIVE VALUE OF SUPERFOODS (Cont.)

MINOR DIETARY CONSTITUENT	FOUND IN THIS FOOD	PROTECTS AGAINST
lectins, saponins, phytates, tannins, pectin, protease inhibitors, antioxidants	legumes, seeds	fats, carcinogens, bile acids, free radicals, tumor cells, viruses, oncogenes, may reverse DNA damage
carageenan, guar gum, fucoidan, alginic acid, beta-sitosterol, antioxidants, antibiotics, sulfated saccharides	seaweed	bacteria, virus, fungi, toxic metals, toxic chemicals, tumor cells bile acids, free radicals, intestinal parasites, radioactive strontium, nicotine

Seaweed also has shown promise in counteracting the many harmful effects of nicotine.[105] If seaweed can offset the damage from the toxic drug nicotine, perhaps it can also mitigate the harm from other pollutants.

In many ways, through many MDCs, seaweed protects you from a wide variety of harmful agents in the food and water supply. Seaweed is as high in protein (dry weight) as soybeans, with protein quality nearly equal to animal tissue. Seaweed is rich in calcium, potassium, trace minerals from the sea, and one of the better plant sources of iron. You may have to acquire a taste for these sea vegetables, but the benefits are most worth the effort.

How to use. There are almost as many sea vegetables as there are fish in the sea, so the flavor of seaweed varies with the species; mildly fishy, nutty, beany, sweet, sour, etc. Most seaweed is easiest to use by hydrating it in a small amount of warm water, then cutting it up and using it in a salad or soup. One seaweed dish that we are partial to:

Seaweed Rice Balls:

-Combine 3 cups of cooked brown rice, up to 1 tablespoon of soy sauce, and ¼ cup of nutritional yeast in a bowl and mix.

-Have hydrated sheets of nori seaweed ready in a bowl of warm water.

-Dip hands in bowl of water, scoop out about ½ cup of rice mixture, form into a ball, and wrap in seaweed. You can warm the seaweed rice balls in the microwave or serve cold. They make kind of an oriental taco.

GOOD FOODS: INCLUDE OFTEN IN YOUR DIET

Apples. Most Americans like at least a few of the seven thousand different varieties of apples grown in this country. Apples have an MDC that can kill lethal viruses, like polio. People who eat more apples have fewer colds and upper respiratory tract ailments.[106] Apples also contain potent MDCs, such as caffeic and chlorogenic acids, that can neutralize carcinogens in animal studies.

Alar use is rare these days, and only red apples have any Alar. Best apples are green varieties (Macintosh, Pippin, etc.), or unsprayed, or tree ripened. Avoid shiny apples, due to their wax coating, or wash these apples in mild soap and warm water. Don't give up on apples just because of the Alar incident. They are a potent medicine against pollutants and common diseases. Fresh apples also act as a "toothbrush" to cleanse teeth after a meal, particularly valuable to include in a box lunch. Unfiltered apple juice is also acceptable, since it retains the valuable pectin which binds carcinogens and carries them out of the system. Canned apple products should be of the low-sugar variety. I like to test the sturdiness of my teeth by eating crisp fresh apples in season. We also serve low-sugar jarred apples throughout the year with poultry, fish, and meat entrees.

Apricots. In ancient Hebrew tradition, "apples" were actually apricots. King Solomon requested "apples" (apricots) when he was ill. It was apricots that tempted Eve in the Garden of Eden. Indeed, I would be tempted—fresh apricots have always ranked as one of my favorite foods. The reputedly-long-lived Hunza tribe of mountainous Afghanistan claim apricots as their source of health and longevity (the classic film, *Lost Horizon,* was based on the Shangri-la land of the Hunzas). For some unknown reason, the Nobel laureate G. S. Whipple praised apricots in 1934 as a wonder food "equal to liver in hemoglobin regeneration."

Aside from legend, apricots are a valuable source of beta-carotene, the potent antioxidant that can neutralize toxins and cancer cells. One serving of three medium-size apricots contains 2,800 i.u. of beta-carotene, over half the RDA. Also, dietary studies show that people who eat more fruits and vegetables get less cancer. There may be much more to apricots than the beta-carotene content. Since apricots are a fruit that is usually eaten with the peeling; it would be wise to peel, or thoroughly wash them, or buy organic apricots to avoid the pesticide residues.

Barley. Not only can barley drive down serum cholesterol levels better than oats, it also contains the protease inhibitors (PI) discussed previously with legumes. PIs are proven anticancer, antiviral compounds worthy of your dietary attention. By disposing of the outer wrapper (chaff), grains have the advantage of being relatively free of pesticide residues. Substitute one quarter whole grain barley flour in your cake, cookie, and bread recipes. We pressure cook whole grain barley for five minutes, then add it to most of our soups, stews, casseroles, and even use it as a stand-alone starch instead of rice or potatoes.

Blueberries. Anecdotally, blueberries hold top position in many home-remedy books for curing diarrhea. In scientific studies, blueberries were able to kill food-infection bacteria (especially *E. coli* from fecal contamination) and viruses. Blueberries are so effective against diarrhea that blueberry extract is the active ingredient in Pecarin, a drug sold in Sweden to treat diarrhea.[107] Crushed blueberries were able to destroy nearly 100 percent of the polio viruses in test-tube studies, even when the blueberries were diluted ten times. Both blueberries and blackcurrants contain the MDCs, tannins, and anthocyanosides, that may fight off disease-causing microbes in your food supply. If Oscar awards were given to popular foods, surely blueberry muffins would be a nominee.

Citrus (orange, lemon, lime, grapefruit, tangerine). According to the National Cancer Institute, the year-round availability of citrus products in the United States has been a main factor leading to the reduction in stomach cancer. Epidemiological studies have shown that people who eat more citrus cut their risk for cancer in half. Esophagus and pancreatic cancer are notably low in citrus lovers.[108] Something in citrus (including vitamin C and other unknown MDCs) improved human recovery time from German measles (rubella).[109]

Fortunately, the heavily sprayed citrus peel tends to be discarded. Do not use commercial citrus peels in cooking or for juicing. Oranges that are picked green and then stored in hot warehouses for weeks can lose much of their potent therapeutic value against pollutants. Buy citrus in season.

For vitamin C content choose (best first): navel orange, valencia orange, pink grapefruit, white grapefruit, mandarin orange, tangelo, tangerine, lemon, lime. Do not consume too much orange juice from frozen concentrate, since high-pressure mechanical squeezing of oranges brings much of the peeling's dangerous pesticides into the product. Fresh tree-ripened unsprayed oranges are true antipollution food, while unripened and oversprayed oranges are insipid at best, unhealthy at worst.

Corn. One of the few foods on the American dinner table that is American in origin, corn is notably clean from pesticides because it hides within a heavy overcoat throughout the chemical spraying period. Also, Dr. Pelayo Correa at the Louisiana State University Medical Center has found that diets high in corn show a lower incidence of colon, breast, and prostate cancer. When corn is part of a well-varied diet, it is a valuable addition; when corn becomes a main staple in the diet, unexplained diseases like pellagra (niacin deficiency) and depressed immune system occur. We often use warmed up whole grain corn tortillas to wrap up beans, scrambled eggs, honey and cheese, fish, and nearly anything edible.

Cranberries. For over a century, new Englanders have known of the antibiotic effect of their indigenous cranberry juice against bladder and urinary tract infections. Americans are experiencing a surge in infections of the urinary tract, possibly due to the immune-depressing action of pollutants. Cranberries contain the MDCs hippuric and quinic acid to acidify the urine and assassinate bacteria.

But cranberries have another clever trick to assist the immune system. Dr. Anthony Sobota at Youngstown State University in Ohio was investigating how bacteria adhere to healthy cells to begin their infection. In order to start trouble, bacteria must attach themselves to the host cell, like plugging an electrical cord into a wall outlet. Dr. Sobota found that normal antibiotics are relatively ineffective at preventing this dangerous attachment process. Trying various other substances, he found cranberry juice prevented the bacteria from clinging to the healthy host cells: it somehow fills in the "outlet" on host cells so that the bacteria cannot "plug in" and begin its infection. Actually, even at 30 percent dilution, cranberry juice was ten times more effective than prescription antibiotics at preventing this bacterial adherence.[110]

There is also evidence that cranberry juice fights other viral and bacterial infections in regions beyond the urinary tract.[111] A half cup a day may keep the doctor away, so don't restrict cranberries to just Thanksgiving dinner.

Eggs. You probably thought you would never see a nutritionist recommend eggs again. True, in the 1960s researchers found that cholesterol substances were blocking the arteries of heart disease patients. They made the obvious, but not accurate, conclusion: if you don't eat any cholesterol, then you won't get heart disease. Wrong. Actually, the newest and most complete studies show that total fat intake is much more influential in determining serum cholesterol levels than dietary cholesterol intake.[112] Your liver makes more cholesterol each day than you could eat from eight egg yolks.[113] So eggs are not the culprit in heart disease.

Eggs do have nutritional advantages. They are:

-high in protein, which is essential for a healthy immune and detoxification system
-a decent source of vitamin A and riboflavin
-cheap, available fresh year-round, easy to chew for everyone, and easy to digest.

Even more important, eggs may be rich sources of antibodies to help your body fight off viral infections and generally bolster the immune system.

Robert Yolken, M.D., at Johns Hopkins University Medical School has found that "first foods," or foods designed to sustain newborn animals, can be swarming with immune gifts from the mother. Dr. Yolken found many antibodies present in both milk and egg yolks.[114] This makes perfectly good sense. Human milk is rich in immune factors that help to pass on the mother's accumulated immune competence to her vulnerable newborn infant. Cows and chickens are equally generous with their offspring. Amazingly, 20 to 50 percent of these immune factors survive not only cooking but also the chemical shredder of the human intestinal tract.

Actually, Dr. Yolken found that the amount of antibodies produced in either milk or eggs could be increased by twenty-fold simply by administering a small safe innoculation to the mother cow or chicken who would then produce the antibodies. Our innoculations of the future may come from our food as well as needles. We eat four to five eggs weekly.

Fiber. Fiber is nutritionally valueless: it cannot be digested or absorbed. And because of that, it has a vast ability to protect you from food pollutants. Fiber has the following uses:

- soaks up fat, pollutants, toxic metals, pesticide residues, bile acids, and other carcinogens and carries them out with the feces.
- adds bulk to the stools, which dilutes the poisons in the food supply.
- speeds the rate at which food moves through the intestines. Since there are many natural and synthetic carcinogens in the diet, the less time these poisons have to instigate trouble in the intestines, the better.

A high-fiber diet may be one of he wisest choices Americans can make toward protecting themselves from food pollutants.

In thirty-two out of forty large-scale studies, high-fiber foods lowered the risk for various types of cancer, especially colon cancer.[115] And fiber seems to protect against toxic chemicals in the diet. When scientists fed test animals small amounts of cyclamate, red dye #2, and an emulsifier, all animals died within two weeks; yet if all three toxins were fed along with a high-fiber diet, there was no noticeable harm.[116] A high-fiber diet probably cuts the risk for colon cancer by 90 percent.[117] Fiber may also protect against breast cancer[118] and prostate cancer.[119]

There are two types of fiber: that which dissolves in water (water soluble), and that which does not dissolve in water (water insoluble).

Foods that contain soluble fiber include apples, oats, bananas, carrots, and citrus fruits. These foods are proven to lower the risk for heart disease.

Foods that contain insoluble fiber include lentils, brown rice, wheat products, and wheat bran. These foods are proven to lower the risk for colon cancer.

Foods that contain healthy amounts of both soluble and insoluble fibers include legumes, beans, peas, lentils, and green beans. These foods obviously cover both problems and should be included in the diet often.

The most commonly eaten food in America is white bread, which is practically devoid of fiber. Dr. Dennis Burkitt found that regions of Africa which consume 80 to 100 grams of fiber daily have almost no cancer, heart disease, diabetes, or obesity. The American Cancer Society has recommended that Americans increase their fiber intake from the current 15 grams per day to a healthier 30 grams. A more beneficial goal would be 50 grams daily.

How much fiber in the diet is enough? If your feces float, then you are eating enough fiber; the buoyancy is caused by tiny gas bubbles produced by bacteria which ferment the indigestible fiber. Too much fiber can instigate diarrhea, gas, and bind up precious minerals in the diet. Fiber is found almost exclusively in plant foods, such as:

-whole grains, like wheat, corn, rye, rice, oats, and millet

-seaweeds, like nori, contain guar gum and carageenan

-vegetables, like cabbage, tomatoes, carrots, and onions

-fruits, like citrus, apples, pears, plums, figs, and watermelon

-legumes, like beans, peas lentils, and peanuts

-nuts and seeds, sunflower seeds, walnuts cashews, and Brazil nuts

Figs. Although there is a great deal of far-fetched folklore surrounding figs, there is also some scientific evidence that figs have anticancer therapeutic value. Japanese scientists at the Institute of Physical and Chemical Research in Tokyo found that frozen fig distillate shrunk implanted tumors in mice by an average of 39 percent.[120] The active MDC in figs was identified as benzaldehyde.

When these experiments were repeated on human subjects, the results were even more striking: 55 percent of patients with advanced cancer improved, of which 29 percent went into partial remission, 7 percent went into complete remission, and nearly all fig-treated patients lived longer. Oral doses of figs have provided some success aginst cancer, but injecting the benzaldehyde from figs was more effective. Figs also contain ficins to help digestion. Other MDCs in figs have been shown to kill bacteria and worms in animal experiments.

It is most unfortunate that figs do not travel well, hence making them rare and expensive in most grocery stores. The readers who live in the warmer climates of the U.S. could plant their own fig trees, which are hardy and require little attention except to eat the treasured figs before the birds get there first. Dried figs are a viable option for everyone else.

Fish and fish oil. The pre-twentieth-century doctor regularly prescribed fish oil for everything from skin and joint ailments to consumption (tuberculosis). There is now more science than folklore in the praises for fish.

Prostaglandins are a group of important hormonelike compounds made in that body the have a major impact on health. For instance, all tumor tissue studied is overendowed with arachidonic acid, which is manufactured from dietary fats like beef lard and corn oil.

The active ingredient in fish oil, EPA or eicosapentaenoic acid, is able to interrupt the deadly progression of arachidonic acid production in the body, which has been shown in animal and human studies to slow down or prevent tumor growth. EPA from fish oil has been found to inhibit breast, pancreas, lung, prostate, and colon cancer in animals.[121]

Fish is also rich in protein, B-6, zinc, and other immune-bolstering nutrients. People who eat fish regularly have a lower incidence of many diseases, including harm from pollution. Unfortunately, since we have used our waterways and oceans like open sewers, some fish are among the most polluted of all foods. There are freshwater streams in heavily polluted regions of America where two-thirds of the fish have cancer. Obviously, a cancerous fish is not good food.

For those who do not like to eat fish but wish to share in their chemopreventive value, fish oil capsules can offer a solution. Do not take more than 5 grams daily of EPA, lest you thin out your blood excessively and markedly alter the prostaglandin and clotting systems in the body.

Figure 10C. How Dietary Fats Influence Prostaglandins

linoleic acid (found in plants and animals)

GLA (evening primrose oil)

DHGLA   Prostaglandins 1, PGE

EPA shuts this down

arachidonic acid   Prostaglandins 2
(instigates cancer,   (thromboxane)
and depresses
immune system)

Ginger. A regular performer on the apothecary's list around the world, ginger may offer more than just a glitzy reputation. Ginger has been in Chinese medical books for more than two-thousand years, is included in at least half of all oriental medicines, is used as an aphrodisiac in parts of Africa, as a contraceptive in New Guinea, and is given to children in India for whooping cough. There is some evidence in Japanese research that ginger can interfere with the dangerous DNA changes that signal a tumor cell beginning.

Ginger root looks like a stubby brown carrot and can be purchased in most fresh-produce sections of a grocery store. Peel the ginger root like you would a carrot, place it in a small freezer bag, and store it in the freezer. Whenever you want to add ginger to a meal for spice or have ginger tea, just grate off some shavings of the frozen ginger root. Ginger is a major ingredient in chutney, a delicious condiment that can be used on many foods.

Essentially, ginger offers a healthier alternative to the typical American indulgence in salt, sugar, and fat for seasonings. Although there is no scientific evidence to support the theory that ginger is a contraceptive, don't consume too much of this root if you are trying to get pregnant.

Green tea. In the classic movie, *Bridge over the River Kwai,* the British prisoners of war struck a dignified pose as they quickly dipped their well-used tea bag into the water. No doubt there was little tea flavor from a picosecond of steeping, but the ritual was maintained and life became slightly more tolerable. Though the British have become the world's de facto tea experts, most teas originate in warmer climates, like India.

Many plants contain varying amounts of substances known as polyphenols. Green teas are particularly rich in several types of polyphenols, including tannins, which contribute the astringent flavor, and catechin. Top researchers at the National Cancer Institute are vigorously pursuing studies that show both tannins and catechins to be strong preventers of cancer.

Tannins seem to be able to coat viruses like wrapping them with a straitjacket to prevent the viruses from executing their mission of attaching to healthy cells.[122] Without a host cell to support their parasitic lifestyle, viruses just die. These MDCs in tea are also potent antioxidants to squelch free-radical damage.[123] One or all of the polyphenols (caffeic acid, ellagic acid, ferulic acid, or gallotannic) have been found to block cancer formation in tissue cultures. Mice fed polyphenols and then carcinogens had 40 percent less stomach cancer than the unprotected group.[124] Gallotannic acid in green tea is the most potent anticancer agent ever tested, according to a group of Japanese researchers.[125]

Recall that one of the more common carcinogens in our food and water supply is nitrate or nitrites, which are converted into nitroso compounds in the intestines. Nitrosamines are very carcinogenic. Polyphenols in green tea block nitrosamine formation even better than vitamins C and E.[126] The catechin in green tea may prove as effective as beta-carotene in blocking free-radical destruction that often leads to cancer. Green tea also helps to treat dysentery, which is common from bacterially infected food and water.

There are many varieties of green tea, including peppermint, spearmint, alfalfa, and much more. Green tea steeped for five minutes with some honey and one-eighth teaspoon of vitamin C crystals (500 mg) is a favorite beverage of mine that may offer some potent chemopreventive abilities. The more commonly consumed black teas like orange pekoe may not have the same therapeutic value as green teas. Avoid comfrey tea, which may be more carcinogenic than many dangerous pesticides, and never take comfrey tablets.[127]

Honey. Honey was to the Egyptians what aspirin is to Americans—a commonly used drug. Modern researchers may have found why honey has therapeutic value—it kills bacteria and viruses. Honey is a valuable ointment on open wounds to prevent infection,[128] and may even accelerate wound healing.[129] Honey is able to kill the bacteria that are responsible for many cases of food poisoning: *E. coli*, *Salmonella*, *cholerae*, *Shigella*, and others.

Researchers in Durban, South Africa, gave children with bacterially caused diarrhea either honey and fluids or sugar and fluids. The honey-treated group recovered 40 percent faster.[130] Although experts used to credit honey's antibacterial action to its ability to bind moisture, that is no longer the accepted theory. After the sugar was extracted from a honey preparation, some unknown MDC in honey was able to kill a broad range of bacteria colonies better than streptomycin, and the bacteria did not develop a resistance to the honey antibiotic.

We use honey often as a sugar substitute, although certain physical properties of honey prevent it from being a total sugar substitute. Honey-based syrup on whole grain rice pancakes is a special treat for us; and honey is a major ingredient, along with instant nonfat milk, in our cake frostings.

Although honey in the grocery store is more costly than sugar, you can usually buy honey much cheaper in large cans or from a nearby beehive. Honey has the added benefit of being particularly free of pesticide residue, since bees are so sensitive to poisons that they readily die upon exposure to many pesticides and herbicides. Honey should not be fed to infants under one year of age, since they may develop botulism in their relatively sterile guts from the botulism spores that are sometimes found in honey.

Milk. Milk is a "first food," a gift from mother to infant to protect the helpless child and provide optimum nourishment. Milk may also contain some undetermined MDCs that are powerful anticarcinogens. When Dr. Cedric Garland of the University of California at San Diego looked at the diets of over two thousand men through a twenty-year period, he found that two and a half glasses of milk daily cut the risk for colon cancer by two-thirds.[131] There are a number of ways in which milk may offer cancer protection:

-The high calcium content detoxifies bile acids to prevent their carcinogenic breakdown products. Calcium also binds to dietary fat, which would also lower cancer risk.

-Calcium also seems to "sedate" the cancer prone cells in the colon of high risk patients.

-The antibiotic agents in milk may prevent bacteria from creating carcinogens in the intestines or the general bloodstream.

These same antibiotic properties in milk may also help to reduce diarrhea from food infections. Each year, over 50,000 American children are hospitalized for acute diarrhea from intestinal infections. Some of this problem is caused by flulike viruses and some is caused by food poisoning from bacteria. Milk antibodies may squelch unfriendly bacterial growth in the intestines. Remember that milk contains numerous immune factors passed on from mother to youngster. Much of these immune factors somehow survive the gauntlet of pasteurization, cooking, and digestion.

When researchers exposed mice to a rotavirus that commonly infects the intestines of humans, all sixteen mice developed diarrhea. Eight more mice were fed raw milk and then the rotavirus—none got diarrhea. Eight more mice were fed normal pasteurized milk and then the rotavirus—only one got diarrhea.[132] Another eight mice were given infant formula and then rotavirus—all got diarrhea. Infant formula is exposed to canning heat temperatures that apparently neutralize the immune factors in milk. It is most unfortunate that the ones who need this protection the most, infants, get the least.

If you have lactose intolerance, you can still derive milk benefits by eating yogurt. If you have a milk protein allergy, which is one of the more common food allergies, then you may have to forgo dairy products. I find that milk creates halitosis and excess mucus production in me, but yogurt does not, so I eat my daily bowl of yogurt.

Mushrooms. The typical white mushroom found in American produce sections may contain naturally occurring toxins that are unwise in large quantities. Yet oriental mushrooms (shiitake, oyster, enoki, and tree ear) have been shown to bolster the immune system against infections, cancer, and even autoimmune diseases, like arthritis.

It was the American researcher Dr. Kenneth Cochran of the University of Michigan who initially discovered the antiviral properties of the shiitake (or golden oaks) mushroom. The responsible MDC was found to be lentinan. In followup studies, lentinan was more effective against flu viruses than a powerful prescription antiviral drug.[133] Shiitake mushrooms apparently spur the human immune system to produce more interferon, the anticancer "napalm" that is produced internally.[134] Shiitake lentinan is being tested on leukemia patients in China and breast cancer patients in Japan.

Actually, this food item was not on our menu plan at all until doing the research for this book. Although it is very expensive, we occasionally use it in soups, stir-fry vegetables, and other mixture meals.

Onions. For over six thousand years, onion, and its close cousin garlic, have been prescribed for nearly every ailment known to mankind. Now there may be some evidence why that tradition persisted for so long. Both garlic and onions are members of the allium vegetable family. Although the scientific evidence shows garlic to be the more protective of these two foods, onions are consumed more often and in greater volume in America. The cumulative effect of onions could help against our pollution problem. Onions have been proven to kill viruses and bacteria and to squelch the early stages of cancer growth.

After several thousand years of folklore, Pasteur declared onions a genuine antibiotic. Since then, onions and onion extract have effectively killed various bacteria strains that cause food poisoning.[135] Benzo-pyrenes are the stalwart carcinogens that are found in barbecued, smoked, or overcooked protein foods. Various sulfur-containing MDCs in garlic and onion are able to block the carcinogenic effect of benzo-pyrenes in test animals by stimulating the production of glutathione, a heavyweight scavenger of tumor cells.[136] Next time you can't resist that urge to have a barbecue cookout, make sure that you have a healthy batch of onions with the same meal. Onions and garlic have been shown to lower the risk for stomach cancer.[137] Dental researchers at Harvard found that onion extract not only slowed the growth of cancer cells in the mouth but also reduced the size of the tumors.

Eat onions often, any way you can. Fresh onions can be used in salads, bean salads, grated carrot and cabbage salads, etc. Onion soup is a personal favorite of mine. Another favorite is alternating slices of thin red onion slivers with fresh tomato slices, with a small sprinkling of Italian dressing to wet the mixture. When fried in minimum oil or butter, onions make a nice side dish for fish and beef. Cooked onions pack less of a halitosis punch than raw onions. If you chew a parsley or mint leaf after eating onion food, the odor problem is minimized. Both cooked and raw onions have valuable therapeutic actions.

Spinach. Maybe Popeye was right. Scientists find that spinach has almost three times more carotenoids than carrots, and the carotenoids in spinach are much more varied, which may offer broad spectrum protection. Spinach is also rich in chlorophyll (the green pigment), an independent cancer blocker.[138] *Something* in spinach blocks the formation of carcinogenic nitrosamines in the stomach better than any other food tested.[139] Spinach helps to lower the risk of cancer of the cervix.[140] Once again, commercial spinach is heavily sprayed with pesticides and cannot be purged of these poisons, so choose organic spinach, or soak your commercial spinach leaves for five minutes in lukewarm water.

Turnip. Recall the value of the cruciferous vegetables in preventing cancer. One of the potent MDCs in cruciferous vegetables is glucosinolate, which is found in very high concentrations in rutabagas and turnip greens. Turnip greens are also high in chlorophyll, beta-carotene, other carotenoids, and folic acid, all of which have proven anticancer abilities.

Other foods that offer more benefits than harm, but would not be considered "superfoods," include potatoes (peel them), hot peppers (like red chiles, paprika, Tabasco, etc.), rice, and the panoply of healthy spices (rosemary, thyme, turmeric). Dr. Gary Stoner at the Medical College of Ohio has found that ellagic acid (a component in berries and nuts) is able to substantially reduce the cancer risk from burned meats, alcohol, pickled vegetables, aflatoxins, and nitrosamines. Dr. Zbigniew Walaszek, of the University of Texas, has isolated a potent anti-cancer substance (glucarate) found in cruciferous vegetables, bean sprouts, and other vegetables. Strawberries and tomatoes may help lower the risk for cancer,[141] but are also among the more dangerous produce items in America due to pesticide residues.[142] Eat these foods sparingly as commercial produce or liberally as organic produce.

OPTIMAL EATING

You stand a much better chance against food pollutants if your body is well nourished. Foods provide more than just the officially recognized fifty essential nutrients. As you can see from this chapter, foods can be potent antipollution protectors. Also, by eating an optimally balanced diet, you can better fortify your immune and detoxification systems to ward off pollutants and cancer. With that in mind, let's spend a few minutes on optimal nutrition.

Cardinal Rules of Nutrition. When sailing instructors teach you how to sail, they cannot show you around the world. They show you how to use the instruments of navigation—sextant, compass, and map—and hope you can fare well on your own. So, too, I cannot follow you around for the rest of your life and make nutritional decisions for you; but I can condense the volumes of nutrition information into several easy-to-follow rules that become your navigation instruments in choosing the right foods.

Eat foods in as close to their natural state as possible. Refining often adds questionable agents (like food additives, salt, sugar, and fat), removes valuable nutrients (like vitamins, minerals, and fiber), and always raises the cost of the food.

Eat a wide variety of food. Though some foods do have potent chemo-protective value, they usually also contain other less desirable substances. By eating a variety, you derive benefits from the desirable food ingredients and avoid building up a toxicity from too much of the undesirable ingredients.

Eat small, frequent meals: nibbling is better than gorging. Nibbling helps the digestive and cardiovascular system, helps prevent overeating, and extends lifespan and prevents energy sags that occur in "gorgers."

Minimize your intake of fat, salt, sugar, cholesterol, alcohol, caffeine, processed luncheon meats, and most food additives. In small amounts, these are probably relatively harmless. In normal American amounts, they may be dangerous. A diet high in sugar has been shown to lower various human immune factors like mitogens and lymphocytes.[143] All types of sugar, even natural sugars from fruit, depressed the Pac-Man ability of human immune factors to devour bacteria.[144] In animal studies, there was a dose dependent relationship between sugar intake and immune rsponse: the more sugar in the diet, the lower the overall production of antibodies.[145] People who consume high sugar diets are more predisposed toward cancer of the colon and breast.[146] While the average American gets 18 percent of their calories from refined sugar, cutting that number in half would measurably improve our overall health while fortifying natural defenses against food pollutants.

Maximize your intake of fresh vegetables, fruit, legumes, fish, poultry, clean water, and low-fat dairy products. These foods should form the bulk of your diet.

Balance your calorie intake with calorie expenditure to avoid overweight. By pinching the skin behind the arm (triceps region) you can get a general idea of your fitness level: less than an inch of skinfold thickness means that you are in good shape; more than two inches in skinfold thickness means you need to lose fat tissue.

Make sure that you get enough protein. Protein is a basic build-

Figure 10D: The exchange System of Meal Planning

Approved by every major U.S. health organization, the Exchange System provides everyone with a simple but accurate method of achieving a "balanced diet". "Exchange" means that, within a group, one selection may be exchanged for another to provide nearly identical calories and macronutrients. Use the sample exchange patterns given below to become familiar with this valuable eating guide.

VEGETABLES:	FRUIT	BREADS &	MEAT/PROTEIN
½ cup each	apple, small	STARCHES	(Low Fat)
asparagus	apple j. ⅓ c.	bread, 1 slice	lean beef, lamb, pork,
bean sprouts	applesauce	bagel, ½	poultry, veal, fish, 1
beets	apricots, 2	English muffin, ½	oz.
broccoli	banana, ½ small	hamburger bun, ½	clams, oyster,
brussels sprouts	cherries, 10	tortilla, 1 at 6″	scallops, shrimp, 5
cabbage	dates, 2	bran flakes, ½ c.	lobster, salmon, tuna,
carrots	grapefruit, ½	puffed cereal, 1 c.	crab, ¼ c.
cauliflower	grapes, 12	cooked cereal, ½ c.	cottage cheese, ¼ c.
celery	grape j., ¼ c.	grits, ½ c.	farmer's cheese, 1 oz.
cucumber	mango, ½	rice or barley, ½ c.	beans, peas, lentils,
eggplant	nectarine, 1	pasta cooked, ½ c.	plus 1 bread, ½c.
green pepper	orange, 1	popcorn, 3 c.	(Medium Fat)
greens:	orange j., ½ c.	cornmeal, 2 T.	organ meats, 1 oz.
beet	papaya, ⅓	flour, 2½ T.	mozzarella, 1 oz.
chard	peach, 1 med.	wheat germ, ¼ c.	canadian bacon, 1 oz.
collards	pear, 1 small	crackers:	parmesan cheese, 3 T.
dandelion	persimmon, 1	arrowroot, 3	egg, 1
kale	pineapple, ½ c.	graham, 2 squares	peanut butter
mustard	pineapple j. ⅓ c.	matzoth, 2	(plus 2 fats), 2 T.
spinach	plums, 2	oyster, 20	medium fat beef,
turnip	prunes, 2	pretzels, 25 small	lamb, pork, veal,
mushrooms	prune j., ¼ c.	rye water, 3	fish, 1 oz.
okra	raisins, 2T.	saltines, 6	(High Fat)
onions	tangerine, 1	soda, 4	hamburger, steak,
rhubarb	watermelon, 1 c.	beans, peas, lentils ½	lamb breast, spare
rutabaga		c.	ribs, duck, capon,
sauerkraut	———————	baked beans, ¼ c.	goose, most cheeses,
squash, summer	FATS	corn, ⅓ c.	cold cuts,
string beans	margarine, butter, oil,	corn on cob, 1 small	frankfurters,
tomatoes	lard, bacon fat,	lima beans, ½ c.	sausage, salami, 1
tomato juice	mayonnaise, 1 tsp.	parsnips, ⅔ c.	oz.
turnips	avocado, ⅛	peas, ½ c.	
veg. juice	nuts, small, 20	potato, 1 small	MILK
zucchini	nuts, large, 6	potato, ½ c.	skim, non fat,
	heavy cream, cream	squash, ½ c.	buttermilk, non fat
	cheese, salad	yam, ¼ c.	yogurt, 1 c.
	dressing, 1 T.		low fat milk or yogurt,
	bacon, 1 strip		(plus 1 fat), 1 c.
	olives, 5 small		whole milk or yogurt,
			(plus 2 fats), 1 c.

GUIDE TO EXCHANGE SYSTEM

(grams)					Sample exchange pattern calories/day			
GROUP	P	F	C	CALORIES	1000	1200	1900	2400
MILK (non fat)	8	—	12	80	2	2	3	4
VEGETABLES	2	—	5	25	4	4	7	7
FRUIT	—	—	10	40	3	4	7	10
BREADS	2	—	15	70	3	5	8	11
MEAT/PROTEIN								
LOW FAT	7	3	—	55	5	5	5	5
MEDIUM FAT	7	5½	—	77	(= 1 protein + ½ fat exchange)			
HIGH FAT	7	8	—	100	(= 1 protein + 1 fat exchange)			
FATS	—	5	—	45	3	3	8	10

FREE
chicory, endive
lettuce, parsley
radishes, watercress
spices, vanilla
artificial sweeteners
vinegar, water, coffee,
tea

ing block for the immune and detoxifying systems, as well as other critical functions throughout the body.

Whenever possible, get your nutrients "with a fork and spoon." This means that food should be the mainstay of any quality nutrition program. However, in the next chapter you will see some of the proven merits of certain nutrients. Supplements should be used in addition to, never in lieu of, good eating habits.

EXCHANGE PROGRAM

Many people ask the obvious question: "So how do I choose the right foods? I don't have time to calculate amounts of nutrients from various food groups. Give me something easy." And here it is: see previous page for the exchange system.

SAMPLE MENU

I often get the question: "Alright, you are the nutritionist and expert on safe eating. So what do *you* eat?" Just to show you that I practice what I teach and that safe eating can be easy, tasty, and inexpensive; here is a recent day of dining for myself.

Breakfast: One cup of oatmeal with teaspoon of honey and teaspoon of butter. One slice of whole wheat toast with butter and jam. One cup of yogurt with tablespoon of wheat germ and some fruit preserves. Two fresh oranges, peeled and cut up. Postum hot beverage with honey.

Lunch: Bowl of tomato and barley soup. Tuna fish sandwich with onions and sprouts on whole wheat bread. Butterscotch pudding (basic ingredients are milk and eggs). Two cups of cranberry tea with vitamin C crystals and honey.

Dinner: Baked chicken. Slices of fresh tomato mixed with thin slices of red onions. Pressure cooked brown rice. Ginger cookies (whole wheat flour and ginger). Chicory hot beverage.

CHAPTER 11

Nutrients that Increase Your Tolerance of Toxins

*T*hroughout human history, people worshipped and feared that which they did not understand. They worshipped the sun, fire, giant whirlpools, etc. They offered sacrifices to the gods during plagues, eclipses, earthquakes, and droughts. As science slowly unravels the mysteries of life, we try to deal with problems pragmatically rather than hysterically. Rather than trembling in fear of a typhoid outbreak, we now know that poor sanitation causes it. We didn't offer burnt sacrifices to deal with typhoid, we built indoor plumbing and the problem stopped.

Similarly, cancer has long been considered a capricious and wrathful Grim Reaper. Victims cried out "Why me!" Cancer-free people often worried "When will it be me?" No longer. Scientists have exposed the demon cancer for what it really is. We know what causes cancer. After decades of research by brilliant scientists and billions of dollars invested, many cancers (like lung, liver, brain, and pancreas) remain resistant to treatment—but up to 90 percent of all cancer can be prevented through optimal nutrition.[1] Which means that by lowering our intake of toxins and increasing our intake of antitoxin nutrients, cancer could become a plague of the past to be found only in history books, like the bubonic plague.

Can nutrition really help to shield us from pollutants in the food and water supply? You bet. Starting with the 1982 landmark book, *Diet, Nutrition, and Cancer,* the National Academy of Sciences recognized the strong preventive role of nutrition against cancer. In 1988, the Surgeon General of the United States published an extensive book with hundreds of studies outlining the major preventive role of nutrition against cancer.[2] Shortly thereafter, the prestigious National Academy of Sciences issued *Diet and Health*, with hundreds of studies showing the nutrition-cancer link.

Doctors Newberne and Connor at the prestigious Massachusetts Institute of Technology find that nutrients offer an untapped reservoir of protection against pesticides, aflatoxins, and many other poisons in our food supply.[3] Dr. Bruce Ames of the University of California at Berkeley is similarly in favor of using antioxidant nutrients, like vitamins E, C, beta-carotene, selenium, and glutathione to shield us from the plethora of toxins in our food.[4] Since these have been shown to protect against cancer and our polluted era increases the risk for cancer, shouldn't we match pollutants against equally impressive antioxidant supplements?[5] There are dozens of studies in this chapter to support the idea that nutrients can provide us with a coat of armor against pollution.

One study serves as a beacon of hope because it was designed to mimic the American diet and lifestyle. Researchers fed animals either a high-cancer-risk diet, which is the typical American food pattern, or low-risk diet (with nonextreme variations in fat, fiber, protein, vitamins A and E, and selenium). Each group of animals were then exposed to long-term low intake of a carcinogen, which is what happens to all of us. Twenty-nine percent of the high-risk group got cancer, a statistic that is nearly identical to the 30 percent rate that is seen in Americans. Only 4 percent of the low-risk group got cancer.[6] If we can extrapolate this date, it would seem that we could cut cancer incidence from 990,000 new cases each year down to 132,000 or less with the measures outlined in this book.

"Ignorance of the law is no excuse!" is a favorite expression of a police officer writing a traffic ticket. The same applies to cancer.

By using the laws to your advantage, you can cut your cancer risk by 90 percent. Take heart. There is hope that, even though we have recklessly polluted our food and water, we can protect ourselves enough to live through the crisis. This chapter details scientifically proven nutrients that buffer the impact of pollution on your body. Use them wisely.

WHY ARE SUPPLEMENTS SUCH A CONTROVERSIAL AREA?

What I am basically recommending is the judicious use of nutritional supplements to help fend off the effects of pollutants; yet the supplement controversy rages on. While there is an abundance of evidence that supports the use of supplements, there are high-visibility professional health groups who oppose that viewpoint. How can the experts be so at odds at interpreting what should be scientific facts?

There are a number of explanations to help the reader understand the confusion. When nutritionists began their work in the earlier part of this century, malnutrition was blatant: clinical scurvy from a low intake of vitamin C, goiter from low iodine intake, rickets from low intake of vitamin D, pellagra from low niacin intake, and so on. Each nutrient seemed to have its own distinct deficiency condition, which was unlike any other disease. Then things got complicated.

The 1980s have brought about a radically new mentality that grinds noisily against those traditional principles of nutrition. New research shows that a long-term low intake of a nutrient may not yield an immediate and obvious clinical condition, like scurvy, but it does produce a health problem decades later. Long-term low intake of vitamins E, C and A, and selenium may eventually lead to cancer: Does that mean that cancer is a deficiency symptom of these valuable nutrients? Low intake of chromium may lead to heart disease: Is heart disease a symptom of chromium deficiency? No in each case, because both cancer and heart disease have numerous other inciting factors. So although low vitamin E intake can bring on cancer, cancer is a condition that can be caused by many factors; vitamin E does not have its own unique deficiency condition.

Low intake of calcium, magnesium, and vitamin D may lead to osteoporosis. Low intake of vitamin C can lead to gallstones, heart disease, hypertension, and premature aging. Americans are currently experiencing an incredible rise in the incidence of cataracts. It has been well established in both animal and human studies that long-term low intake of antioxidant nutrients (C, E, beta-carotene) provides fertile grounds for cataracts.[7] Do we then call cataracts the clinical deficiency symptom of antioxidants? If so, how can we tie them together when it takes decades for the problem to develop?

The problem is that traditional nutrition deals with immediate and obvious clinical deficiency conditions, yet modern science shows us that you don't need to be dying of scurvy to be suffering from a vitamin C deficiency. The death certificate may read "cancer," but the real cause of death may have been low intake of protective nutrients that could have prevented cancer. We cannot deny the overwhelming facts that much of our health woes center around suboptimal intake of nutrients. Too many free radicals (from pollutants) or low intake of antioxidant nutrients probably cause many cases of arthritis, cataracts, Parkinson's disease, cancer, heart disease, and much, much more.[8]

The reader may ask, "If the evidence is so impressive, then why doesn't the government and medical establishment do something nutritionally to prevent all of these health woes?" Two big reasons. First, no one really understands how these nutrients slow down damage. Scientists are often reluctant to endorse anything until they can fully explain it. Yet we do not fully understand genes, psycho-active drugs, electricity, healing, fusion, the medicinal value of garlic, or how a seed sprouts, but that does not stop us from using these mysteries for our betterment. Second, the risk/benefit model with drugs and surgery is so different from nutrients. In many instances, the most dramatic and potentially helpful drugs (like chemotherapy) and surgery (like open-heart surgery) also carry with them the highest risk. Many of the reigning experts are suspicious of nutrients: "If these substances are so effective, then they must have a comparable toxicity problem." Not so. Nutrients may help—they may even be our only immediate salvation from pollution—but they rarely hurt anyone.[9] Although about 90 million Americans regularly take nutritional supplements, and some do so in radically high amounts, there are only dozens of toxicities reported per year and no deaths. Hence the risk/benefit ratio is obviously in favor of using nutrients to protect ourselves. This radical shift in thinking is difficult for many policy makers.

The ranks are swelling of experts who support the idea of using nutrients to protect against cancer and pollution. The National Cancer Institute has recently established a $12 million annual fund for a sixty-person lab to study the link between nutrition and lowering the risk for cancer.[10] Dr. William Pryor at Louisiana State University notes that cancer, especially in our heavily polluted era, may be a deficiency condition of vitamins E and C.[11] Dr. Anthony Diplock at a major hospital in London says that the evidence warrants doubling the RDA for vitamin C, a three- to five-fold increase for vitamin E, and establishment of a separate RDA for beta-carotene outside of vitamin A.[12] Dr. John Bieri of the National Institute of Diabetes, Digestive and Kidney Diseases in Maryland also has been convinced that a higher intake of vitamins A, C and E, and carotenoids is warranted, based on the overwhelming data.[13] Dr. Sheldon Hendler, M.D., Ph.D., has endorsed an above-RDA daily supplement routine to help protect against the common diseases in America.

It could be that we will never receive some sweeping proclamation from the Surgeon General or the American Medical Association regarding supplement use. We may never need it if people make their own decisions based upon the available information. Doctors Draper and Bird at the Ludwig Institute of Cancer Research in Canada find that the supplement issue may be a moot question. Because, even though most U.S. government agencies and health associations publicly discourage the use of supplements, 71 percent of vegetarians and 57 percent of nonvegetarians in the U.S. take supplements anyway.[14] There even seems to be a professional schizophrenia among health care professionals. Through the official voice of registered dietitians, the American Dietetic Association, denounces the use of supplements, more than 60 percent of dietitians take supplements anyway.[15] (Supplement usage is higher among well-educated Americans.)

CAN'T WE GET ALL THE NUTRIENTS WE NEED FROM A HEALTHY DIET?

That is a trick question. It is always wise to get your nutrients "with a fork and a spoon" whenever possible. If we all lived that "Tarzan" lifestyle, eating large quantities of clean nutrient-dense foods, exercising that food into a lean fit body, avoiding poisons from pollution and drugs, and not being exposed to high levels of stress, then supplements would be unnecessary. Realistically speaking, not everyone can do that. It would be nice if everyone made a concerted effort to eat right, but we don't. Rather than be seriously penalized, supplements can compensate for some of those nutritional misdeeds; and in today's polluted environment, we need all the help we can get from protective nutrients. Supplements, then, are elevated from "useful" to "essential."

Drugs often increase the need for nutrients or decrease the intake of foods that provide nutreints. Ninety-eight percent of older adults in this country take prescription medication. Although older adults constitute 12 percent of the U.S. population, they consume 35 percent of all prescription drugs, with the average older adult taking six different medications. Dr. Jeffrey Blumberg of Tufts University in Boston is finding that drug-induced malnutrition among the elderly is a serious problem in this country. An international expert on immunity, Dr. Ranjit Chandra of Canada, has shown that low intake of nutrients may relate to the typical poor immune response of older adults.[16] Older adults are also among the higher risk groups for developing cancer from food pollutants. Also, one-third of our children are on prescription drugs at any given time.

Swedish officials were able to lower their high incidence of cancer of the esophagus with a national program of providing nutritional supplements.[17] The director of the Japanese National Cancer Center issued a twelve-point program in 1978 to lower the incidence of cancer among Japanese. Eight of the twelve points involved nutrition advice, with one point being "take vitamins in appropriate amounts."[18] Finland began a national program to fortify their bread with selenium to help lower their dreadfully high heart disease and cancer incidence, due in part to the low levels of selenium in Finnish soil. In a large Australian study of 715 people with colon cancer and 727 healthy controls, the use of vitamin supplements substantially lowered the risk for cancer.[19] The Aussies who violated all the nutritional risk factors had a 2000 percent greater risk for colon cancer than the more nutritionally-oriented people. Maybe I'm missing something, but it appears to me that the major skeptical organizations are ignoring the evidence: supplements could provide Americans with a much needed edge against pollution, cancer, and many degenerative diseases.

HOW CANCER IS RELATED TO GENETICS, NUTRITION, AND SUPPLEMENTS

For many years, some health care experts told us that cancer is genetic—some families seem to be more prone toward getting cancer due to some biochemical difference—which certainly makes it seem, once again, like an unavoidable and unjust monster. Scientists now find that cancer is much more influenced by environment (toxins, nutrient intake) than genetics. Dr. Thorkild Sorensen and his associates in Denmark gathered the files on 960 Danes born between 1924 and 1926 who had been adopted. They found that cancer is much more related to environment than genetics. The Danes whose adoptive parent died of cancer had a 500 percent increase in their risk for cancer themselves.[20]

Japanese researchers looked at 115 children of 55 patients with lung cancer and had matched controls to compare their data. The lung cancer patients and their offspring had a definite trend toward lower serum levels of vitamin E and selenium,[21] so perhaps genetic trends of cancer simply show us people who have elevated needs for certain nutrients. According to data from the National Research Council, as least 2.5 percent of the American population cannot get along with RDA levels of nutrients. That leaves at least six million Americans deficient, even if they are consuming 100 percent of the RDA for all nutrients. And many large-scale dietary surveys by the government and various universities show that the average American is eating less than the RDA for a variety of nutrients.[22]

Perhaps cancer is not some unavoidable death sentence from genetics, but rather some quirk in the inherited biochemistry that has a different set of nutrient demands. If those demands are not met, a disease occurs. Hence, even if cancer runs in your family, you can do something to lower your risks. Nutritional supplements offer a nontoxic, inexpensive, easily administered, and scientifically proven way to lower cancer risks.

BUT WHAT ABOUT THE RDA?

The Recommended Dietary Allowance (RDA) is a guideline established by a noted panel of scientists that are appointed by Congress to advise on matters of science and health. By definition, the RDA is designed as "the levels of intake of essential nutrients that, on the basis of scientific knowledge, are judged by the Food and Nutrition Board to be adequate to meet the known nutrient needs of practically all healthy persons."[23]

The RDA does not attempt to bring anyone toward optimal health, nor to fend off the effects of pollution, nor to compensate for the nutrient drain of drugs, alcohol, stress, illness, and tobacco. The RDA is a useful guideline, but not a law to be inscribed in stone. In the words of Dr. Mark Hegsted of Harvard University, the RDA is a "guesstimate of unknown reliability."[24]

The RDA is designed to keep "normal" people in "normal" health. Normal people in this country, based upon statistical averages, get six colds per year, wear glasses, are overweight, are regularly plagued with lethargy, constipation, and mild depression, wear dentures by age forty-five, get sick somewhere in their sixties and die in their seventies of heart disease or cancer. That is "normal."—and not very enviable. The RDA will keep most people from exhibiting blatant symptoms of deficiency, but it will not protect anyone from the ravages of twentieth-century pollution.

Many experts say that the RDA needs to be revised from its current standard which provides for "no visible signs of immediate clinical disease" to a standard that prevents long-term health problems. But if the RDA were to be elevated to more optimal levels of nutrients, there would be a thunderstorm in Washington—because the RDA is the government "yardstick" for the poverty line. Government researchers buy enough groceries for a standard family of four to be able to consume the RDA level of nutrients. Anyone who cannot afford that grocery bill is considered to be poor. So by elevating the RDA, one sweep of the pen would roughly triple the number of Americans living below the poverty line. No politician wants such a calamitous event to occur while they are in office.

And what happens, if, as the evidence already indicates, we need pharmacological doses of nutrients, in pill form to combat the diseases of a polluted society? Do we raise the RDA beyond a level that could be obtained from any diet? Does the government then have to include vitamin pills for recipients of Welfare and Food Stamps? If these nutrients have potent preventive value to them, like drugs, should they be controlled like drugs and only dispensed with a prescription? If a couple hundred dollars worth of supplements could prevent $100,000 worth of a long-term chemotherapy, then should the government dispense supplements to everyone? If the government uses supplements to protect the people from pollutants, then have they admitted complicity in the pollution problem and opened themselves to legal and political attack?

Dr. John Kitzhaber, a physician and president of the state senate in Oregon, has shepherded a bill that would provide cost effective health care to nearly all Oregonians. Dr. Kitzhaber's bill was based on a thorough study by an elite panel of experts, who found that nutrition supplements (food and pills) should be a top priority of any health program because of the effectiveness of nutrition at preventing long-term health problems.[25] I strongly believe that if we passed out broad-spectrum vitamin and mineral supplements in school each morning, there would be less cancer and other health woes. There are many questions that loom on the horizon for politicians and health care administrators. The times they are a changing.

Knowing what we know about computers, it would be foolish not to use them. The same applies for genetic engineering, modern drugs, space technology, and kitchen appliances. Scientists have unveiled a few select mysteries of the universe to allow us to live with less drudgery, higher productivity, and potentially better health. They know that vitamins E, C, and beta-carotene, and selenium are amazingly effective at stimulating a more protective immune system, while also assassinating the saboteurs of free radicals within the body.[26] If we ignore this evidence to the detriment of our health, we might as well give up computers and modern hospitals, too.

THE CASE OF VITAMIN E

Vitamin E provides an excellent example of the need for supplementation in our polluted times. Vitamin E was once referred to as "a vitamin in search of a disease" because long-term low intake of vitamin E did not produce some strikingly distinct deficiency condition. The RDA for vitamin E was originally set at 30 i.u. per day. Yet the National Research Council later realized that few people could obtain 30 i.u. from the typical American diet, and besides, no widespread "scurvylike" condition existed among Americans, which indicated to the NRC that low vitamin E intake was causing us no harm. So they cut the RDA in half, to 15 i.u.[27] The RDA of vitamin E for adult males is 10 i.u. Yet abundant evidence shows us that long-term low intake of vitamin E is strongly linked to cancer, cataracts, heart disease, immune diseases, and other assorted degenerative problems.

A review of the literature finds that vitamin E is nontoxic in doses up to 213 times the RDA.[28] Doses of 100 to 800 i.u. per day have been found effective at treating some conditions (like angina, leg cramps, and premenstrual syndrome) and preventing others (like cataracts, cancer, and heart disease). Meanwhile, the average intake of vitamin E in this country is 11 i.u. With so many proven benefits to supplementation and no risks, the only realistic way to bolster our intake of precious vitamin E is to begin taking rational levels of supplements.

A QUESTION OF BALANCE

As with foods in the previous chapter, I strongly encourage a balanced approach to the supplement use that is outlined in this chapter. Vitamins C and E work better together, so do not take a huge dose of only one of these or avoid either nutrient. Researchers at the University of California at San Diego found that large doses of zinc supplements were not as effective at improving the immune system of older adults as a balanced mineral supplement containing zinc, copper, iron, and manganese.[29]

Since vitamins E, C, and beta-carotene all "prop each other up," that is, regenerate each other's ability to work as an antioxidant, a balanced intake will lead to optimal protection from pollutants. Do not take one nutrient out of context and overemphasize it. Refer to the table at the end of the chapter for recommendations on an "optimal" supplement program for either "normal" toxin exposure or "maximum risk" toxin exposure.

Just like the food chapter, this chapter is subdivided into "supernutrients" first and "protective nutrients" second. The "supernutrient" category is reserved for nutrients that have been well proven in their role to neutralize toxins and stunt cancer.

Experts have argued that since most of our morbidity and mortality in the U.S. comes from degenerative disease (i.e. heart disease, cancer, emphysema) and most degenerative disease is caused by free-radical damage, and free radicals can be slowed down with supplemental antioxidant nutrients, it is foolish to neglect these valuable protectors in our polluted times.[30]

The remaining nutrients are related to a healthy immune system. Don't let your diet and supplement program fall short in any of these categories. Since it is virtually impossible to avoid toxins in the food and water supply, these nutrients help your body to better tolerate them.

SUPERNUTRIENTS AGAINST POLLUTION

Ascorbic acid (C). Two decades ago, the twice Nobel laureate Linus Pauling began advocating large doses of vitamin C to stem the tide of viruses, cancer, and pollution harm. He was ridiculed, pressured out of jobs, and lampooned for years before the scientific world began to accept some of his theories. Today, the scientific evidence indicates that vitamin C may be even more impressive than Dr. Pauling had predicted. Here is a true champion in the war against food and water pollutants. Vitamin C is able to:

quench free radicals, which are the major cause of harm from pollutants

stimulate the immune system in many different categories

bind up carcinogenic nitrosamines in the stomach and elsewhere in the body

chelate toxic metals, like lead, and evict them from the body

reinforce natural barriers against microbes and pollutants.

Vitamin C is the "Marshall Dillon" of the water-soluble fraction of the body, "blasting" free radicals into oblivion, and indirectly helping vitamin E to also maintain law and order in the fat-soluble portion of the body. Vitamin C is able to recharge "spent" or oxidized vitamin E, hence loaning vitamin E "bullets" when it is out of "ammunition."

Because of these many important functions in protecting the body, a low intake of vitamin C seriously elevates the risk for all types of cancer, especially stomach cancer.[31] Women who are deficient in C are at considerable risk for cervical cancer.[32] When researchers matched 374 males with cancer of the larynx against 381 healthy controls, they found that a low intake of C doubled the risk for cancer, even after adjusting for smoking and drinking.[33] Although beta-carotene is considered the reigning champion at protecting the lungs from cancer, a study of 1253 lung cancer patients in Louisiana found that vitamin C was even more important than beta-carotene in lung cancer prevention.[34]

One of the more dangerous and common pollutants in our water supply is nitrates from fertilizer runoff, which join with amino acids in the stomach to form potent carcinogens called nitrosamines. Nitrosamines are considered the leading suspect in cancer of the stomach, and may have something to do with cancers elsewhere in the body. Vitamin C supplements (1000 to 2000 milligrams daily) were able to thwart the formation of nitrosamines in human subjects.[35] Supplements of C in lab animals prevented the liver damage that commonly occurs from nitrosamines.[36] Vitamin C and retinoic acid supplements (a form of vitamin A) were able to block the cancerous effects of benzopyrenes, which are products from burned protein food.[37] So if you cannot resist charring your meat on the barbecue grill, make sure you have an extra gram of vitamin C at that meal. There is even some evidence that vitamins C and B-12 together form a synergistic and formidable duo against cancer cells.[38]

For centuries it has been known that a severe deficiency of C (scurvy) often led to serious infections. Vitamin C is indeed a kingpin in maintaining a stalwart immune system. Of all nutrients examined to date, serum vitamin C and zinc most closely relate to a competent immune system.[39] Vitamin C is intimately involved in:

-maintaining natural barriers, like skin and colla-
gen, against pollutants and microbes
-stimulating the output of secretions, like
immunoglobulins, interferon, and cytokines, that kill
invading microbes and cancer cells
-maximizing the gobbling abilities of soldiers in the
immune system, like leukocytes and neutrophils.[40]

Supplements of 1000 milligrams per day of vitamin C boosted
the immune response (IgA, IgM, C3) in healthy students.[41] Supplements of 500 milligrams per day boosted T lymphocytes
response in elderly subjects.[42] Massive supplements of vitamin
C (50,000 to 200,000 milligrams daily) have been shown to sup-
press the symptoms brought on by the AIDs virus.[43] Sick people
and those exposed to high levels of pollution are able to tolerate
higher supplemental doses of C, yet too much C can blunt the
immune system in some sensitive individuals.

One of the most desolating pollution issues in America today
is lead poisoning, especially of young children. Lead toxicity
tampers with all systems in the body, but is most obvious in lowering intellect and creating behavioral problems in the developing nervous system. Vitamin C may help out in the war against
heavy metal pollution because it is a potent chelating agent, so
that it ensnares the metal ion in a cage and carries it out of the
system.[44]

For many years, high dose vitamin C was discouraged by scientists because it could lead to "rebound scurvy." That is, if you
took mega-doses for months, then suddenly ceased taking any
supplements, you could begin developing scurvy within a few
weeks since the body had adjusted to abnormally high intake of
C. New data finds that theory to be gibberish. Researchers have
never been able to create "rebound scurvy" in lab settings.[45] The
recommendations for vitamin C intake given at the end of this
chapter are safe for all people, but I would encourage pregnant
women to stay well below 5 grams daily and for other people to
be alert to any changes in bowel habits. In some sensitive individuals, high intake of vitamin C creates diarrhea or intestinal

distress. Just reduce your intake until you no longer have the symptoms.

Food sources: primarily fruits and vegetables; kiwifruit, sweet peppers, broccoli, cauliflower, kale, tomatoes, oranges, grapefruit, lemons, strawberries, papaya, asparagus, spinach, cantaloupe

Beta-carotene and vitamin A. Carotenoids, including beta-carotene, were also discussed in the previous chapter, though I offer some additional information here. In the billion-dollar hunt for some drug to prevent cancer, most researchers have tried to find something that will quench the wrecking balls in life—free radicals. Beta-carotene is considered by scientists to be "the most effective quencher of singlet oxygen [free radicals] thus far discovered."[46] You cannot buy better cancer or pollution protection, at any price from any drug company, than beta-carotene.

It is fascinating to trace the antioxidant talents of carotenoids. There are five hundred or more different carotenoids that work with the green pigment chlorophyll in plants to capture the energy of the sun. Photosynthesis is a high-charged reaction in which electrons are jumping all over the place from the sun's energy. The plant is able to convert some of this electron energy into making sugar. However, this is a dangerous reaction since the supercharged electrons could easily destroy the surrounding tissue just like free radicals do.

Carotenoids are given the responsibility of preventing damage to the surrounding plant by absorbing the excess electrons. Capturing nuclear energy is a dangerous but potentially profitable reaction. The soft, porous metal lead lines the reactors to absorb the dangerous subatomic particles that go flying outward. So, too, carotenoids act like a shield of sponges to absorb the excess electrons from photosynthesis. This is a talent we are desperately in need of in our polluted and cancer-riddled age.

Beta-carotene is the best studied of the super antioxidants, with splendid evidence showing that it can lower the risk of most types of cancer.[47] So important is vitamin A in preventing cancer that serum levels of vitamin A are like a crystal ball in predicting who will get cancer: the lower the level of serum vitamin A and/or beta-carotene the greater the risk for cancer.[48] People with the highest levels of plasma beta-carotene cut their cervical cancer risk by 80 percent over the low beta-carotene people.[49] Scientists find that the lower the serum levels of beta-carotene and vitamin E, the higher the risk for lung cancer.[50] Two carotenoids (beta-carotene and canthaxanthin) were even effective at *reversing* tumor growth in animals.[51] Numerous studies show that vitamin A and/or beta-carotene may be able to reverse cancer.[52]

Betel nuts are chewed by East Indian men like Americans chew tobacco, and they are as carcinogenic. Researchers gave injections of 400,000 i.u. of vitamin A weekly to men with obvious signs of early mouth cancer from betel nuts. The men kept chewing their poison, but the vitamin A caused remission of most abnormal tissue growth.[53] If vitamin A can both prevent and reverse cancer when humans are exposed to a known carcinogen, then it merits special attention as a shield against twentieth-century pollutants in the food supply.

Beta-carotene is to the immune system what water is to desert flowers: a must for any signs of life to appear. Beta-carotene protects the gobblers in the immune system from being damaged by their own poisons. It enhances the activity of T and B lymphocytes, stimulates T-cell function, elevates the tumor-killing abilities of natural killer cells, and in general revs up the body's ability to protect itself from outside invasion.[54] In only two weeks, supplements of beta-carotene improved immune function (helper T-cells, the "battle managers" of the immune system) in ten healthy men.[55] Modest supplemental doses of beta-carotene have been shown to boost the human immune system[56] and especially helper T cells.[57]

Less than a decade ago, beta-carotene was considered no more than an occasional stand-in for vitamin A. Now, scientists find that beta-carotene has talents that vitamin A does not have, including beta-carotene's role in stimulating the immune system to kill cancer cells and also its potent antioxidant abilities.[58] For that reason, many scientists feel that we should distinguish between beta-carotene and vitamin A, having a separate RDA for each nutrient.

Beta-carotene is the plant version of vitamin A and must be converted into vitamin A in the body. For that reason, preformed vitamin A (as from liver) is potentially toxic, while the raw materials to make vitamin A (as beta-carotene) is almost completely nontoxic. It takes about 500,000 i.u. daily of preformed vitamin A for long periods to instigate toxicity, which includes hair loss, headaches, skin problems, etc.[59] Pregnant women should not take more than 25,000 i.u. of preformed A. Although the safety record of beta-carotene is flawless,[60] I would still advise women to avoid taking more than 50,000 i.u. per day while pregnant. As with many other nutrients, the symptoms of deficiency and excess of vitamin A are similar: birth defects, skin and hair problems, abnormal growth.

Food sources:
● preformed A, possibly toxic: liver, fish liver oil
● beta-carotene, nontoxic: dark green vegetables (like broccoli, peas, kale, spinach), orange and yellow vegetables (like squash, carrots, pumpkin, sweet potatoes), orange fruits (like apricots, cantaloupe, papaya, peaches), watermelon, cherries

Vitamin E. This is another crucial element in protecting the body against pollution and cancer. Both vitamins E and C have been shown to detoxify an entire group of carcinogenic chemicals from industry (polycyclic hydrocarbons) by binding to these poisons and rendering them neutral.[61] These same chemicals are produced when you burn your meat on the barbecue grill. Vitamin E to the rescue.

Finnish researchers examined 20,000 people over ten years and came to the unavoidable conclusion that low serum levels of vitamin E significantly elevate the risk for cancer.[62] Another Finnish study looked at 313 cancer cases over a six-year screening period and once again found that low levels of serum vitamin E elevated the risk for many types of cancer.[63] Vitamin E supplements (1600 i.u./day) even prevented the normal hair loss that occurs when giving cancer patients the potent chemother-apy agent, Adriamycin.[64]

Cancer of the colon is on the increase in America and is likely due to the toxins in our food supply combined with a high fat diet. Vitamin E supplements were able to block 79 percent of the formation of carcinogenic compounds in the colon.[65] Low intake of vitamin E has been closely associated with cancer of the bowels,[66] breast,[67] lungs,[68] and other tissues. Vitamin E sup-plements are also a potent weapon against the carcinogenic nitrosamines that form in the stomach.[69]

Vitamin E is the only fat-soluble antioxidant in the body. A deficiency of E can leave the entire fat-soluble portion of the body to degenerate into "free-radical heaven" with no E to stop the destruction.[70] Free-radical destruction in the fat portion of the body(lipid peroxidation) is largely responsible for cancer and aging. And in order for vitamin E to be effective at stopping trou-ble in the fatty sections of the body, it needs to have optimal levels of vitamin C in the water soluble portion of the body to recharge it.[71]

In order to stop free-radical damage, vitamins C and E must be oxidized in place of the host tissue, kind of like a secret ser-vice agent throwing his body in front of the president to catch an assassin's bullet. Yet an active version of one can recharge the other and send it back into the fracas, so that an excess of vita-min C can partially substitute for a slight deficiency of vitamin E.[72] This is just one of many examples of synergistic action between nutrients. They act like sticks in a bundle: enough of them together and they are unbreakable, yet each one by itself is easily broken.

A deficiency of vitamin E stunts the immune system.[73] Vita-min E acts like a bulletproof vest for soldiers in the immune sys-tem, protecting them from free-radical damage so that they can carry out their mission. Also, immune warriors (like neutrophils) carry with them bags (lysosomes) full of strong poisons (lyso-zymes) to douse the invader cell or cancer cell. Vitamin E acts as a "double wrapping" around the poison bags to make sure that they kill the invader, not the immune soldier.[74] Older adults may need above-normal levels of vitamin E intake just to maintain adequate immune function.[75] High-dose vitamin E supplements increased immune functions in test animals.[76]

The safety record of vitamin E is impressive. Long-term consumption of 3200 i.u. per day (much higher than recommended in this book) has resulted in no side effects in humans.[77] However, the reason that vitamin E supplements have been helpful at eliminating the "hot flashes" of menopause[78] is because vitamin E has some ability to substitute for estogen in women. Therefore, if you are trying to get pregnant, do not take more than 100 i.u. daily of vitamin E.

Paradoxically, the National Research Council keeps lowering the RDA on vitamin E, since they see no widespread deficiency symptoms from our low intake of this nutrient. What could be more widespread than nearly one million new cases of cancer discovered each year, along with a serious epidemic of heart disease and cataracts that are also related to long-term low intake of this wonder nutrient?

Food sources: Wheat germ oil, wheat germ, cold processed vegetable oils (soy, corn, cottonseed, safflower, sunflower, olive), mayonnaise, margarine, egg yolk, butter, liver, nuts. The heat processing and hydrogenation that most American oils are exposed to kills much of the vitamin E.

Selenium. The evidence is overwhelming that selenium is a true champion in defending the body against pollution, cancer, and microbe attacks. Selenium works closely with vitamin E to produce more of the protective GSH (glutathione peroxidase) that patrols the body in search of saboteurs. Researchers from Johns Hopkins University found that the greatest predictor of someone getting pancreatic cancer (a nasty variety with very low survival rate) was low serum selenium levels.[79]

A low selenium diet increases the risk for many types of cancer, including those of the esophagus, stomach, liver, lung, skin, breast, and other sites.[80] In a study that encompassed 10,000 Americans over five years, low selenium levels in the blood were found to double the risk for cancer.[81] When lab animals were given supplements of selenium and a high- or low-fat diet, then exposed to one of the most potent carcinogens known (DMBA, found in tobacco smoke), the selenium provided cancer protection regardless of the level of fat intake.[82]

Researchers in South Africa found that the extreme variation in rates of esophageal cancer were due to selenium: higher blood selenium levels lowered the risk for cancer of the esophagus considerably.[83] Professors from the University of California and Cornell University in New York have reviewed at least fifty-five different scientific studies showing the potent anticancer activity of selenium.[84]

Selenium may not only prevent cancer, but may slow down tumor cells once they occur. Selenium has been shown to improve the efficiency at which the cell can repair itself after the DNA has been damaged by toxins;[85] supplements were able to stunt tumor growth by 93 percent in animal studies.[86] In another experiment, selenium supplements provided test animals with the ability to shrink their implanted tumors by an average of 50 percent.[87] At high enough levels of intake, selenium is like a "heat seeking missle" in its selective toxicity for tumor cells.[88]

Dr. Gerhard Schrauzer, a noted expert in this field, estimates that our current intake of about 30 to 100 micrograms of selenium daily (depending on the soil) is a major cancer risk for our polluted times, and recommends an intake of 250 to 300 micrograms daily.

In only twenty-five years, selenium has been promoted from the FDA's status of "toxin" to being recently assigned an RDA by the National Academy of Sciences.[89] Selenium is able to stimulate the overall immune system to maintain a vigilance over toxins and tumor cells.[90] Low selenium status retards the animal's ability to respond to an invading virus,[91] lowers general immune functions, and may even permanently lower immune functions in future generations.[92] Selenium is a true ally in the war against food and water pollution.

While nutrients always have a lower toxicity than drugs, preformed vitamin A and selenium are the two nutrients most likely to create a toxicity problem. According to the National Research

Council, an adult would need to take more than 2400 micrograms daily for extended periods before any possibility of toxicity symptoms could occur.[93] The amounts recommended at the end of the chapter are well below this level. Still, do not overdo a good thing. A little selenium could be a major ally in your war against pollution, but too much could become more of a problem than a solution.

Food sources: It is difficult to determine one's selenium intake from food since the selenium concentration in the soil will dictate the selenium levels in the plants and animals raised in that area. Brazil nuts, soybeans, tuna, seafood, meat, and whole grains are good selenium sources. Selenium is a nutrient that is so importantly protective against toxins, and so evasive in the food supply, that I strongly encourage selenium supplements.

Folic acid. This is one of the more unsung heroes of the B vitamin complex. Folic acid (a.k.a. folate, folacin) is involved in new cell growth, which includes building immune factors and repairing DNA that has been attacked by toxins. Low folic acid intake greatly increases the risk for cervical cancer.[94] Folate supplements (10 milligrams daily) were able to reverse the precancerous condition in the cervix for a significant number of women tested.[95] A low intake of folic acid, which is common in America, can depress the immune system.[96]

Although the evidence is not as overwhelming with folic acid as it is for the nutrients listed above, its biochemical functions lead me to believe that folic acid is a potent protector against pollution and cancer.

Food Sources: liver, eggs, asparagus, whole wheat, green leafy vegetables, salmon, beans, broccoli, sweet potatoes.

Pyridoxine (B-6). B-6 is basically involved in creating and rearranging amino acids, which are the building blocks of many immune soldiers and protective enzyme systems. People who are deficient in B-6 at the time of exposure to a toxin are at much greater risk for getting cancer.[97] Women with low B-6 status were much more likely to develop cancer of the cervix.[98]

Of all the B vitamins, B-6 is the most directly related to immune function. A deficiency of B-6 will reduce the immune system output of crucial soldiers, including T and B lymphocytes, immunoglobulins, neutrophils, and others.[99]

Scientists have always accepted the fact that older adults experience a general decline in their immune functions, which makes them more vulnerable to infections and cancer. Well-fed healthy older adults were given supplements of B-6 at twelve times the RDA and found to have measurably improved immune functions.[100] Perhaps instead of accepting this decline in immune function, older adults may have an elevated need for B-6 and other immune nutrients.

There have been isolated reports of people developing a tingling in their extremities when taking large doses of B-6 (3,000 mg/day) for extended periods, but B-6 appears to be quite safe in long-term doses of less than 500 mg daily.[101]

Food sources: Soybeans, liver, bananas, lamb, kidney, chicken, steak, poultry, tuna, fish, legumes, potatoes, oatmeal, wheat germ.

Amino acids are the building blocks of proteins, kind of like beads (amino acids) on a necklace (protein). There are twenty-two different amino acids, of which ten are essential and must be included in the diet. Several of these amino acids seem to have a hand at building a healthy immune system and scouting the body for poisons to neuturalize. Cysteine, methionine, and glutathione are all sulfur-bearing amino acids with potent abilities to detoxify poisons. Arginine and ornithine are capable of stimulating a stronger immune system.

GSH is the consummate "Robo-Cop" in the body, defending us against any and all invaders with considerable effectiveness. GSH is made up of cysteine, glutamic acid, and glycine, and requires vitamin E and selenium for its assembly-line production. Scientists at Cornell University found that cysteine supplements improve the production of GSH:[102] These have been shown to reduce heavy metal toxicity, to prevent and even reverse cancer, and to neutralize a wide variety of toxins.[103] Cysteine was able to protect lab animals from harm done by radiation.[104]

When exposed to realistic levels of toxic aldehydes (which occur from smoking, drinking, smog, fatty diets, and pollution), 90 percent of the test animals died. Yet, when first supplemented with cysteine, thiamin, and vitamin C, and then exposed to identical levels of toxins, none of the test animals died.[105] GSH is one of the more exciting scientific discoveries of our polluted age, since it shows us how to bolster our protective mechanisms in the body. GSH protects your body from a variety of toxins:[106]

> -acetaldehyde pollution (smoking, drinking, air pollution)
> -aflatoxins, which are potent cancer causing agents[107]
> -quenches free radicals, which are the instigators of cancer and aging
> -can recycle other spent antioxidants (like vitamins C and E)
> -detoxifies and eliminates poisons (like DDT and lead)
> -stimulates the immune system to devour invaders (like bacteria, virus, and cancer cells)
> -helps to repair liver damage (e.g., from aflatoxins)
> -provides cancer protection of beta-carotene calibre
> -protects against radiation damage
> -protects against the possible harm done by excess production of stress chemicals
> -protects the eyes to lower the risk of cataracts
> -is nontoxic and completely safe in reasonable supplement levels.

Actually, some substances do not become toxic until the liver tries to rearrange the chemical structure of the invading substance. The resulting product can sometimes be more lethal than the original, as is the case with many herbicides, pesticides, benzene, plastics, and petroleum derivatives. GSH then neutralizes the "Frankenstein" that is created by the liver. GSH and gluta-thione can render harmless an impressive list of toxins in our food and water supply.

However, long-term intake of high doses of cysteine supplements may lead to kidney stones. In order to avoid that complication, take supplements of glutathione rather than cysteine. Glutathione is a complex amino acid that contains cysteine, but is not broken down into toxic by-products that can create kidney stones. Glutathione also bolsters the immune system by helping in the production of warriors, called lymphocytes. Although your body produces survival levels of GSH internally, in our polluted times extra GSH from glutathione supplements can provide an edge against the unavoidable poisons in our food and water supply. The problem with glutathione is price: one kilogram (2.2 pounds) costs about the same as an ounce of gold ($450 at early 1989 price). You can safely take up to 1 gram daily of glutathione, although 250 mg will provide significant pollution protection.

Another sulfur-bearing amino acid, methionine, was able to reduce mercury concentrations while enhancing weight gain in test animals that were purposefully poisoned with mercury.[108] Ornithine is another amino acid that is capable of stimulating a stronger immune system.[109] However, the best amino acid for immune stimulation is arginine, which improves lymphocyte output,[110] overall immune function,[111] and stunts the growth of tumor cells.[112]

Food sources: Since amino acids are building blocks of protein, the best sources of amino acids are high protein foods: egg white, dairy, meat, poultry, and fish. However, it may be impossible to obtain the protective levels of certain amino acids from foods. Amino acid supplements can be of value to some people.

Fat. This subject provides a perfect example of the lightning pace at which nutrition is advancing. While in my undergraduate nutrition studies, my professors spoke briefly of the essential fatty acid (linoleic acid) but never of the problems of a high fat diet. While in my master's studies, teachers began talking about the problems of a high fat diet. While in my doctorate studies, professors began speaking of the role certain fats, like omega-3 fats, may play in regulating important bodily functions. Dietary fat is no longer a nonissue.

While Americans eat plenty of fat, we rarely eat the right amount or type of fat. Since many pollutants are fat soluble, and most pollutants get more concentrated as they ascend up the food chain, a diet high in animal fat can be quite dangerous. There is an abundance of evidence showing that a high-fat diet is a primary risk factor toward many types of cancer. Obesity (high-fat body) substantially increases the risk for several types of cancer.[113]

It is well documented that the nutrients listed in this chapter stimulate the immune system. However, there is some puzzling and contradictory evidence that "undernutrition without malnutrition," or eating sparingly of high nutrient-density foods, also bolsters the immune system and extends lifespan. Animals fed half the calories (but adequate vitamins and minerals) had a stronger immune system and lower incidence of disease than their well-fed peers.[114] Anorexic humans showed above-average immune systems while two-thirds of them had not had an infection in that previous year.[115] This "undernutrition without malnutrition" means going hungry most of the time and thus it appeals to few people; but it also contradicts much of the other evidence presented in this book that shows how optimal levels of supplements can protect against cancer and pollutants. Perhaps the reason "undernutrition without malnutrition" works is because fat in both the diet and body are brought to a bare minimum during starvation. Excess fat in both the body and/or the diet are true risk factors toward a host of health problems.

There was some preliminary evidence in the late 1970s that polyunsaturated fats, or PUFAs such as found in corn, soy, and safflower oil, could lower the levels of fat in the blood to prevent heart disease. Then reality hit. These same PUFAs also are vulnerable to oxidative "rusting" (lipid peroxidation) if there aren't enough antioxidants to protect them. PUFAs also encourage a prostaglandin pathway that seems to induce tumors. Researchers now find that tumors have a higher level of a certain PUFA (linoleic acid) than healthy cells.[116] Although a deficiency of the essential fatty acid, linoleic acid, can lower immune capabilities,[117] a diet high in linoleic acid also weakens the immune system.[118] Dr. Michael Bennett at the University of Texas found that monounsaturated fats, such as found in olive oil, seem to support a healthier immune system in humans.[119] For many reasons, olive oil has become the oil of choice among nutritionists.

The importance of fats goes beyond eating either too much, too little, or proper amounts of the essential fatty acid of linoleic acid. There are some recently discovered fats that are crucial for full protection from pollution and cancer. Fish oil contains a unique type of fat, omega-3 fats (eicosapentaenoic acid, mercifully shortened to EPA), that bolsters the immune system in humans.[120]

In a Chinese study matching 309 childhood leukemia victims against 618 healthy controls, researchers found that long-term intake of cod liver oil provided major protection against leukemia.[121] In animals studies, fish oil cut colon cancer rates by 80 percent compared to a corn oil diet.[122] When scientists looked at diet and breast cancer incidence in twenty-one countries around the world, they found that fish consumption was the second most important factor in preventing breast cancer, after total fat intake.[123] In spite of their atrocious diet that is high in fat and low in fiber, Eskimos have a very low incidence of breast and colon cancer, probably due to their regular intake of fish.[124]

Conclusive evidence from the National Institutes of Health shows that the higher the EPA intake, the less invasive cancer cells become.[125] Fish oil may even be able to reverse some types of cancer.[126] In animal studies, fish oil supplements *reduced* tumor growth from implanted breast cancer.[127] For a better understanding of the importance of EPA in dictating cancer-protective prostaglandin pathways, see Figure 10C.

There is so much evidence supporting the need for EPA that several reputable scientists have suggested that we establish an RDA for this critical nutrient.[128] Even Harvard Medical School puts out a newsletter entitled "n-3 News" all about this wonder fat.

The only side effect of consuming excessive fish oil is that it thins out the blood, reducing clotting abilities. If you are planning on surgery, stop intake of fish oil. Other than reduced clotting abilities, the news on fish oil is exciting and most welcome. I take a tablet of fish oil at each meal, which totals 540 mg per day of EPA.

Another special fatty acid, gamma-linolenic acid (a.k.a. GLA or evening primrose oil), may also hold promise in bolstering your immune system against food pollutants. GLA supplements were able to prevent the changes in cell structure of bone marrow that can lead to leukemia or bone cancer.[129] GLA was also able to reverse the deterioration of cancer cells in human tissue cultures (in vitro).[130] When the special fats of GLA and EPA were added to human cancer cells that were growing alongside of normal cells, the normal cells (fibroblasts) overwhelmed the cancer cells.[131] GLA also supressed tumor growth in human tissue cultures better than the body's own prostaglandin system (PGE1)[132]

When rats were given supplements of GLA, transplanted breast tumors did not grow.[133] GLA supplements were able to double the mean survival time of human cancer patients.[134] GLA bolsters the immune system and cancer fighting capabilities in the body, which can be a definite survival edge in our polluted times.

Although GLA supplements are expensive, they may be worth the money for some people. By taking EPA and GLA supplements together in a 4 to 1 ratio, you can enhance the effectiveness of these special fatty acids while encouraging healthy prostaglandin pathways.

Food sources:

-Foods that are rich in saturated fat, and hence are more harmful than beneficial: lard, hydrogenated fat, beef marbling, butter, ice cream, cream cheese, cheese, palm oil, coconut oil, stick margarine, bacon.

-Best sources of the valuable EPA: salmon, haddock, tuna, sardines, cod, menhaden.

-Best source of valuable GLA: evening primrose (a plant native to Canada and northern Europe).

OTHER VALUABLE ANTIPOLLUTION NUTRIENTS

Protein. While the average intake of protein in America is too high (about 100 grams per day), some people do not get enough protein in their diet. Most of the "soldiers" in the immune and detoxifying systems are composed of protein building blocks. Therefore, it should not be surprising that a protein deficiency depresses the immune system.[135] Most adults need about 1 gram of protein per kilogram of body weight per day. Which means that a 150-pound person would need 68 grams of protein daily. If you are not getting enough protein in your diet, then take protein supplements, which are usually powdered egg or milk that is mixed in with water to form a drink.

Food sources: egg white, milk, cheese, chicken, fish, turkey, pork, and other animal tissue. Vegetarians can create a high quality protein by matching grains (wheat, rice, oats, etc.) with legumes (beans, peas, lentils, peanuts). In general, animal food is higher in quality and quantity of protein than plant food, but a well-planned vegetarian diet can provide optimal amounts of protein.

Pantothenic acid. This B vitamin is crucial for proper functioning of the immune system. Excess stress quickly depletes pantothenic acid supplies. Low intake of pantothenic acid has been shown to depress the immune system response.

Food sources: royal bee jelly, liver, kidney, heart, egg yolk, bran, fish, whole grain cereals, cauliflower, beans, nuts, cheese, sweet potatoes.

Riboflavin (B-2). A deficiency of riboflavin can depress antibody response in the immune system. A riboflavin deficiency causes precancerous lesions in the esophagus of humans.[136]

Food sources; brewer's yeast, kidney, liver, heart, milk, broccoli, wheat germ, almonds, cottage cheese, yogurt, tuna, salmon, macaroni, brussels sprouts, asparagus, eggs, green leafy vegetables.

B-12 (cyanocobalamin). Low intake of B-12 is unlikely among meat-eating Americans, but can occur in strict vegetarians. However, as many people age, they lose the ability to absorb the large complex molecule of vitamin B-12. Hence, older adults are at risk for B-12 deficiency, which can reduce the gobbling abilities (phagocytosis) and bacteria-killing talents of the immune system.

Food sources; Liver, oysters, poultry, fish, beef, pork, clams, eggs, animal foods in general. Some B-12 in spirulina, some types of seaweed, miso (fermented soybean paste), tempeh (fermented whole soybeans), and brewer's yeast grown in B-12 medium.

Bioflavonoids. The more than five hundred different types of bioflavonoids act as helpers along with carotenoids in the photosynthesis process in plants. Quercetin and rutin are among the more commonly available bioflavonoids in supplement form. Although bioflavonoids have fallen from favor with most American researchers, European scientists have found that bioflavonoids boost the immune attack on bacteria and viruses.[137]

Bioflavonoids are also quite useful against pollution as:

-antioxidants to slow down pollutants
-chelating agents to imprison toxic minerals and carry them out of the body
-stimulants to the liver's detoxifying enzyme systems
-inhibitors of the carcinogenic nitrosamines found commonly in the food and water supply.[138]

Food sources: Exclusively in plant food. White rind of citrus fruit, vegetables, whole grains, (especially buckwheat), legumes, honey.

Vitamin D. Although fifteen to thirty minutes of sunshine daily will allow your body to make its own vitamin D, many elderly people in America are still deficient in this nutrient. When researchers examined sixty-three elderly men and women, 30 percent were found to have poor immune response *and* low vitamin D levels in their serum. After two months of supplementation with vitamin D, the immune responses returned to healthy levels.[139]

Food sources: Fish liver oil, fortified milk, high-fat fish (salmon, herring, sardines), sunshine on skin, butter, eggs. Caution: vitamin D supplements beyond 1000 i.u. daily could be toxic for some people.

Calcium. Grandmother used to make soap by combining a mineral (like lye, which is sodium or potassium hydroxide) with saturated fat (from duck, beef, or bear fat). The same chemical reaction can take place in your intestines and serve a very protective purpose of preventing colon cancer.[140] When calcium ions combine with roaming molecules of fat or bile acids, they form a happy couple (called a soap) and are carried out of the intestines with the feces. Though the calcium is not absorbed into the body, by grabbing trouble makers in the bowels and escorting them out of the body, a high calcium diet may save many people from colon cancer.[141]

One of the breakdown products of digestive bile is deoxycholic acid, a likely carcinogen. Calcium supplements in lab animals were able to neutralize the presence of deoxycholic acid in the intestines.[142] In people with a family history of colon cancer, calcium supplements (1,250 milligrams/day) were able to reverse the abnormal cells, called colonic crypts, that forewarn of cancer.[143] Another study showed that a combined low intake of calcium and vitamin D increased the risk for colon cancer by 250 percent.[144] People who drink soft water, in which calcium is removed, have a higher incidence of colon cancer.[145] Vitamin D is necessary for calcium absorption and metabolism.

Food sources: Cooked bones (as in canned salmon), collards, yogurt, turnip greens, broccoli, milk and dairy products, kale, tempeh and tofu (soy products), hard water (contains dissolved salts of calcium and magnesium).

Magnesium. A deficiency in this vital mineral can depress all sorts of immune functions, including a main reservoir of immune soldiers (the thymus). A low intake of magnesium increases the risk for cancer. Animals fed supplemental magnesium have a lower rate of cancer from induced tumors.[146]

Food sources: Soybeans, buckwheat, shrimp, wheat germ, almonds, cashews, Brazil nuts, whole grains, molasses, clams, cornmeal, spinach, oysters, crabs, peas, bananas, potatoes, oatmeal, salmon, milk, liver, beef, green vegetables, and hard water. Ideal ratio of calcium to phosphorus to magnesium would be 2:2:1.

Zinc. Zinc is crucial to the manufacture and repair of DNA as well as other detoxifying enzymes, like GSH and SOD. Zinc also competes with toxic minerals, like lead and cadmium, for absorption sites. Hence, ideal amounts of zinc in the diet will discourage the absorption of these poison metals. Serum zinc levels are markedly lower in patients with cancer of the esophagus, lungs, and prostate.[147] Zinc and vitamin C supplements together were able to lower the amount of lead absorbed by factory workers.[148] Animals that were given protective levels of zinc supplements and then exposed to toxins get fewer tumors.[149]

Yet other studies have found that low zinc intake slows down tumor growth. How can we reconcile such a conflict of evidence? Sheldon Hendler, M.D., Ph.D., and expert in nutritional medicine, has proposed that if zinc competes with the toxic mineral cadmium for absorption, the net effect is less cancer; while if limited amounts of both zinc and selenium compete for absorption sites, the net effect could be an elevated cancer risk because less of the critical selenium would be absorbed. Of these two minerals, selenium is the cancer-prevention heavyweight. If zinc is able to "bump" selenium "off the flight," then the net effect could be unfavorable.

We have spent much of the book talking about the carcinogenic effects of food and water pollutants, yet another equally important area is the elevated risk for birth defects from pollutants. Zinc is a key nutrient during fetal growth and seems to be able to mitigate the damaging effects of toxins during pregnancy. Zinc supplements can blunt the harmful effects of alcohol on the fetus.[150] In test animals, zinc supplements even prevented birth defects when the infamous drug Thalidomide was given to pregnant animals.[151] Since both alcohol and Thalidomide are among the worst offenders during fetal growth, it could be that zinc provides an "edge" against pollutants during pregnancy.

Although a deficiency of zinc can seriously hamper the immune system, so too can an excess (greater than 150 milligrams daily).[152] Older adults are quite likely to be zinc deficient. Zinc supplements have been shown to improve the vulnerable immune system of older adults.[153] Humans also get fewer infections when taking zinc supplements.[154]

Food sources: Oyster, herring, clams, wheat germ, bran, oatmeal, liver, nuts, beef, lamb, peas, chicken, carrots. Zinc levels in the soil, which vary widely, will strongly dictate zinc levels in food grown on that soil.

Copper. Copper may be one of the rising stars among the protective nutrients listed in this chapter. Researchers found that various nutrients, including copper, manganese, zinc, selenium, retinoids, and riboflavin, all help to reduce the DNA damage done by the dietary toxin, aflatoxin. Yet, copper seemed to excel at preventing aflatoxin damage.[155] Low intake of this trace element may depress various aspects of the immune system.[156]

Food sources: Shellfish (shrimp, lobster, abalone, oyster), liver, cherries, nuts, cocoa, gelatin, whole grain cereals, eggs, poultry, beans, peas. Copper intake should be balanced with zinc in a 1 to 10 ratio of copper to zinc.

Iodine. Iodine controls the ever-critical accelerator in the body that determines how fast basal metabolism occurs. A low intake of iodine can impede immune abilities. Women with low iodine levels in the blood were much more likely to have either precancerous lesions, fibrocystic breast disease, or other abnormal growths indicative of cancer. The abnormal cells abated when iodine supplements were given.[157]

Food sources: Iodized salt, ocean seafood (iodide is not found in freshwater fish), foods grown on high-iodide soil, milk (since iodide-based detergents are used to cleanse dairy equipment).

Iron. The role of iron in the human body extends well beyond the oxygen carrying function in the blood. An iron deficiency, which is common among menstruating women and growing children, can depress the immune system.[158] With as little a 10 percent decrease in iron intake, there can be measurable drops in immune functions.

Food sources: Pork liver, cast iron cookware (iron leaches into the food), cream of wheat, clams, beef, pork, veal, chicken, fish, spinach, asparagus, prunes, raisins, nori seaweed. Chelated iron (bound in a protein complex) is much better absorbed than elemental iron.

Vanadium. Although vanadium is known to be essential in the diets of humans, not much is known of its specific functions in the body. Researchers at the University of New Hampshire found that lab animals protected with vanadium supplements remained cancer-free longer after having tumors implanted.[159] Vanadium is lost in food refining, which means that many Americans may be deficient in this potentially important trace mineral.

Food sources: Black pepper, vegetable oils, olives, gelatin.

Chromium. Chromium takes on a ubiquitous role in the immune system, since it is involved in shuttling glucose molecules across the cell membrane so that sugar can be used for fuel. Many Americans consume low levels of chromium and suffer heart disease, diabetes, or cataracts as symptoms. In animal studies, chromium supplements (in the form of GTF, or glucose tolerance factor) improved the immune system.[160]

Food sources: Brewer's yeast, liver, meat, cheese, legumes, beans, peas, whole grains, black pepper, molasses.

Carnitine. Carnitine is not an essential nutrient, since humans can make some, but probably not enough, carnitine internally. Its primary role is to act like a "shovel" to load fat into the cell "furnace" to create energy. Yet carnitine supplements also bolster the immune system.[161]

Food sources: Sheep, lamb, beef, chicken. Almost exclusively found in animal products.

Dimethyl glycine DMG (pangamic acid). Once touted as a super energy nutrient for athletes, DMG may not guarantee any gold medals, but 120 milligrams daily of DMG has been shown to improve immune functions in humans.[162]

Taurine. Taurine is an unusual amino acid since it prefers to participate in reactions rather than become part of the structure of the body. In lab animals, taurine supplements improved the abilities of the immune system.[163]

Food sources: Mother's milk, shellfish, meat, animal foods.

Coenzyme Q (ubiquinone). CoQ is not required in the diet, but is important in the body's production of energy. Energy is required by all cells, including the immune system. Supplements of CoQ (30 to 60 mg/day) have been shown to bolster the immune system in humans. [164]

Nucleic acids. Damage to the cell's DNA blueprints are the beginning of cancer and birth defects. Even in a healthy person not exposed to any outside toxins, there is a certain amount of damage and repair going on in the DNA throughout the body. Supplements of the nucleic acids of RNA, DNA, and the raw materials (such as orotic acid) to make nucleic acids have shown some promise in repairing the damage done to DNA by pollutants.

Supplements of nucleic acid lowered the incidence of breast tumors in lab animals.[165] Another group of animals that were given injections of RNA followed by tumors induced through toxic chemicals lived much longer than the control group.[166] Intravenous solutions of a nucleic acid solution (Poly A/Poly U) improved the longevity of human breast cancer patients.[167] Supplements of orotic acid improved the status of both humans and animals exposed to pollutants.[168] Orotic acid may become a conditionally essential nutrient when we are exposed to poisons: lab animals given injections of orotic acid followed by exposure to harmful levels of radiation had considerably less damage.[169]

If you go back to our chapter on "tough humans," you may recall that each cell takes up to 10,000 "hits" per day on broken DNA that must be repaired. This is like trying to staple down roof shingles in the midst of a hurricane with shingles being constantly ripped off. Perhaps nucleic acid supplements provide more readily available "roofing shingles" to encourage the repair process and prevent defective cells from deteriorating into cancer.

Food sources: Metabolically active parts of plants and animals, like seeds, nuts, green leafy vegetables, liver.

SOD. Superoxide dismutase is an enzyme system in the body that is given heavy responsibilities in the area of neutralizing poisons. SOD is an excellent antioxidant in the body, but oral supplements of SOD would probably be chopped into unrecognizable pieces by the digestive enzymes. However, injections of SOD have increased the lifespan of animals with implanted tumors.[170]

RECOMMENDED SUPPLEMENT INTAKE

The following program is designed to provide your diet with supplemental help via nutrients that are proven to lower the risk of pollutants. You should be able to find an inexpensive multiple vitamin and mineral supplement that will contain most of these nutrients so that you need only take one or two pills at each meal. This supplement program is convenient, inexpensive, non-toxic, and effective. If you cannot find a supplement from your local pharmacy or health food store that provides the following recommended levels of nutrients, then contact the mail order vitamin firms listed in the appendix. Once again, I have no vested interest in any of the companies or products mentioned in this book.

You will note that there are two supplemental intake levels: normal exposure to toxins and maximum exposure. The maximum protection is for people who:

Live near heavy industry or farming
Work near carcinogens
Have a genetic predisposition toward cancer
Have a reason to believe that your community is heavily polluted.

All other people should be protected with the "normal" supplemental levels.

Figure 11A: THE THERAPEUTIC PROTECTIVE VALUE OF SUPER NUTRIENTS

NUTRIENT	PREFERRED FORM	AMOUNT	NORMAL PROTECTION	MAXIMUM PROTECTION	US RDA *	POSSIBLE TOXICITY
			DAILY INTAKE LEVELS			
A	beta-carotene	RE	2000–3000	3000–20,000	1000	?
D	cholecalciferol	IU	200	400	400	2000
E	d-alpha tocopherol	IU	100–200	200–800	10	2000?
K	phytonadione	mcg	100	200	80	1000
B-1	thiamin-HCL	mg	5–10	10–100	1.5	?
B-2	riboflavin	mg	5–10	10–100	1.7	?
B-3	niacinamide	mg	20–50	50–1000	20	3000
B-6	pyridoxine-HCL	mg	5–10	10–100	2	500
B-12	cobalamin	mcg	10–20	20–1000	2	?
folacin	folic acid	mcg	400–800	800	200	15,000?
biotin	biotin	mcg	300	300–1000	300	?
C	ascorbic acid	mg	100–500	500–10,000	60	20,000
pantothenic acid	Ca-pantothenate	mg	10–30	30–1000	10	?
choline	bitartrate	mg	250	250–1000	NS	?
calcium	carbonate	mg	200–400	400–1500	1200	4000
potassium	chloride	mg	300–1000	1000–2000	NS	10,000?
magnesium	oxide/chelate	mg	200–400	400–800	350	2,000
zinc	gluconate or picolinate	mg	15–20	20–60	15	400
iron	fumarate/chelate	mg	10–20	20–60	18	100
copper	gluconate or chelate	mg	1–2	2–10	2	50
iodine	potassium iodide	mcg	150	150–1000	150	?
manganese	gluconate/ chelate	mg	5–10	10–15	NS	30?
chromium	picolinate/yeast	mcg	100–200	200–600	NS	?
molybdenum	Na-molybdate	mcg	100–200	200–600	NS	2000
selenium	yeast	mcg	100–200	200–1000	75	2500?
silicon	Na-trisilicate	mg	10	10–20	NS	?
carnitine	L-carnitine	mg	—	500–1000	NS	26,000
glutathione (𝕤)		mg	—	250–1000	NS	?
arginine	L-arginine	mg	—	1000–3000	NS	?
EPA	eicosapen- taenoic acid	mg	600	600–1800	4 to 1 ratio	10,000
GLA	gamma-lino- lenic acid	mg	150	150–450		
bioflavonoids	rutin	mg	100	100–500	NS	1000
CoQ	ubiquinone	mg	30	30–60	NS	?

* may change with the new RDAs (1990)
𝕤 expensive, optional
? unknown, not established
NS none stated

CHAPTER 12
Mind and Exercise to Increase Your Tolerance of Toxins

Galen Clark came to Yosemite Valley to die. By his own admission, he had been a failure as a father, husband, and businessman. Now, at age forty-two, he was coughing up blood in the later stages of tuberculosis. When his doctor told him he had six months to live, Galen decided to spend his last days on earth in his favorite place on earth. Galen's first chore was to carve his own tombstone. That done, he proceeded to plant trees, prevent erosion, and protect this precious valley that he loved so much. However, death didn't come six months later, but rather fifty-four years later, when he was just shy of his ninety-sixth birthday in the year 1910. The joy of living amid the beauty of Yosemite and finally feeling useful must have inspired his immune system to round up and destroy all of the mycobacteria that causes tuberculosis.

Mind healing was once a domain of the shaman and country physician. *Real* scientists shunned the "voodoo" of mind healing. Norman Cousins's book, *Anatomy of an Illness*, articulately described his recovery from a very painful and degenerative skeletal disorder, ankylosing spondylitis. Cousins used positive emotions, which he metamorphically classified as "laughter," along with high doses of vitamin C to heal himself. Cousins tolerated nearly a decade of verbal lampooning while teaching at UCLA

Medical School before his hunches bore fruit in credible labs around the world. In the last decade, mind healing has evolved from a circus sideshow to a topic worthy of a Harvard medical textbook,[1] and an appropriately arcane name (psychoneuroimmunology or PNI) is now implemented in the best hospitals and medical schools around the country, including Harvard, UCLA, and Duke.

You may be wondering what PNI has to do with Safe Eating. Quite a bit, actually. While it is true that Americans are being bombarded with a staggering collection of poisons in our food, water, and air supply, there is now overwhelming evidence that negative emotions enhance the toxicity of the many poisons that we eat. We have built-in protective mechanisms that, within reason, can shield us from toxins and cancer. Those protective mechanisms are commanded by the mind. Negative emotions, like hate, guilt, depression, anxiety, low self esteem, lack of purpose, and lack of love or touch can blunt the protective systems. Conversely, positive emotions, like love, forgiveness, joy, laughter, play, control, sense of accomplishment, involvement, and touch can all stimulate the immune system.

The solution to our pollution issue becomes more of a mosaic of pieces, rather than one "magic bullet" to stop the problem. There are physical ways of fighting food pollution through specially protective foods and nutrients, and there are also metaphysical (meaning "beyond physical") ways to improve your tolerance of toxins through mental and physical exercises.

In my thousands of nutrition lectures, I have met many well-intentioned people who were acutely aware of the toxins in the food and water supply. These people could enumerate the poisons, their chemical structures, and the lab studies proving the toxicity of these agents, and, as a result, were often funereal in spirit: they felt like rats being dipped in poison, with a sense of futility and no control. These damaging emotions were more lethal than the poisons in the food supply. This brief chapter is very critical for the reader: a positive outlook may very well be more protective against pollution than large doses of beta-carotene—which is quite a concession from a nutritionist.

You may follow all of the recommendations in the previous chapters about minimizing intake of tainted food while maximizing intake of protective nutrients; but if you are depressed, angry, anxious, worried, and generally in an unhealthy mental state, your efforts may not be enough. It is the jokester who enjoys life and feels useful who is more likely to survive this food pollution issue, not the "puranoid" (cross between a purist and a paranoid) who skittishly avoids any food that may be contaminated with poisons.

With the quantities of pollutants dumped into our food and water supply, the reader may ask "Why doesn't everyone get cancer or some other illness since we are all eating poisons?" Our immune and detoxifying systems can chemically neutralize a certain limited amount of poisons; but if the mind is a positive force on the immune system, our tolerance of toxins is amplified. It is like being on a screened-in porch on a steamy August night: the nearly invisible screen protects you from the blood-thirsty mosquitos waiting outside. However, if a rip occurs in the screen, you are suddenly exposed to the predatory onslaught of bugs. Positive mental health is like keeping that bug screen intact. Negative mental health stabs holes in the screen to allow the mosquitos (poisons and cancerous cells) to wreak havoc.

Although there is an abundance of scientific evidence to support the statements in this chapter, it becomes even more poignant when it happens to your own good friends. Jeff and Judy (not their real names) were a seemingly happily married couple in their fifties. Jeff found out he had cancer of the prostate that had spread (metastasized) to other parts of the body. Jeff had been a smoker for decades, a regular drinker just shy of overindulgence, and didn't watch his diet or exercise program. He was a prime candidate for cancer in his fifties. He attended some PNI programs at a cancer clinic to discover any mental blocks that might hamper healthy functioning of the immune system. He found out that he wanted to be free of his marriage. Jeff left Judy. Jeff started to get better. Judy had been the picture of health prior to this situation—never smoked, drank wine only sparingly, and was a jovial person who radiated life. Judy's health began a downhill slide. A year later, Judy was found to have metastatic brain cancer and died within two weeks. Jeff's cancer has disappeared.

Jeff and Judy represent a growing body of data that shows the incredible power of the mind to kill or cure. Two scientists, Eric Peper and Ken Pelletier, have found over four hundred cases in the medical literature of spontaneous remission from cancer. When Doctors Elmer and Alyce Green analyzed these four hundred people, they found that hope and positive feelings were the only common factors that allow people to "beat the odds" on cancer.[2]

A BRIEF HISTORY OF PSYCHONEUROIMMUNOLOGY

Spiritual and philosophical leaders were first in this area. The biblical axiom, "a merry heart doeth good like a medicine," is an example of the beginnings of PNI. Shamans, priests, medicine men, and country doctors regularly practiced PNI because there were few medicines to treat the patient. So the healer used PNI to stimulate the patient's brain to direct internal healing. Today, we know that the mind can actually produce many medicines to stimulate the immune system or blunt pain.

Epidemics show the link between mind and body. Plagues have a notorious knack of following a war. If you draft the farmers, then burn the fields to induce malnutrition, then mix soldiers from distant lands thoroughly so that foreign pathogens are introduced to vulnerable people, and then add the final blasting cap element of stress that is inherent in wartime—voila, you have the beginnings of the Black Death, which killed about 75 million people or half the known world back in A.D. 1347. The 1918 flu epidemic followed a similar course just on the coattails of World War I, killing 21 million people worldwide.

A noted physician of his time, Sir William Osler, stated that "the care of tuberculosis depends more on what the patient has in his head than what he has in his chest." In 1918, a Japanese researcher published an article which illustrated the link between "mental excitation" and the course of tuberculosis.[3]

Scientists have found that PNI explains:

the link between loss of a spouse and depressed immune function.

lowered immune functions in medical and dental students during exam time.

why a seventeen-year study involving over two thousand men found that depression doubles the risk for death from cancer.

increased rate of mononucleosis among military cadets at exam time.

why outbreaks of rheumatoid arthritis follow stressful periods of life.

that social networking improves longevity; or, simply put, "loneliness kills."

the link between personality (type A) and heart disease.

why negative life events increased the risk for trench mouth and depressed immune function.[4]

why women under the stress of separation or divorce showed depressed immune functions and an increased risk for Epstein-Barr virus or mononucleosis.[5]

The early names in PNI are also impressive. Though many people equate the Russian researcher Ivan Pavlov with training dogs to salivate at the sound of a bell, Pavlov's real contribution was introducing the link between mind and body. In the earlier part of this century, a noted physician at Harvard University, Dr. Walter Cannon, emphasized a balanced mind-body approach to healing. Dr. Hans Selye found that rats that were tied down developed ulcers, elevated blood pressure, depressed immune functions, and other physical symptoms. Let's just ponder how Selye's work relates to Americans. Many Americans feel "tied down" with no control in their life. Fifty-eight million Americans have high blood pressure, one of the most common ailments in this country. The most profitable drug in America is Tagamet (cimetidine), used to treat ulcers. And the escalating incidence of immune problems is equally indicative of that emotionally-trapped sensation that many people are expressing with physical problems.

PNI is no longer the leper of science. Doctors Locke and Horning-Rohan have compiled a text of over 1300 scientific studies published since 1977 showing the strong link between mind and body.[6] Some of the harshest critics of PNI have recently proclaimed a change of heart. Dr. David Spiegel, a Stanford psychiatrist who was the consummate critic of PNI, found that eighty-six women with advanced breast cancer who received his therapy to help relieve their fears lived an average of thirty-seven months longer than their peers who received no psychiatric therapy.[7] Doctors Robert Ornstein and David Sobel, a psychologist and a physician respectively, started their research careers looking for hard facts on the brain. Today they are more impressed with the healing ability of pleasure.[8] Ornstein and Sobel find that "medical terrorism, health dread, and healthism" are all appropriate descriptors that speak of high-tech science propagating fear in the individual. The immune-depressing consequences of "health dread" or "puranoids" are far worse than the bacteria or toxins.

Today, PNI is a fully accredited science with labs, professors, textbooks, monthly journals, grant money, hospitals, and medical schools willing to say it works.

HOW DOES IT WORK?

We know more about outer space than we do about the human mind. Physically, the brain is rather unimposing: three pounds in weight, about one quart in volume of wrinkled gray gelatinous matter. In structure the brain resembles your two clenched fists held together at the knuckles.[9] The brain is composed of mostly fatty material and water. Yet this unimposing organ has some impressive inner workings. There are somewhere between 50 billion and 100 billion brain cells that each come near (but do not touch) one thousand or more other brain cells, like intertwined tree roots from nearby trees.[10] These limitless "connections" where the brain cells approach one another are the storage sites of memory and behavior. The human mind has more memory capacity than the most sophisticated computer. Scientists have speculated that if you tried to duplicate the human brain with a computerlike instrument, it would be as high as the World Trade Center in New York and cover the state of Texas.

There are over fifty known chemicals, called neuropeptides, that communicate across the gap between brain cells. Now, here comes the link between the mind and immune system. The neuropeptides that bridge the gap between brain cells also communicate directly with immune cells. Some neuropeptides reflect the worried state of the mind, and will go on to depress the immune system. Other neuropeptides (like endorphins and enkephalins) reflect a happy mind, and will stimulate a healthier immune system or sedate pain. The net effect: Thought directly influences your ability to tolerate poisons and resist cancer. Neuropeptides link up with immune factors like a cowboy straddling a horse. The two together make or break your defenses against pollution.

One of the main links between the mind and body is the hypothalamus, which is a tiny wishbone-looking nerve ending near the center of the brain. Your moods are directly reflected in the chemical output of the hypothalamus, which then heavily influences the immune system. Scientists have been able to stimulate different parts of the hypothalamus in lab animals, which resulted in raising or lowering immune functions.[11]

Another PNI link was discovered by Dr. Hans Selye who found that stress hormones (catecholamines) blunt the immune system.[12] Put quite simply, fear and worrying kill. Mentally handicapped individuals do not worry. The result of their anxiety-free life is that they have only one-fourth the cancer rate of the population at large.[13] In spite of the fact that nearly all of the criminally insane are chain smokers, have poor diets and atrocious health habits, they also have a lower incidence of cancer than the general population.

A number of noted authorities, including the Harvard professor Dr. Alexander Leaf, have investigated the lifestyle habits of people around the world who live a long and vigorous life. Many of these people who live for a century drink their own strongly brewed alcohol and smoke their homegrown rolled up tobacco.[14] These centenarians probably derive their unusual longevity from genetics, a cleaner environment, low-fat diet, more exercise, less stress, and respect for their advancing years.

I am not endorsing the regular consumption of poisons, but rather am emphasizing the importance of healthy emotions to keep the immune system operating at peak efficiency. You can process a limited amount of poisons if the mind is up to it. It used to be good advice to keep your mind focused on the positive. In our heavily polluted times, it may be mandatory.

Figure 12A: PSYCHONEUROIMMUNOLOGY

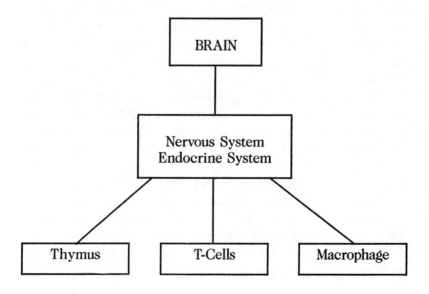

HOW WELL CAN THE MIND GUIDE THE IMMUNE SYSTEM?

With awesome precision. PNI researchers began with the general notion that positive moods encourage a healthy immune system. But the latest data in this area sends shivers down my spine. The mind is more like a general directing a diverse and well-trained army: the mind decides not only whether to go into battle, but which regiments, and how many, and where they go.

Endorphins and enkephalins are the "rivers of pleasure" that the mind releases during times of joy, exercise, music, childbirth, and injury (to blunt the pain). Endorphins were found to increase the T-cells ability to proliferate.[15] Enkephalins spurred on a more vigorous attack by T-cells against cancer.[16] The higher the enkephalin output, the greater the percentage of active T-cells.[17] Now I understand why the only times I get sick anymore are when I am under high stress and do not take the time to relax.

The Russian scientist Pavlov trained dogs to salivate at the sound of a bell that was associated with mealtime. Dr. Robert Ader of the Rochester Medical Center has found that immune bodies can be similarly trained to associate one stimulus (like a bell) with another stimulus (like mealtime). Dr. Ader injected rats with a lethal chemical which depressed immune function, as most xenobiotics do. He then combined the poison with a harmless solution of saccharin to see if the immune system would adjust to the pairing of the poison-placebo combination. Later, he gave injections of just saccharin and found the immune system was devastated as though it were pure poison.[18] According to this startling work, even after you switch from commercial strawberries laced with the carcinogenic pesticide captan, your immune system will still be devastated by the harmless organic strawberries, until the "conditioned behavior" wears off.

We may be able to use Dr. Ader's principle to our advantage. Another study found that pairing saccharin with a potent toxin to treat an immune disease (lupus erythematosus) taught the immune cells to recognize the chemical pair as lethal. Later, injections of just saccharin had the same benefit without any need for the toxin.[19] The upshot of this research is that our immune system is more than just a "dumb" collection of immune soldiers. The immune soldiers can learn chemical associations, which is just another reason to get the unnecessary poisons out of our food supply.

Dr. Howard Hall and his colleagues at Pennsylvania State University used hypnosis on twenty healthy subjects to see if guided imagery could increase overall immune function. The subjects were brought into a relaxed condition, then told to imagine that their immune bodies were like powerful sharks hunting down and destroying the weak and confused germs. Within only one week, the younger subjects showed a significant increase in three different immune parameters.[20] The older subjects exhibited a slightly less pronounced immune response. Many scientists feel that immunity gradually deteriorates as we age. However, you may remember from chapter 11 that vitamin B-6 and other nutrients could stimulate even the aging immune system into healthier protection.

And it appears that our mind can do more than just improve general immune functions. Dr. Barbara Peavey gathered sixteen subjects who were under stress and had depressed immune functions. She measured the ability of the subjects' neutrophils to ingest debris, then put the subjects through a program of relaxation assisted by biofeedback. The newly recharged neutrophils were much more aggressive at eating "junk" in the bloodstream.[21]

The mind does more than just start or stop an avalanche of immune functions. The mind may be more like an archer, who decides exactly which arrow to use, where to send it, and how many arrows will be launched. Sixteen healthy graduate students at Michigan State University were selected for their ability to creatively imagine. The subjects were shown slides of neutrophils and lectured on the function of various fractions of the immune system. Then the group was asked to imagine that their neutrophils could easily squeeze through blood-vessel walls, go to the site of accumulated garbage, and engulf the debris. All sixteen subjects registered a drop in white blood cell count, with the average person experiencing a 60 percent drop in *neutrophils* that had left the bloodstream for the tissue—just as instructed.[22] In a similar follow-up study, the subjects were asked to visualize their neutrophils becoming more active but staying in the bloodstream—and that's where they stayed.

There is metaphorical significance to many of the mind-body links. I have worked with many women who developed breast cancer in the wake of marital problems. In one case study, a woman got ovarian cancer after she did not report her husband for his sexual molestation of her daughter and niece. Loneliness, often depicted with a broken heart, can precipitate heart disease. Impatient, overbearing people (type A) are often represented as being heartless, and they often die of a heart attack. Researchers found a close link between the immune factors and personality profiles: the most positive and purposeful people had the most positive and purposeful immune systems.[23] Cancer victims who visualized their immune "warriors" as Knights of the Round Table or valiant Vikings had good success in shrinking tumors, while people who pictured their immune "warriors" as passive clouds or snowflakes had poor success in this microscopic war within.

Many of us have been mesmerized by the inexplicable, but well documented, abilities of certain mystics to walk on hot coals, to stop their heartbeat, to coil themselves into tiny containers and slow respiration to hibernation levels. Yet, apparently, all of us have similar potential. If the immune system is a well-orchestrated army, as it appears to be, then the mind is the four-star general commanding the battle.

WHICH EMOTIONS ENCOURAGE A HEALTHY IMMUNE SYSTEM?

Laughter. Humor is basically "fooling the mind," coming up with the unexpected punch line. John Kennedy called a sense of humor "the balancing stick that allows us to walk the tightrope of life." The grim German existentialist, Friedrich Nietzsche, claimed that "the most acutely suffering animal on earth invented laughter."[24] Laughter allows us to peacefully co-exist with the many incongruities and absurdities of life: "Hillbilly puts a quarter into a parking meter and exclaims, 'Gol darn. I just lost a hundred pounds.'" Laughter allows us to tolerate the macabre and dismal: "Yes, Mr. Smith, this is your doctor speaking. I have bad news and worse news. The bad news is that you have only twenty-four hours to live. The worse news is that I tried to reach you yesterday." Laughter allows us to press on when we would like to quit: "We've got to do something about this water pollution issue. My kid's got a squirt gun that jams."

A sense of appropriate timing is most crucial when using laughter to help heal sick people, but laughter has been used successfully as part of the physician's healing tools[25] and as nursing treatment in intensive care units.[26] Biochemically, laughter produces endorphins that provide relief from pain, bring euphoria, and stimulate the immune bodies to ostracize invading tumor cells and pathogens. Humor is an extremely subjective tissue, but I would encourage you to pursue books, movies, audiotapes, whatever that you consider to be funny. A carrot and a Marx Brothers film each day may be just the ticket to keep pollutants and cancer from ruining your life.

Love. People need people. Find others who you can share your love with. Love life, nature, work, art, music; and, most importantly: love yourself.

Joy. In the words of Bobby McFerrin's unique Grammy-award-winning song, "Don't worry. Be happy."

Relaxation. Biofeedback scientists can now document the physical changes that take place when you relax. General tension depresses the immune system, while relaxation allows a healthy immune system to repel invaders. One method commonly used for relaxation goes as follows:

Sit in a comfortable chair in a quiet room by yourself (some people find that soft instrumental music in the background enhances the relaxation). Do not lie down or you may fall asleep. Close your eyes and visualize a luminescent white cloud enveloping your feet. All cells that this white cloud touches are relaxed and invigorated. With mental imagery, picture the white cloud slowly moving its way up your body until all muscles are totally relaxed and your breathing is slow and rhythmical. Now picture a pleasant scene that you have experienced: a day in the mountains, a beach setting, a picnic near a waterfall or river, etc. The more realistically you can re-create the scene in your imagination, the greater the relaxation value. Spend at least five minutes daily using this relaxation technique.[27]

Forgiveness. Hatred and vengeance do no harm to the offender, they only put shackles on the offended. Many people have reasons to be hurt and angry—but anger is like termites in wood. With slow and silent progression, termites and anger devour the host. Anger cripples your mind and immune system. Forgiveness is never easy, but it is mandatory. There are a number of techniques in Dr. Harold Bloomfield's book, *Making Peace With Your Parents,* or there are trained counselors who can help you release your anger and purge your mind and immune system of "termites."

Sense of purpose. Notice how children almost insist on wanting to participate and help adults. We are all born with an inherent need to contribute. Though many of us obscure this drive as we mature, the need to do something worthwhile still smolders in every soul. Through work, volunteer work, raising a family, joining consumer action groups, and others, we can all feel like we are doing something positive for mankind.

Control. Dr. Hans Selye found that animals who were tied to a table developed many physical problems, including a compromised immune system. We need to feel some control in our lives. Obviously, we cannot dictate the weather nor many aspects of work and family life, but we need some control. Prisoners of war report that they would invite the guards into their cell, even though they really had no choice. By making it an invitation rather than a forced entry, the POWs exerted some control in an otherwise untenable situation. By following this book, you will feel more control in your life, since you are no longer a hapless victim in the food pollution issue. Those people who feel helpless are more likely to have a helpless immune system.

Right-brain playtime. Music, crafts, nature gazing, art, photography, kite flying, games, and fun are all functions of the right hemisphere of the brain. Americans have a tendency to overemphasize the importance of the left brain, with its language, math, and logical abilities. Yet the right brain apparently houses some potent immune stimulant abilities. Enjoy some right-brain playtime every day.

EXERCISE

Exercise may provide that essential edge against pollution by stimulating the immune system to be more productive and protective. Exercise increases basal metabolism, which accelerates the excretion of poisons via the lungs and skin; improves the mind's tolerance of stress, which indirectly helps the immune system; and burns up fat from both body stores and the blood, which minimizes the hiding places for fat-soluble pollutants.

Selye found that test animals died from stress when exposed to noise, electric shock, bright lights, and other common elements of life in the big city. Yet when another set of animals were given a daily workout (treadmill running) during the same torture test, they neither died nor even showed any untoward effects from these stresses.[28] Exercise may be the only way to tolerate the hectic pace of the modern professional person or parent.

Medical experts now find that the "dis-eases" which are common to Americans may be directly caused by "dis-use" of the body.[29] A study of over 17,000 Harvard alumni showed that exercise is a noteworthy life extender.[30] One hour of exercise increased both interferon and interleukin-1 levels in nonathletes.[31] After only five minutes of exercise, natural killer cells in humans were spurred into action.[32] Exercise also bolsters the output of endorphins, which saddle up with the immune factors and increase the effectiveness of the immune system.

Too much or too little exercise apparently have the same results: a depressed immune system. Nationally ranked cross-country skiers showed depressed immune functions.[33] Thirteen percent of the 2,300 runners in the Los Angeles marathon got a cold within a week, compared with only 2 percent of those runners who trained for but did not run the marathon.[34] Runners who put in sixty miles per week doubled their risk for infections compared to runners who did twenty miles per week.

Personally, I find that if I don't get my three workout sessions each week I get more tired, sick more often, and my mind doesn't function as well. Exercise is considered one of the most effective and uncomplicated ways to better tolerate stress, increase immune response, reduce fatty levels in the blood, and improve overall physical and mental health.

Exercise is always more beneficial if you enjoy it. Biking, stationary biking, brisk walking, rowing machines, cross-country machines, weight lifting, basketball, karate, jazzersize, aerobics, and swimming are among the myriad exercise routines that help to fortify the immune system against pollution. For best results, work out for at least forty-five minutes at least three times each week. Strive for routines that improve strength, aerobic ability of the heart and lungs, and flexibility. And do see your physician before beginning any fitness program.

Combining exercise and laughter, the comedian Robert Orben says: "Why does everybody knock smoking? If it weren't for coughing, some people wouldn't get any exercise at all!"

THE INTERWOVEN MIND AND BODY

Dr. Selye started his career as a scientist interested only in cold hard facts, but ended his productive years more as a philosopher, interested in meshing the mental and physical needs of the human body. Although I certainly don't put myself on a parallel with Selye, I, too, began my career interested in the hard cold biochemistry of nutrition, yet have evolved into a part-time armchair philosopher. We should all avoid confusing our hunches with facts, but I have a hunch that seems to effectively weave the physical and metaphysical principles of this chapter.

There are two sets of rules in life: the physical, and the metaphysical. Most of us live by the physical rules: poisons can kill us, we have certain nutrient needs, we bleed when we are cut by a sharp object, we get burned by walking on hot coals, we need sleep, we lack control over many bodily functions, etc. Yet there are a select few people who seem to transcend these physical laws and live by a more spiritual set of rules: love, forgiveness, hope, helping others, appreciating and developing your talents, realizing the connectedness of all life with a higher power. These spiritual people live by a spiritual set of rules: they don't bleed when cut, they don't necessarily need food, they don't get burned when walking on hot coals, they can control most of their bodily functions, they don't need much sleep, they don't get sick. We choose the rules that our lives are governed by: physical or metaphysical.

I have met and read about too many people who do not comply with the laws of nature, medicine, nutrition, and biochemistry. Spiritually elevated people seem to be able to live in a sea of filth and disease, like Mother Teresa, and never develop the expected ailments. Apparently, metaphysical laws supersede physical laws. We have only begun to recognize the importance of a healthy mind to protect and maintain a healthy body.

PARTING COMMENTS

There is a common theme running through mankind's existence: the need to exterminate "the outside enemy," whatever that is. Bacteria, insects, and Communists have each fallen into this category. The Romans once considered Christians to be "the enemy." The Spanish Inquisition once considered non-Christians to be "the enemy."

Once bacteria had been linked to disease, nineteenth-century scientists considered bacteria to be "the enemy" and set out feverishly to exterminate all bacteria, which we now know is neither wise nor possible. However, the famous French scientists, Claude Bernard and Louis Pasteur, both felt that illness hovered about continuously, but could not take root unless the terrain (the body) was receptive.[35] Essentially they were saying that we need to concentrate on our insides, not focus on an outside enemy.

After the first exuberant batch of farmers had blasted insects with the newly invented DDT, the farmers felt that they could soon alleviate mankind of this menace forever. We now know that idea to be both unwise and impossible.

Hitler tried to convince an entire nation that the Jews were "the enemy." For the past three decades, the Cold War in America pictured Communists as "the enemy." Today we see that alleged enemy, communism, crumbling; while the real enemy throughout that period was our own pollution (much of it created under the guise of national security) and reckless economic policies. In every era, we seem to try to point out some enemy—but we have met the enemy, and it is us.

The moral of this story ties in with this entire book, food pollution, and psychoneuroimmunology: the enemy is not out there, it is within us. We can clean up our food, water, air, and environment for a healthier nation. We can "clean up" our mind for a healthier and happier existence. We, as individuals or as a community, can be our own best friend, or our own worst enemy. Our choice. May you make the right choice and enjoy a long and vigorous life.

APPENDIX

resources, organizations, mail order forms, consumer action groups, etc. to support your efforts at Safe Eating

ORGANIZATIONS WORKING ON ENVIRONMENTAL AND PESTICIDE ISSUES

National Coalition Against the Misuse of Pesticides, 530 7th St. SE, Washington, DC 20003. 202-543-5450

National Coalition to Stop Food Irradiation, Box 59-0488, San Francisco, CA 94159. 415-566-2734

New York Public Interest Research Group, 9 Murray St., New York, NY 10007. 212-349-6460

Food and Water, 3 Whitman Dr., Denville, NJ 07834. 201-625-3111

Natural Resources Defense Council, 90 New Montgomery St., Ste. 620, San Francisco, CA 94105. 415-777-0220

Dept. of Health & Human Services, Public Health Service, Food and Drug Administration, HFF-420, 200 C St. SW, Washington, DC 20204

Environmental Defense Fund, 1616 P St. NW, #150, Washington, DC 20036. 202-387-3500

Environmental Policy Institute, 218 D St. SE, Washington, DC 20003. 202-554-2600

Environmental Protection Agency: Pesticides in general, 800-858-7378; Insecticides and rodenticides, 703-557-2200; Fungicides and herbicides, 703-557-1640

Environmental Task Force, 1012 14th St. NW, Washington, DC 20005. 202-842-2222

Izaak Walton League of America, 1701 N. Fort Myer Dr., #1100, Arlington, VA 22209. 703-528-11818

National Wildlife Federation, 1412 16th St. NW, Washington, DC 20036. 202-797-6800

Natural Resources Defense Council, 122 East 42nd St., New York, NY 10168. 212-949-0049

U.S. Public Interest Research Group, 215 Pennsylvania Ave. SE, Washington, DC 20003. 202-546-9707

World Wildlife Fund/Conservation Foundation, 1255 23rd St. NW, Washington, DC 20037. 202-293-4800

Environmental Action Foundation, 1525 New Hampshire Ave. NW, Washington, DC 20036. 202-745-4871

Environmental Policy Institute, 218 D St. SE, Washington DC 20003. 202-544-2600

Rachel Carson Council, Inc., 8940 Jones Mill Rd., Chevy Chase, MD 20815. 301-652-1877

Concern, Inc., 1794 Columbia Rd. NW, Washington, DC 20009

Northwest Coalition for Alternatives to Pesticides, PO Box 1393, Eugene, OR 97440. 503-344-5044

NRDC Toxic Substances Information Line. 800-648-6732 (212-687-6862 in NY state)

Pesticide Hotline, National Pesticide Telecommunications Network. 800-858-7378

US Environmental Protection Agency, Public Information Center, 401 M St. SW, Washington, DC 20460. 202-475-7751

US Public Interest Research Group, 215 Pennsylvania Ave. SE, Washington, DC 20003. 202-546-9707

Americans for Safe Food, Center for Science in the Public Interest, 1501 16th St. NW, Washington, DC 20036. 202-332-9110

National Toxics Campaign, Consumer Pesticide Project, 10 Gold Mine Dr., San Francisco, CA 94131

Public Citizen, 215 Pennsylvania Ave. SE, Washington, DC 20003. 202-546-4996

Appropriate Technology Transfer for Rural Areas, PO Box 3657, Fayetteville, AR 72702. 501-575-7570, 800-346-9140

Agroecology Program, University of California, Santa Cruz, CA 95064. 408-429-4140

BioIntegral Research Center, PO Box 7414, Berkeley, CA 94707. 415-524-2567

California Certified Organic Farmers, PO Box 8136, Santa Cruz, CA 95061. 408-423-2263

Committee for Sustainable Agriculture, PO Box 1300, Colfax, CA 95713. 916-346-2777

Rodale Institute, 222 Main St., Emmaus, PA 18098. 215-967-5171

Sustainable Agriculture Program, Agronomy Extension, University of California, Davis, CA 95616. 916-752-8667

Texas Department of Agriculture, PO Box 12847, Austin, TX 78711. 512-463-7534

NATIONAL ORGANIZATIONS WITH SOME LOCAL GROUPS ACTIVE ON PESTICIDE ISSUES

League of Women Voters, 1730 M St. NW, Washington, DC 20036. 202-429-1965

National Audubon Society, 801 Pennsylvania Ave. SE, Washington, DC 20003. 202-547-9009

Sierra Club, 730 Polk St., San Francisco, CA 94109. 415-776-2211

ATTRA, PO Box 3657, Fayetteville, AR 72702. 800-346-9140

Richard Wiles, Board on Agriculture, National Academy of Sciences, 2101 Pennsylvania Ave. NW, Washington, DC 20418

Garth Youngberg, Executive Director, Institute for Alternative

Agriculture, 9200 Edmonston Rd., #117, Greenbelt, MD 20770. 301-411-8777

Jayne Maclean, National Agriculture Library, Alternative Farming Systems, Information Center—USDA, Beltsville, MD 20705. 301-344-3755

Jeff Tryens, National Center for Policy Alternatives, 200 Florida Ave. NW, #400, Washington, DC 20009. 202-387-6030

Paul F. O'Connell, Deputy Administrator, USDA, Cooperative States Research Service, 901 D St., Ste. 342, Washington, DC 20251-2200. 202-447-2860

Neill Schaller, USDA/CSRS, Low Input Sustainable Agriculture Program, 14th & Independence Ave. SW, Suite 342, Washington, DC 20251-2200. 202-447-3640

STATE OR REGIONAL ORGANIZATIONS TO JOIN OR WRITE TO FOR MORE INFORMATION

Audubon Naturalist Society, 8940 Jones Mill Rd., Chevy Chase, MD 20815. 301-652-9188

California Agrarian Action Project, PO Box 464, Davis, CA 94617. 916-756-8518

Center for Rural Affairs, Box 405, Walthill, NE 68067. 402-846-5428

Delaware Valley Toxics Coalition, 125 S. 9th St., Ste. 700, Philadelphia, PA 19107. 215-627-7100

Kansans for Safe Pest Control, RR 5, Box 163, Lawrence, KS 66046. 913-748-0950

American Defender Network, Box 911, Lake Zurich, IL 60047. 312-381-1975

Madison Audubon Society, 111 King St., Madison, WI 53703. 608-256-0565

Massachusetts Audubon Society, Inc., South Great Rd., Lincoln, MA 01773. 617-259-9500

New Jersey Coalition for Alternatives to Pesticides, PO Box 627, Boonton, NJ 07005. 201-334-7975

Newton County Wildlife Association, PO Box 189, Jasper, AR 72641. 501-446-2211

Northwest Coalition for Alternatives to Pesticides, PO Box 1393, Eugene, OR 97440. 503-344-5044

Protect our Environment from Sprayed Toxics, 1 Cathance Lane, Cooper, ME 04638. 207-454-8029

Rhode Island Group for Alternatives to Spraying Pesticides, RR 1, Box 689, Exeter, RI 02822. 401-397-4433

Texas Center for Policy Studies, PO Box 2618, Austin, TX 78768. 512-474-0811

Western Washington Toxics Coalition, 4516 University Way NE, Seattle, WA 98105. 206-632-1545

Citizens for a Better Environment, 33 East Congress St., #523, Chicago, IL 60605. 312-939-1530

City of Durham Environmental Coordinator, 101 City Hall Plaza, Durham, NC 27701. 919-683-4137

County of Suffolk, Dept. of Health Services, Environmental Pollution Control, 15 Horseblock Place, Farmingville, NY 11738. 516-451-4634

INFORM, 381 Park Ave. S., New York, NY 10016. 212-689-4040

Institute for Local Self-Reliance, 2425 18th St. NW, Washington, DC 20009. 202-232-4108

Rural New England, Inc., PO Box 786, Waldoboro, ME 04572. 207-832-6825

South Branch Watershed Assoc., RD 1, Rt. 31, Lebanon, NJ 08833. 201-782-5513

Southwest Research and Information Center, Box 4524, Albuquerque, NM 87106. 505-262-1862

Spokane County Engineers, Public Works Building, North 811 Jefferson St., Spokane, WA 99260. 509-456-3600

Water Pollution Control Federation, 601 Wyeth St., Alexandria, VA 22314-1994. 703-684-2400

FOR MORE INFORMATION ON AGRICULTURE AND IPM

Rodale Press, 33 East Minor St., Emmaus, PA 18049. 215-967-5171

Natural Gardening Research Center, Highway 48-PO Box 149, Sunman, IN 47041. 812-623-3800

Necessary Trading Co., New Castle, VA 24127. 703-864-5103

Nitron Industries, 100 W Rock St., PO Box 400, Fayetteville, AR 72702. 800-835-0123 (AR: 501-521-0055)

Reuter Laboratories, Inc., 8450 Natural Way, Manassas Park, VA 22111.

David Pimentel, PhD, Office of Natural Resources, Dept. of Agriculture, PO Box 12847, Austin, TX 78711. 512-463-7506

Terry Gips, International Alliance for Sustainable Agriculture, 1701 University Ave., #202, Minneapolis, MN 55414. 612-331-1099

Diane Matthews-Gerringer, Rodale Research Center, RDD 1, Box 323, Kutztown, PA 19530. 215-683-6383

Bio-Integral Resource Center, PO Box 7414, Berkeley, CA 94707. 415-524-2567. Has a catalog of IPM publications, videos, and technical staff support.

FOR MORE INFORMATION ON HEALTH AND SAFE EATING

American Academy of Environmental Medicine, PO Box 16106, Denver, CO 80216

Center for Science in the Public Interest, 1501 16th St. NW, Washington DC 20036. 202-332-9110

Community Health Improvement Program, Harvard School of Public Health, 677 Huntington Ave., Boston, MA 02115. 617-732-1265

Americans for Safe Food, Center for Science in the Public Interest, 1501 16th St. NW, Washington, DC 20036. 202-332-9110

Public Citizen Health Research Group, 2000 P St. NW, Washington, DC 20036. 207-293-9142

Americans for Safe Food, 1501 16th St. NW, Washington, DC 20036

Clean Water Action Project, 317 Pennsylvania Ave. SE, Washington, DC 20003

Community Nutrition Institute, 2001 S St. NW, Ste. 530, Washington, DC 20009

Environmental Action, 1525 New Hampshire Ave. NW, Washington, DC 20036

Food Research and Action Center, Ste. 500, 1319 F St. NW, Washington, DC 20004

Institute for Food and Development Policy, 145 9th St., San Francisco, CA 94103

National Coalition Against the Misuse of Pesticides, 530 7th St. SE, Washington, DC 20003

Natural Resources Defense Council, 122 E. 42nd St., New York, NY 10168

Public Voice for Food and Health Policy, 1001 Connecticut Ave. NW, Suite 522, Washington, DC 20036

Coalition for Alternatives in Nutrition and Health Care, Box B-12, Richlantown, PA 18955

Consumers United for Food Safety, Box 22988, Seattle, WA 98122

Health and Energy Institute, 236 Massachusetts Ave. NE, Ste. 506, Washington, DC 20002

National Coalition to Stop Food Irradiation, Box 590488, San Francisco, CA 94159

New York Public Interest Research Group, 9 Murray St., New York, NY 10007

People for Responsible Management of Radioactive Wastes, Colleen McGrath, 146 Mills St., Morristown, NJ 07960

Vermont Alliance to Protect Our Food, Box 237, Vergennes, VT 05491

U.S. General Accounting Office, PO Box 6015, Gaithersburg, MD 20877. 202-275-6241

FOR LEGAL ASSISTANCE

California Rural Legal Assistance, 1900 K St., Ste. 200, Sacramento, CA 95814. 916-446-1416

Doug Parker, Institute of Public Representation, Georgetown University, 25 E St. NW, Washington, DC 20001. 202-662-9535

FOR LEGISLATIVE EFFORTS TO LOBBY FOR ENVIRONMENT ISSUES

David Baker, Friends of the Earth, 530 7th St. SE, Washington, DC 20003. 202-543-4312

Craig McDonald, Director, Public Citizen's Congress Watch, 215 Pennsylvania Ave. SE, Washington, DC 20003. 202-546-4996

FOR GROUPS OF WORKERS WHO ARE OCCUPATIONALLY EXPOSED TO POLLUTANTS

Jordan Barab, American Federation of State, County, and Municipal Employees, 1625 L St. NW, Washington, DC 20036. 202-452-4800

Debbie Berkowitz, Food and Allied Service Trades AFL-CIO, 815 16th St. NW, Ste. 408, Washington, DC 20006. 202-737-7200

Migrant Legal Action Program, 2001 S St. NW, Washington, DC 20009. 202-462-7744.

Pesticide Education Center, Marion Moses, M.D., 942 Market St., #709, San Francisco, CA 94102. 415-391-8511

United Farm Workers of America, AFL-CIO, LaPaz, Keene, CA 93570

FOR MAIL ORDER FIRMS THAT SELL SEEDS, FRUIT TREES, AND GARDENING IMPLEMENTS

W. Atlee Burpee Co., 300 Park Ave., Warminster, PA 18991
Research for Better Gardens, Hwy 48, PO Box 149, Sunman, IN 47041
Earl May Seed & Nursery L.P., 208 N. Elm St., Shenandoah, IA 51603. 800-831-4193
Stark Bros. Nurseries, Louisiana, MO 63353. 800-325-4180
Henry Field's Seed & Nursery Co., Shenandoah, IA 51602. 605-665-9391
Burgess Seed & Plant Co., 905 Four Seasons Rd., Bloomington, IL 61701

FOR MAIL ORDER FIRMS THAT SELL ORGANIC FOOD

Arjoy Acres, HCR Box 1410, Payson, AZ 85541. 602-474-1224
Eagle Agricultural Products, Pr. 4, Box 4-B, Huntsville, AR 72740
Pine Ridge Farms, PO Box 98, Subiaco, AR 72865. 501-934-4565
Mountain Ark Trading Company, 120 South East Ave., Fayetteville, AR 72701. 800-643-8909
Ahler's Organic Date Garden, PO Box 726, Mecca, CA 92254-0726. 619-396-2337
Blue Heron Farm, PO Box 68, Rumsey, CA 95679. 916-796-3799
Dach Ranch, PO Box 44, Philo, CA 95466. 707-895-3173
Gold Mine Natural Food Company, 1947 30th Street, San Diego, CA 92102. 800-647-2927 CA (800-647-2929 elsewhere in U.S.)
Gravelly Ridge Farms, Star Route 16, Elk Creek, CA 95939. 916-963-3216
Great Date in the Morning, PO Box 31, Coachella, CA 92236. 619-398-6171

Green Knoll Farm, PO Box 434, Gridley, CA 95948. 916-846-3431

Lundberg Family Farm, PO Box 369, Richvale, CA 95974. 916-882-4551

Marin Organic Network, PO Box 7037, Corte Madera, CA 94939. 415-285-6907

Mendocino Sea Vegetable Company, PO Box 372, Navarro, CA 95463. 707-895-3741

Sleepy Hollow Farm, 44001 Dunlap Road, Miramonte, CA 93641. 209-336-2444

Timber Crest Farms, 4791 Dry Creak Rd., Healdsburg, CA 95448. 707-433-8251

Van Dyke Ranch, 7665 Crews Rd., Gilroy, CA 95020. 408-842-5423

Weiss' Kiwifruit, 594 Paseo Companeros, Chico, CA 95928. 916-343-2354

Wiggin Farms, Rt. 1, Box 17, Arbuckle, CA 95912. 916-476-2288

Old Mill Farm School of Country Living, PO Box 463, Mendocino, CA 95460. 707-937-0244

Giusto's Specialty Foods, Inc., 241 East Harris Ave., S. San Francisco, CA 94080. 415-873-6566

Star Route, Box 3, Capay, CA 95607. 916-796-4111

Jaffe Bros., PO Box 636, Valley Center, CA 92082-0636. 619-749-1133

Lee Anderson's Covalda Date Co., PO Box 908, Coachella, CA 92236. 619-398-3441

Living Tree Centre, PO Box 797, Bolinas, CA 94924. 415-868-2224

Joe Soghomonian, 8624 S. Chestnut, Fresno, CA 93725. 209-834-2772

West Valley Produce Co., 726 S. Mateo St., Los Angeles, CA 90021. 213-627-4131 or 629-1656

Be Wise Ranch, Bill Brammar, 9018 Artesian Rd., San Diego, CA 92127. 619-756-4851

Ecology Sound Farms, 42126 Road 168, Orosi, CA 93647. 209-528-3816

Sun Mountain Research Center, 35751 Oak Springs Dr., Tollhouse, CA 93667. 209-855-3710

G & J Farms, Gregory F. Gaffney, 4218 W. Muscat, Fresno, CA 93706. 209-268-2835

Malachite Small Farm School, ASR Box 21, Gardner, CO 81040. 719-746-2389

Butterbrooke Farm, 78 Barry Road, Oxford, CT 06483. 203-888-2000

Tabard Farm Potato Chips, 1739 N St. NW, Washington, DC 20036. 202-785-1277

Maverick Ranch Beef, 402 N. Pine Meadow Dr., DeBary, FL 32713-2307. 305-668-6361

Starr Organic Produce Inc., PO Box 561502, Miami, FL 33256-1502. 305-262-1242

Nu-World Amaranth, PO Box 2202, Naperville, IL 60540. 312-369-6819

The Green Earth, 2545 Prairie Ave., Evanston, IL 60201. 800-322-3662

Brown Company, PO Box 69, Tetonia, ID 83452. 208-456-2500 or 456-2629

Frontier Cooperative Herbs, PO Box 299, Norway, IA 52318. 319-227-7991

Paul's Grains, 2475-B 340 St., Laurel, IA 50141. 515-476-3373

Fiddler's Green Farm, RR1, Box 656, Belfast, ME 04915. 207-338-3568

Johnny's Selected Seeds, Foss Hill Rd., Albion, ME 04910. 207-437-9294

Maine Coast Sea Vegetables, Shore Rd., Franklin, ME 04634. 207-565-2907

Organic Foods Express, 11003 Emack Rd., Beltsville, MD 20705. 301-937-8608

Tuscarora Valley Beef Farm, PO Box 15839, Chevy Chase, MD 20815. 301-588-5220

Smile Herb Shop, 4908 Berwyn Rd., College Park, MD 20740. 301-474-4288 or 474-8495

Baldwin Hill Bakery, Baldwin Hill Rd., Phillipston, MA 01331. 617-249-4691

Nassopoulos Family Groves, 195 Whiting St., Hingham, MA 02043. 617-749-1866

Haypoint Farm, Box 292, Sugar Island, Star Route, Sault Ste. Marie, MI 49783. 906-632-1280

Roseland Farms, 27427 M-60 West, Cassopolis, MI 49031. 616-445-8987

Specialty Grain Company, Box 2458, Dearborn, MI 48123. 313-561-0421

Eugene and Joan Saintz, 2225 63rd St., Fennville, MI 49408. 616-561-2761

American Spoon Foods, 411 E. Lake St., Petoskey, MI 49770. 616-347-9030

Country Life Natural Foods, 109 Oakhaven Ave., Pullman, MI 49450. 616-236-5011

Diamond K Enterprises, RR I, Box 30, St. Charles, MN 55972. 507-932-4308

Living Farms, Box 50, Tracey, MN 56175.

Mill City Sourdough Bakery, 1566 Randolph Ave., St. Paul, MN 55105. 612-698-4705

Natural Way Mills, Inc., Rt. 2, Box 37, Middle River, MN 56737. 218-222-3677

Midheaven Farms Beef, Rt. 1, Box 404, Park Rapids, MN 56470. 218-732-4866

Morningland Dairy, Rt. 1, Box 188-B, Mountain View, MO 65548. 417-469-3817

M & M Distributing, R.R. 2, Box 61A, Oshkosh, NE 69154. 308-772-3664

Stapleman Meats, Rt. 2, Box 61A, Belden, NE 68717. 402-985-2470

Water Wheel Sugar House, Rt. 2, Jefferson, NH 03583. 603-586-4479

Bread Alone, Rt. 28, Boiceville, NY 12412. 914-657-3328

Community Mill and Bean, RD 1, Rt. 89, Savannah, NY 13146. 315-365-2664

Four Chimneys Farm Winery, RD 1, Hall Rd., Himrod, NY 14842. 607-243-7502

Hawthorne Valley Farm, RD 2, Box 225A, Ghent, NY 12075. 518-672-7500

Deer Valley Farm, RD 1, Guilford, NY 13780. 607-764-8556

Chesnok Farm, RD 1, Marshland Rd., Apalachin, NY 13732. 607-748-3495

Millstream Marketing, 1310-A East Tallmadge Ave., Akron, OH 44310. 216-630-2700

Herb Pharm, PO Box 116, Williams, OR 97544

R. Ransdell, PO Box 155, Broadbent, OR 97414. 503-572-5564

Dutch Country Gardens, Box 1122, RD 1, Tamaqua, PA 18252. 717-668-0441

Krystal Wharf Farms, RD 2, Box 191A, Mansfield, PA 16933. 717-549-8194

Garden Spot Distributors, Rte. 1, Box 729A, New Holland, PA 17557. 800-292-9631 PA, 717-354-4936 local, 800-445-5100 northeastern U.S.

Neshaminy Valley Natural Foods, 421 Pike Road, Huntingdon Valley, PA 19006. 215-364-8440

Rising Sun Distributors, PO Box 627, Milesburg, PA 16853. 814-355-9850

Walnut Aces, Penns Creek, PA 17862. 717-837-0601

Genesee Natural Foods, Rt. 449, Genesee, PA 16923-9414. 814-228-3200 or 228-3205

J. Francis Co., Rt. 3, Box 54, Atlanta, TX 75551. 214-796-3364

Stanley Jacobson, 1505 Doherty, Mission, TX 78572. 512-585-1712

Aquaculture Marketing Service, 356 W. Redview Dr., Monroe, UT 84754. 801-527-4528

Teago Hill Farm, Barber Hill Rd., Pomfret, VT 05067. 802-457-3507

Hill and Dale Farms, West Hill-Daniel Davis Rd., Putney, VT 05346. 802-387-5817

Jordan River Farm, Huntly, VA 22640. 703-636-9388

Blue Ridge Food Service, Rt. 3, Box 304, Edinburg, VA 22824. 703-459-3376

Golden Angels Apiary, PO Box 2, Singers Glen, VA 22850. 703-833-5104

Kennedy's Natural Foods, 1051 West Broad St., Falls Church, VA 22046. 703-533-8484

Natural Beef Farms Food Distribution Company, 4399-A Henninger Ct., Chantilly, VA 22021. 703-631-0881

Golden Acres Orchard, A.P. Thomson, Rt. 2, Box 2450, Front Royal, VA 22630. 703-636-9611

Homestead Organic Produce, Bill Weiss, Rt. 1, 2002, Road 7 NW, Quincy, WA 98849. 509-787-2248

Farmers' Wholesale Cooperative, PO Box 7446, Olympia, WA 98507. 206-754-8989

Cascadian Farm Star Route, Rockport, WA 98283. 206-853-8175

The Meat Shop, Inc., 6522 Freemont Ave. N., Seattle, WA 98103. 206-789-5834

Hardscrabble Enterprises, Inc., Paul and Nan Goland, Route 6, Box 42, Cherry Grove, WV 26804. 304-567-2727

Brier Run Farm, Rt. 1, Box 73, Birch River, WV 26610. 304-649-2975

Joel Afdahl, Rt. 1, Box 271, Hammond, WI 54015. 715-796-5395

Nokomis Farm and Bakery, 3293 Main St., East Troy, WI 53120. 414-642-9393

Oak Manor Farms Tavistock, Ontario N0B 2R0 Canada. 519-934-4565

FOR STATE ORGANIZATIONS ON IPM/LISA AGRICULTURE

California Agrarian Action Project, PO Box 464, Davis, CA 95617. 916-756-8518

California Certified Organic Farmers, PO Box 8136, Santa Cruz, CA 95061. 408-423-2263

Demeter Association, West of the Mississippi, 4214 National Ave., Burbank, CA 91505. 818-363-7312

Demeter Association, East of the Mississippi, PO Box 6606, Ithaca, NY 12851

Farm Verified Organic Program, Mercantile Development Inc.,

274 Riverside Ave., PO Box 2747, Westport, CT 06880.
203-226-7803

Natural Organic Farmers Association, PO Box 335, Antrim, NH 03440. 603-588-6668

NOFA-Vermont, 15 Barre St., Montpelier, VT 05602. 802-223-7222

NOFA-Massachusetts, 21 Great Plain Ave., Wellesley, MA 02181

NOFA-Connecticut, 100 Rose Hills Rd., Branford, CT 06405

NOFA-New York, PO Box 454, Ithaca, NY 14851

Ohio Ecological Food and Farm Association, 7300 Bagley Rd., Mt. Perry, OH 43769. 614-448-3951

Organic Crop Improvement Association, 125 W. Seventh St., Wind Gap, PA 18091. 215-863-6700

Organic Food Network, c/o American Fruitarian Society, 6600 Burleson Rd., PO Box 17128, Austin, TX 78760-7128. 512-385-2841

Organic Food Production Association of North America, c/o Judith Gillan, PO Box 31, Belchertown, MA 01007. 413-323-6821

Organic Growers of Michigan, c/o Lewis King, 3031 White Creek Rd., Kingston, MI 48741. 517-683-2573

The Organic Network—Eden Acres, Inc., 12100 Lima Center Rd., Clinton, MI 49236. 517-456-4288

Tilth Producer's Cooperative, 1219 East Sauk Rd., Concrete, WA 98237. 206-853-8449

Ozark Organic Growers Association, HCR 72, Box 34, Parthenon, AR 72666. 501-446-5783

CA Certified Organic Farmers, PO Box 8136, Santa Cruz, CA 95061-8136. 408-423-2263

William Liebhardt, Director Sustainable Agriculture Research and Education Program, Agronomy Extension, University of California-Davis, Davis, CA 95616. 916-752-2379

Steve Gliessman, University of California-Santa Cruz, Santa Cruz, CA 95064

Bob Scowcroft, Executive Director, California Certified Organic Farmers, Box 8136, Santa Cruz, CA 95061. 408-423-2263

Kevin Martin, Executive Director, Committee for Sustainable

Agriculture, PO Box 7037, Corte Madera, CA 94925. 415-285-6907

Helen J. Davis, Marketing and Consumer Affairs, Colorado Dept. of Agriculture, 1525 Sherman St., Denver, CO 80203. 303-866-2811

Rocky Mountain Institute, 1739 Snowmass Creek Rd., Snowmass, CO 81654-9199. 303-927-3128

Colorado Organic Producers Association, 23242 Hwy. 371, Lajara, CO 81140. 719-274-5230

NOFA-Connecticut, 51 Mott Hill Rd., East Hampton, CT 06424. 203-267-4289

Farm Verified Organic, c/o Mercantile Development Inc., PO Box 45, Redding, CT 06875

Kansas Organic Producers, Inc., 307 South Hillside, Wichita, KS 67211. 316-682-0747

Don Klor, Illinois Sustainable Agriculture Society, Rt. 1, Box 58A, Buffalo, NY 62515

Iowans for Organic Food Standards, 22 East Court St., Iowa City, IA 52240

Dennis Keeney, Director, Leopold Center for Sustainable Agriculture, Iowa State University, Ames, IA 50011. 515-294-8066

Rep. David Osterberg, Iowa Legislature, State Capitol, Des Moines, IA 50319. 515-281-3221

University of Maine Agriculture, Experiment Station, Room 1, Winslow Hall, Orono, ME 04469-0163

Nancy Ross, Director, Maine Organic Farmers and Gardeners Association, Box 2176, Augusta, ME 04330. 207-622-3118

Ammie Chickering, Dept. of Food and Agriculture, 142 Old Common Rd., Lancaster, MA 01523. 508-792-7712

John Pontius, Small Scale Agriculture Program, Draper Hall, University of Massachusetts, Amherst, MA 01003. 413-545-1921

Ron Kroese, Executive Director, Land Stewardship Project, 14758 Ostlund Trail, Marine, MN 55047. 612-433-2770

Yvonne Buckley, Executive Director, Organic Growers & Buyers Association, PO Box 9747, Minneapolis, MN 55440. 612-636-7933

Richard E. Gauger, Coordinator, Sustainable Agriculture Loan Program, Minnesota Dept. of Agriculture, 90 West Plato Blvd., Saint Paul, MN 55107. 612-331-1099

Terry Gips, International Alliance for Sustainable Agriculture, 1701 University Ave., SE, Minneapolis, MN 55414. 612-331-1099

Missouri Alternatives Center, Rt. 2, Box 237, Clark, MO 65243. 800-433-3704

Zane R. Helsel, Agronomy Dept., 214 Waters Hall, Columbia, MO. 314-882-2004

Warren Sahs, Institute of Agriculture and Natural Resources, Dept. of Agronomy, Lincoln, NE 68583. 402-472-2811

Center for Rural Affairs, PO Box 405, Walthill, NE 68067. 402-846-5428

Natural Organic Farmers Association, Rt 1, Box 78A, Andover, NH 03216. 603-648-2521

NOFA-New Jersey, RD 1, Box 263A, Titus Mill Rd., Pennington, NJ 08534. 609-737-9183

NOFA-New York, RD 31, Box 134A, Port Crane, NY 13833. 607-648-3696

David Stern, Natural Organic Farmers Association, Box 149, Rose Valley Farm, Rose, NY 14542. 315-587-9787

Cornell Cooperative Extension, Cornell University, Ithaca, NY 14853

R.H. Miller, Head, Dept. of Soil Science, School of Agriculture and Life Sciences, University of North Carolina, Box 7619, Raleigh, NC 27695-7619

Kate Havel, Carolina Farm Stewardship Association, Route 3, Box n494, Siler City, NC 27344. 919-663-2429

Northern Plains Sustainable Agriculture Society, Rt. 1, Windsor, ND 58493. 701-763-6287

Carolina Farm Stewardship Assoc., Rt. 1, Box 667, Franklinville, NC 27248

Fred Kirschenmann, Northern Plains Sustainable Agriculture Society, RR 1, Box 73, Windsor, ND 58493. 701-763-6287

Clive A. Edwards, Director, Sustainable Agriculture Program,

Dept. of Entomology, Ohio State University, 1735 Neil Ave., Columbus, OH 43210-1220. 614-292-8209

Ohio Ecological Food and Farm Association, 7300 Bagley Rd., Mt. Perry, OH 43769. 644-448-3951

Organic Crop Improvement Assoc. International, 3185 Township Rd., 179, Bellefontaine, OH 43311. 513-592-4983

Kerr Center for Sustainable Agriculture, PO Box 588, Poteau, OK 74953. 918-647-9123

Oregon Tilth, PO Box 218, Tualatin, OR 97062. 503-692-4877

Susan Raleigh, Director of Consumer Affairs, Texas Dept. of Agriculture, Box 12847, Austin, TX 78711. 512-463-7602

Vermont Organic Farmers, 116 State St., Montpelier, VT 05602. 802-828-2427

Enid Wonnacott, RR 1, Box 177, Richmond, VT 05477. 802-434-4435

John Luna, Extension Entomologist, Virginia Polytechnic, Blacksburg, VA 24061. 703-231-4823

The Virginia Assoc. of Biological Farmers, PO Box 252, Flint Hill, VA 22627

Vern Hedlund, Chief, Food Section, State Dept. of Agriculture, 406 General Administrative Bldg., Olympia, WA 98504. 206-753-5042

R.I. Papendick USDA/ARS, Land Management/Water Conservation Research, Room 215, Johnson Hall, Washington State University, Pullman, WA 99164-6421

Margaret Krome, Director, Sustainable Agriculture Program, Wisconsin Rural Development Center, Box 504, Black Earth, WI 53513-0504. 608-767-2539

Wisconsin Natural Food Assoc., Inc., 6616 CTH I, Waunakee, WI 53597

Wisconsin Organic Growers Association, Rt. 2, Box 110, Boyceville, WI 54725

Kenneth Rineer, Coordinator, Sustainable Agriculture Program, Wisconsin Dept. of Agriculture, Trade, and Consumer Protection, Box 8911, Madison, WI 53708. 608-267-3319

Ray Field, Professor, University of Wyoming College of Agriculture, Dept. of Animal Science, Box 3684, University Station, Laramie, WY 82071. 307-766-2224

INTERNATIONAL PESTICIDE ALERT ORGANIZATIONS

Dr. Issa Beye, Environment Liaison Centre Int'l., PO Box 72461, Nairobi, Kenya. 254-2-24770

Dr. Abou Thiam, Environment and Development Action in the Third World (ENDA-TM), BP3370, Dakar, Senegal. 221-224229, 221-216027

Ms. Sarojini Rengam, Int'l. Organization of Consumers Unions, PO Box 1045, 10830 Penang, Malaysia. 604-371396, 604-371318

Mr. Bert Lokhorst, PAN Europe, Stevinstraat 115, 1040 Brussels, Belgium. 32-2-2300776

Ms. Pilar Perez de Sevilla, Fundacion Natura, Casilla 243, Quito, Ecuador. 593-2-249-780

Ms. Monica Moore, Pesticide Action Network North America Regional Center, PO Box 610, San Francisco, CA 94101. 415-541-9140

ORGANIC WHOLESALERS

For a listing of stores and producers who handle hormone-free animal products, send $.50 plus a self-addressed stamped envelope to: CSPI/Hormone-Free Beef, 1501 16th St. NW, Washington, DC 20036

The following distributors require a large minimum order and are more appropriate for group orders or for buying clubs. For a comprehensive listing of distributors servicing your area, consult the *1988 Organic Wholesalers Directory and Yearbook*, published by the California Action Network. The directory can be ordered for $19.00, plus $1.75 for shipping and handling, from: CAN, P.O. Box 464, Davis, CA 95617. 916-756-8518

Blooming Prairie Warehouse, 2340 Heinz Rd., Iowa City, IA 52240. 319-337-6448

Clear Eye Warehouse, RD 1, Box 89, Savannah, NY 13146. 315-365-2816

Common Health Warehouse, 1505 N. 8th St., Superior, WI 54880

D.A.N.C.E., 510 Kasota Ave., Minneapolis, MN 55414. 612-378-9774

Federation of Ohio River Cooperatives, 320 Outerbelt, Ste. E., Columbus, OH 43213. 614-861-2446

Genessee Natural Foods, Rt. 449, Genessee, PA 16923. 814-228-3200

Hudson Valley Federation, PO Box 367, Clintondale, NY 12515. 914-883-6848

Michigan Federation of Food Cooperatives, 727 W. Ellsworth #15, Ann Arbor, MI 48104. 313-761-4642

Mountain Warehouse, 305 S. Dillard St. SW, Durham, NC 27701. 919-682-9234

Neshaminy Valley Natural Foods, 421 Pike Rd., Huntington Valley, PA 19006. 215-364-8440

North Coast Cooperative, 3134 Jacobs Ave., Eureka, CA 95501. 707-445-3185

Northeast Cooperatives, 5 Cameron Ave., Cambridge, MA 02140. 617-354-3544

North Farm Cooperative Warehouse, 204 Regas Rd., Madison, WI 53714. 608-241-3995

Nutrasource, 4005 Sixth Ave. S., Seattle, WA 98108. 206-467-7190

Orange Blossom Cooperative Warehouse, 210 SE 5th Ave., Gainesville, FL 32601. 904-372-7061

Ozark Cooperative Warehouse, PO Box 30, Fayetteville, AR 72702-0030. 501-521-COOP

Tucson Cooperative Warehouse, 1716 E. Factory Ave., Tucson, AZ 85719. 602-884-9951

MAIL ORDER VENDORS OF NUTRITIONAL SUPPLEMENTS

Bronson Pharmaceuticals, 4526 Rinetti Lane, La Canada, CA 91011-0628. In CA 800-521-3323, outside CA 818-790-2646

Nutri Guard Research, Box 865, Encinitas, CA 92024. In CA 800-426-6374, outside CA 800-433-2402

Vitamin Research Products, 2044 Old Middlefield Way, Mountain View, CA 94043. In CA 800-541-8536, outside CA 800-541-1623

Notes

INTRODUCTION

[1]. Schauss, A. *Diet, Crime, and Delinquency.* p.32. Berkeley: Parker House, 1981.
[2]. Roark, A. C., Los Angeles Times. p.14. *Good Health Magazine,* Oct.8, 1989.
[3]. *FDA Consumer.* July/Aug. 1984, p.12.

CHAPTER 1: FUEL FOR THE OPTIMIST

[1]. *Food Marketing Institute, 1987 Trends.* p.32.
[2]. Paddock, R. C. *Los Angeles Times.* Part I, p.3, June 1, 1989.

CHAPTER 2: HUMANS ARE TOUGH CREATURES

[1]. Groves, P., Schlesinger, K., *Biological Psychology.* p.26. Dubuque, IA: WC Brown, 1982.
[2]. Center for Disease Control. *Journal of the American Medical Association,* vol.255, p.3224, June 20, 1986.
[3]. Ames, B. *National Association of Water Companies: Water,* vol.27, no.4, p.20, winter 1986.
[4]. Tierney, J. *Hippocrates,* p.29, Jan.1988.
[5]. Brochure by the U.S. Department of Health, Education and Welfare Public Service, *Everything Doesn't Cause Cancer,* National Institutes of Health.

6. *The Economist,* p.97, Mar.21, 1987.

7. Ames, B. N. *Environmental and Molecular Mutagens,* vol.16, p.66, sup., 1989.

8. Ames, B. N. *Science,* vol.221, p.1256, Sept.1983.

9. Quillin, P. *Healing Nutrients.* Chicago: Contemporary Books, 1987. *passim.*

10. Ames, B. N. *Environmental and Molecular Mutagenesis,* vol.14, sup.16, p.66, 1989.

11. Ahmed, A. K., et al. *Elements of Toxicology and Chemical Risk Assessment.* Washington, D.C.: Environ Corp., 1988. *passim.*

12. DeBruin, A. *Biochemical Toxicology of Environmental Agents.* p.2. Holland: Elsevier Press, 1976.

13. State of California, Dept. of Health Services. *Pesticides: Health Aspects of Exposure and Issues Surrounding Their Use.* p.13, 1988.

14. Ames, B. N., et al. in *Molecular Biology of Aging: Gene Stability and Gene Expression,* edited by R. A. Sohol, et al. p.137. NY: Raven Press, 1985.

CHAPTER 3: WHAT FOOD POLLUTANTS DO TO OUR HEALTH

1. Roark, A. C. *Los Angeles Times, Good Health Magazine,* p.14, Oct.8, 1989.

2. Cohen, M. N. *Health and the Rise of Civilization.* New Haven, CT: Yale University Press, 1989.

3. Berry, C. L. *Human Toxicology,* vol.7, no.5, p.433, Sept.1988.

4. American Cancer Society, *Cancer Facts & Figures-1988,* ACS, NY, 1989.

5. Galler, J.R. (ed.), *Nutrition and Behavior.* p.175. NY: Plenum Press, 1984.

6. Fan, A., and Jackson, R. J. *Regulatory Toxicology and Pharmacology,* vol.9, p.158, 1989.

7. Natural Resources Defense Council. *Intolerate Risk: Pesti-*

326 • NOTES

cides in Our Children's Food. p.3. New York: NRDC, Feb.1989.

8. Nelson, H. *Los Angeles Times,* part I, p.3, Apr.23, 1987.
9. *Los Angeles Times,* part I, p.6, Feb.10, 1985.
10. National Center for Health Statistics. *Health: United States, 1988.* p.27, Dept. Health and Human Services, publ. # 89–1232. Washington, DC: U.S. Govt. Printing Office, 1989.
11. *Journal of the American Medical Association,* vol.256, p.1141, 1986.
12. Regenstein, L. *How to Survive in America the Poisoned.* p.20. Washington, DC: Acropolis Books, 1986.
13. Blair, A., et al. *American Journal of Epidemiology,* vol.110, p.264, 1979; see also Burmeister, L., et al. *American Journal of Epidemiology,* vol.118, p.72, 1983.
14. Moses, M. *American Association of Occupational and Health Nurses,* vol.37, no.3, p.115, Mar.1989; see also p.131 for review article.
15. Pins, K. *Des Moines Register.* Nov.16, 1986.
16. Lowengart, R., et al. *Journal of National Cancer Institute,* vol.79, p.39, 1987.
17. Gold, E., et al. *American Journal of Epidemiology,* vol.109, no.3, p.309, 1979.
18. Infante, P.F., et al. *Scandinavian Journal of Work, Environment and Health,* vol.4, p.137, 1978.
19. Pratt, C. B., et al. *Cancer,* vol.40, p.2464, 1977.
20. Shu, X. O., et al. *Cancer,* vol.62, no.3, p.635, Aug.1, 1988.
21. Schwartz, D. A., et al. *Scandinavian Journal of Work, Environment, and Health,* vol.12, p.51, 1986.
22. Taylor, R. B. *Los Angeles Times,* part I, p.3, Dec.31, 1987.
23. *International Agency for Research on Cancer,* vol.30, 1983.
24. National Research Council. *Diet and Health,* p.484. Washington, DC: National Academy of Sciences, 1989.
25. Vaughan, T. L. *Journal of Occupational Medicine,* vol.26, p.676, 1984; see also Rita, P., et al. *Environmental Research,* vol.44, p.1, 1987.
26. Sharp, D. S., et al. *Annual Review of Public Health,* vol.7, p.441, 1986.

27. McGrath, C., et al. (eds.) *Pesticides: A Community Action Guide,* Washington, DC: Concern, Inc., 1985.
28. Wiles, R. *The Nation,* Oct.5, 1985.
29. Wilson, C. *Los Angeles Times,* part I, p.3, Aug.18, 1985.
30. National Center for Health Statistics. *Health: United States, 1988,* p.150, Dept. Health and Human Services, #89–1232, Public Health Service, U.S. Govt. Printing Office, Mar.1989.
31. Wright, J. W. (ed.) *The Universal Almanac,* p.226. Kansas City: Andrews & McMeel, 1989.
32. U.S. Bureau of the Census. *Statistical Abstract of the United States: 1985,* 105th ed., p.843, Washington, DC, 1984.
33. Surgeon General. *Nutrition and Health,* p.142. U.S. Dept. of Health and Human Services, #017–001–00465–1. Washington, DC: U.S. Govt. Printing Office, 1988.
34. Stini, W. A. *Federation Proceedings,* vol.40, p.2588, Sept.1981.
35. Murphy, R. S., et al. *Environmental and Health Perspectives,* vol.48, p.81, 1983.
36. Bailar, J. C., and Smith, E. M. *New England Journal of Medicine,* vol.314, p.1226, 1986.
37. Robinson, D. *Parade,* p.14, June 14, 1987.
38. Davis, D. L., and Schwartz, J. *Lancet,* vol.i., p.633, Mar.19, 1988.
39. Newell, G. R., et al. *Seminars in Oncology,* vol.16, no.1, p.3, Feb.1989.
40. Epstein, S. S. *The Politics of Cancer.* San Francisco: Sierra Club Books, 1978.
41. Howe, G. R., et al. *Journal of the National Cancer Institute,* vol.64, p.701, 1980.
42. National Cancer Institute. *Cancer Rates and Risks,* p.40, U.S. Dept. of Health and Human Services, #85–691. Washington, DC, 1985.
43. Hoover, R. *Journal of the National Cancer Institute,* vol.79, p.1269, 1987.
44. National Research Council. *op.cit.,* p.595.
45. Kurihara M., et al. (eds.) *Cancer Mortality Statistics in the World,* Nagoya, Japan: University of Nagoya Press, 1984.

46. National Research Council. *Regulating Pesticides in Food.* Washington, DC: National Academy Press, 1987.

47. *Cancer Facts and Figures: 1988,* p.6, American Cancer Society, NY, 1988.

48. Hendler, S. S. *The Complete Guide to Anti-Aging Nutrients,* p.27. NY: Simon & Schuster, 1985.

49. Hanson, M. R., and Mulvihill, J. J. *Cancer in the Young,* p.3. NY: Arthur Levine Publ., 1982.

50. National Cancer Institute. *Cancer Statistics Review 1973–1986,* p.III-20, U.S. Dept. Health and Human Services, National Institute of Health pub. #89-2789, Washington, DC, May 1988.

51. Stahnke, N., and Zeisel, H. J. *European Journal of Pediatrics,* vol.148, no.7, p.591, June 1989; see also *Canadian Medical Association,* vol.139, no.9, p.877, Nov.1988.

52. Weiss, B. *Toxicology and Industrial Health,* vol.4, no.3, p.351, Sept.1988.

53. Fan, A. M., and Jackson, R. J. *Regulatory Toxicology and Pharmacology,* vol.9, p.158, 1989.

54. Surgeon General. *Healthy People: The Surgeon's Report on Health Promotion and Disease Prevention.* p.68, pub.#79-55071A, Washington, DC, 1979.

55. Witkin, M. J. *Trends in Patient Care Episodes,* U.S. Dept. Health and Human Services, #154, Sept.1980.

56. Ross, D. M., et al. *Hyperactivity.* p.3, NY: John Wiley & Sons, 1982.

57. *U.S. News and World Report,* p.13, Nov.20, 1989.

58. Wheater, R. H. *Journal of the American Medical Association,* vol.253, p.2288, Apr.1985.

59. Littlewood, J. T., et al. *Lancet,* vol.i, p.558, Mar.12, 1988.

60. Wurtman, R. J. *Lancet,* p.1060, Nov.1985.

61. Nation, J. R., et al. *Neurotoxicology,* vol.8, no.4, p.561, 1987.

62. Bellinger, D., et al. *New England Journal of Medicine,* vol.316, p.1037, Apr.23, 1987; see also Raloff, J. *Science News,* p.333, Nov.22, 1986.

63. Schwartz, J., et al. *Pediatrics,* vol.77, p.281, 1986.

[64]. Bellinger, D., et al. *New England Journal of Medicine,* vol.316, p.1037, Apr.23, 1987.

[65]. Raloff, J. *Science News,* p.333, Nov.22, 1986.

[66]. Galler, J. R. (ed.) *Nutrition and Behavior,* p.175. Plenum Press, NY, 1984.

[67]. Ritz, E., et al. *Advances in Nephrology,* vol.17, p.241, 1988.

[68]. Needleman, H. L. *American Journal of Public Health,* vol.79, no.5, p.643, 1989.

[69]. Jayson, M. I., et al. *Understanding Arthritis and Rheumatism.* NY: Pantheon Books, 1974.

[70]. Darlington, L. G., et al. *Lancet,* vol.i, p.236, Feb.1, 1986.

[71]. Paldy, A., et al. *Science of the Total Environment,* vol.73, no.3, p.229, July 15, 1988.

[72]. Forman, M. B., et al. *New England Journal of Medicine,* vol.313, no.18, p.1138, Oct.1985.

[73]. Willett, W., et al. *New England Journal of Medicine,* vol.310, p.633, Mar.1984.

[74]. Breneman, J. *Basics of Food Allergy.* Springfield, IL: C. C. Thomas, 1984.

[75]. Weissman, J. D. *Choose To Live.* NY: Grove Press, 1988.

[76]. Olson, L. *Journal of Pesticide Reform,* Summer, 1986.

[77]. Bellina, J. H., and Wilson, J. *YOU CAN HAVE A BABY.* NY: Bantam Books, 1985.

[78]. Cimons, M. *Los Angeles Times,* p.A41, Dec.3, 1989.

[79]. Edmonds, L. D., et al. *Temporal Trends in the Incidence of Malformation in the United States,* p.1ss, vol.24, no.2ss, 1985.

[80]. *Los Angeles Times,* p.2, Sept.24, 1989.

[81]. *Journal of Food Protection,* vol.48, p.887, 1985.

[82]. Rodriguez, C. A., et al. *Journal of Pediatrics,* vol.107, p.393, 1985.

CHAPTER 4: PESTICIDES: THE FALLEN ANGEL

1. Carson, R. *Silent Spring*. NY: Fawcett Crest, 1962, p.29.
2. Dover, M. *Technology Review*, p.53, Nov.1985.
3. Pimentel, D., et al. *BioScience*, vol.28, no.12, p.772, Dec.1978.
4. Meadows, D. *Los Angeles Times*, p.m4, Nov.19, 1989.
5. *The Economist*, p.97, Mar.21, 1987.
6. McGrath, C., et al. (eds.) *Pesticides: A Community Action Guide.* p.12, Washington DC: Concern, Inc., 1985.
7. Metcalf, R. L., and W. H. Luckman. *Introduction to Pest Management*. NY: John Wiley Publishers, 1982. *passim*.
8. Hanson, B. *The Amicus Journal*, p.3, Summer 1989.
9. Moses, M. *American Association of Occupational and Health Nurses*, vol.37, no.3, p.115, Mar.1989.
10. State of California, Dept. of Health Services. *Pesticides: Health Aspects of Exposure and Issues Surrounding Their Use.* Hazard Evaluation Section, Berkeley, CA, June 1988.
11. Kim, Y. *Cornell Chronicle*. June 26, 1986, p.17.

CHAPTER 5: OUR WIDESPREAD POLLUTION

1. U.S. Bureau of the Census. *Statistical Abstract of the United States: 1985,* 105th ed., Washington, DC 1984.
2. Epstein, S. S., et al. *Hazardous Waste in America.* p.iv. San Francisco: Sierra Club Books; 1982.
3. Brownlee, S. *U.S. News and World Report.* Aug.21, 1989, p.52.
4. State of California, Dept. Health Services. *Pesticides: Health Aspects of Exposure and Issues Surrounding Their Use.* Hazard Evaluation Section, Berkeley, CA, June 1988.
5. Johnston L. *Environmental Action.* Jan./Feb.1987, p.8.
6. Brown, M. H. *Discover.* Nov.1987, p.42.
7. Mosher, M., and G. Moyer. *Nutrition Action Newsletter.* Center for Science in the Public Interest, Nov.1980.

[8]. Rogan, W. J., et al. *New England Journal of Medicine.* vol.302, p.1450, 1980.

[9]. Allen, J. R., et al. *Food and Cosmetics Toxicology.* vol.15, p.401, 1977.

[10]. Thurston, F. E. *American Family Physician,* p.203, Jan.1988.

[11]. Rogan, W. J., et al. *American Journal of Public Health,* vol.76, no.2, p.172, Feb.1986.

[12]. Magnuson, E. *Time.* Oct.14, 1985, p.76.

[13]. *Los Angeles Times.* July 3, 1988, part 1, p.28.

[14]. *Milwaukee Journal.* p.3a, Oct.1, 1989.

[15]. *Newsweek.* Aug.1, 1988, p.44.

[16]. Mott, L., and K. Snyder. *Pesticide Alert.* San Francisco: Sierra Club Books, 1987.

[17]. Eaton, W. J. *Los Angeles Times.* Jan.15, 1989, part 1, p.4.

[18]. Jacobs, P. *Los Angeles Times.* Aug.13, 1989, part 1, p.3.

[19]. Ehrlich, E., et al. *Business Week.* p.154, Sept.25, 1989.

[20]. Bruske, E. *Los Angeles Times.* p.e12, Oct.22, 1989.

CHAPTER 6: SHOULD WE CALL IT "GOVERNMENT IN ACTION" OR "GOVERNMENT INACTION"?

[1]. Government Accounting Office. *Federal Regulation of Pesticide Residues in Food.* GAE/T-Rced-87-21, Apr.30, 1987.

[2]. Shodell, M. *Science.* p.43, Oct.1985.

[3]. Personal communication with Rabbi Langer of San Diego, California, 1989.

[4]. Food and Drug Administration. *Residues in Foods-1987.* FDA, Washington, DC.

[5]. Center for Science in the Public Interest. *Pesticide Residues in Meat.* Washington, DC.

[6]. Long, P. J., and B. Shannon. *Nutrition: An Inquiry into the Issues.* p.387. Englewood Cliffs, NJ: Prentice-Hall, 1983.

[7]. Isaac, K., and S. Gold. *Eating Clean.* p.85. Center for Study of Responsive Law, Washington, DC, 1987.

[8]. National Coalition Against the Misuse of Pesticides, *Pesticides and You,* vol.9, no.3, p.1, Aug.1989.

[9]. National Center for Health Statistics. *Health: United States, 1988.* Dept. Health and Human Services, publ.#89–1232, U.S. Govt. Printing Off., Washington, DC, Mar. 1989.

[10]. Fan, A. M., and Jackson, R. J. *Regulatory Toxicology and Pharmacology.* vol.9, p.158, 1989.

[11]. Skeets, K., et al. *U.S. News and World Report.* p.53, Sept.18, 1989.

[12]. Montgomery, A. *Nutrition Action.* vol.14, no.5, p.1, June 1987.

[13]. Meadows, D. H. *Los Angeles Times.* part 5, p.3, Dec.4, 1988.

[14]. Foran, J. A., et al. *American Journal of Public Health.* vol.79, p.322, 1989.

[15]. Ershoff, B. H. *Journal of Food Science.* vol.41, p.949, 1976.

[16]. *Nutrition Action Health Letter.* vol.14, no.10, p.3, Dec.1987.

[17]. General Accounting Office. *Pesticides: Need to Enhance FDA's Ability to Protect the Public from Illegal Residues.* Washington, DC, 1986.

[18]. Barnhill, M., and B. Barrett. *Glendale Daily News.* p.1, Dec.23, 1986.

[19]. GAO. *Pesticides: EPA's Formidable Task to Assess and Regulate Their Risks.* Apr.1986.

[20]. Allman, W. F. *Science.* p.14, Oct.1985.

[21]. Milbourn, M. A. *Glendale Daily News.* p.12, Jan.13, 1988.

[22]. Bashin, B. J. *Harrowsmith.* p.41, Jan.1987.

[23]. Mott, L., and K. Snyder. *Pesticide Alert.* p.62. San Francisco: Sierra Club, 1987.

[24]. Hearne, S. A. *Harvest of Unknowns.* p.13, Natural Resources Defense Council, NY, 1984.

[25]. GAO. *Better Regulation of Pesticide Exports and Pesticide Residues in Imported Foods is Essential,* CED-79-43, June 22, 1979, p.iii, 39.

[26]. West, K. *Glendale Daily News,* p.6, Jan.28, 1988.

[27]. Quinn, L. *Glendale Daily News,* p.3, Apr.23, 1988.

CHAPTER 7: WHAT'S IN THE FOOD?

[1]. Beck, M., et al. *Newsweek.* p.16, Mar.27, 1989.

[2]. *Lancet*, vol.i, p.1387, June 13, 1987.

[3]. *Safe Food Gazette,* p.3, Americans for Safe Food, Washington, DC.

[4]. Saunders, J. C. *Veterinary Record.* vol.123, p.464, 1988.

[5]. Zuckerman, S. *Nutrition Action Healthletter,* p.8, Jan.1985.

[6]. Spika, J. S., et al. *New England Journal of Medicine,* vol.316, no.10, p.565, 1987.

[7]. Markus, C. K., et al. *American Journal of Cardiology.* vol.63, p.1154, May 1989.

[8]. Blume, E., and Jacobsen, M. *Nutrition Action Health Letter,* vol.13, no.10, p.1, Nov.1986.

[9]. *Hippocrates.* p.28, Nov.1988.

[10]. Institute of Food Technologists. *Food Technology,* p.109, Dec.1986.

[11]. McGivney, W. T. *Seminars in Nuclear Medicine,* vol.18, no.1, p.36, Jan.1988.

[12]. *Los Angeles Times,* part 1, p.2, July 24, 1988.

[13]. Piccioni, R. *The Ecologist,* p.48, vol.18, no.2, 1988.

[14]. Bhaskaram, C., and Sadasivan, G. *American Journal of Clinical Nutrition.* vol.28, no.2, p.130, 1975.

[15]. Levina, A. I., and Ivanov, A. E. *Bulletin of Experimental and Biological Medicine.* vol.85, no.2, p.236.

[16]. Ralston Purina Company. Final Report: Contract 53-3K06-1-29, Animal Feeding Study for Irradiation Sterilized Chicken, June 1983.

[17]. Food and Drug Administration. Federal Register, vol.49, no.31, p.5715, Feb.14, 1984, docket no.81N-0004.

[18]. Schindler, A. F., et al. *Journal of Food Protection,* vol.43, no.1, p.7, 1980.

[19]. deWolff, F. A. *Human Toxicology,* vol.7, p.443, 1988.

[20]. *Nutrition Reviews,* vol.34 p.347, 1976.

[21]. Harris, T. *Press Enterprise, Riverside,* p.1, Dec.4, 1988.

[22]. Lai, D. Y. *Nutrition Report,* vol.7, no.1, p.8, Jan.1989.

[23]. *San Diego Union,* p.2, July 27, 1985.

24. Willett, W., et al. *New England Journal of Medicine*, p.1159, Nov. 13, 1980.

25. Quillin, P., and Reyonlds, A. G. *The La Costa Book of Nutrition*. p.149. NY: Pharos Books, 1988.

26. Fan, A. M., and Jackson, R. J. *Regulatory Toxicology and Pharmacology*, vol.9, p.158, 1989.

27. *Nutrition Action Health Letter*, vol.15, no.3, p.3, Apr.1988.

28. Mitchell, C. P., and Jacobsen, M. F. *Tainted Booze*. Center for Science in the Public Interest, Washington, DC, 1987.

29. Long P., et al. *Nutrition: An Inquiry into the Issues.* p.389. Englewood Cliffs, NJ: Prentice-Hall, 1983.

30. *The Nutrition Times*, vol.2, no.1, p.1, Jan.1987.

31. *San Diego Tribune*, D-1, May 18, 1981.

32. Wheater, R. H. *Journal of the American Medical Association*, vol.253, p.2288, Apr.1985.

33. Folkers, K., et al. *Hoppe-Seylers Zeitschrift Fur Physiologische Chimie*, vol.365, p.405, Mar.1984.

34. Yudkin, J. *The Nutrition Report*, vol.7, no.8, p.1, Aug.1989.

35. FDA, Docket no., 75F-0355, U.S. Dept. of Health, Washington, DC, 1980.

36. Wurtman, R. J., *Lancet*, p.1060, Nov.1985.

37. Zapsalis, C. *Food Chemistry and Nutritional Biochemistry.* p.1061. NY: John Wiley, 1985.

38. Ames, B. N. *Science*, vol.221, p.1256, 1983.

39. Kronhausen, E., and Kronhausen, P. *Formula for Life.* p.355. NY: William Morrow, 1989.

40. *Journal of Food Protection*, vol.48, p.887, 1985.

41. Blume, E. *Nutrition Action Health Letter*, p.1, June 1986.

42. Young, F., and Skinner, K. J. *FDA Consumer*, June 1987.

43. Ryan, C. A., et al. *Journal of the American Medical Association*, vol.258, p.3269, Dec.11, 1987.

44. Barnhill, M., and Barrett, B. *Glendale Daily News*, p.11, Dec.22, 1986.

45. Barnhill, M. *Glendale Daily News*, p.18, Dec.21, 1986.

46. *Food Technology*, vol.42, no.4, p.2, Apr. 1988.

47. *Glendale Daily News*, p.5, Nov.14, 1989.

SAFE EATING • 335

48. USDA, Food Safety Inspection Service-9, Foodborne Bacterial Poisoning, 1980.
49. Caster, W. O., et al. *International Journal for Vitamin and Nutrition Research,* vol.54, p.371, 1984.
50. Rodricks, J. V. *FDA Consumer,* Oct. 1980.
51. Berry, C. L. *Journal of Pathology,* vol.154, p.301, 1988.
52. *Nutrition Action Health Letter,* vol.3, no.2, Mar.1987.
53. Hobbs, B. *Food Poisoning and Food Hygiene.* 2nd ed. London: Edward Arnold Press, 1968.
54. National Research Council. *Regulating Pesticides in Food.* p.78, Washington, DC: National Academy Press, 1987.
55. Mott, L., Snyder, K. *Pesticide Alert.* San Francisco: Sierra Club Books, 1987.
56. *Newsweek,* p.22, Mar.27, 1989.
57. *Health Research Group Health Letter,* p.13, July 1986.
58. Scott, J. *Los Angeles Times,* p.57, magazine part 2, Oct.8, 1989.
59. National Research Council. *Diet and Health.* p.481, National Academy of Sciences, Washington, DC, 1989.
60. U.S. GAO, *Seafood Safety: Seriousness of Problems and Efforts to Protect Consumers,* GAO/RCED-88-135, Aug.1988.
61. Young, F. E. *Consumer's Research.* p.10, Aug.1989.
62. Puzo, D. P. *Los Angeles Times,* p.H1, Oct.12, 1989
63. Sibbison, J. *Bestways,* p.16, Mar.1989.
64. Zamula, E. *Dairy and Food Sanitation,* p.502, Oct.1987.
65. *New England Journal of Medicine,* vol.315, p.582, Aug.28, 1986.
66. *New England Journal of Medicine,* vol.314, p.707, 1986.
67. Brownlee, S. *U.S. News and World Report,* p.52, Aug.21, 1989.
68. Lefferts, L. *Nutrition Action Health Letter,* vol.15, no.8, p.5, Oct.1988.
69. *Developmental Psychology,* vol.20, p.523, 1984.
70. Kaizer, L., et al. *Nutrition and Cancer,* vol.12, p.61, 1989.
71. Foran, J. A., et al. *American Journal of Public Health,* vol.79, p.322, Mar.1989.

[72]. *Newsweek,* p.44, Aug.1, 1988.

CHAPTER 8: WHAT'S IN THE WATER?

[1]. Hand, D. *American Health,* p.48, May 1988.
[2]. Magnuson, E., et al. *Times,* p.76, Oct.14, 1985.
[3]. Quillin, P., and Reynolds, A. G. *The La Costa Book of Nutrition.* p.74. NY: Pharos Books, 1988.
[4]. Zemla, B. *Nutrition and Cancer,* vol.11, p.1, 1988.
[5]. Isaac, K., and Gold, S. *Eating Clean,* p.65, Center for the Study of Responsive Law, Washington, DC, 1987.
[6]. Darst, G. *Glendale Daily News,* p.11, Jan.6, 1988.
[7]. Russell, H. H., et al. *Western Journal of Medicine,* vol.147, p.615, Nov.1987.
[8]. Boyd, S., et al. *Drinking Water.* p.13. Washington, DC: Concern, Inc., 1986.
[9]. Cantor, K. P., et al. *Journal of the National Cancer Institute,* vol.79, no.6, p.1269, Dec.1987.
[10]. Bagnell, P. C., and Ellenberger, H. A. *Canadian Medical Association,* vol.117, p.1047, 1977.
[11]. *Los Angeles Times,* p.2, Sept.24, 1989.
[12]. Peterson, J., *Science News,* p.103, Feb. 16, 1985.
[13]. Burlison, N. E., et al. *Environmental Science Technology,* vol.16, p.627, 1982.
[14]. Braithwaite, R. A., and Brown, S. S. *Human Toxicology,* vol.7, p.503, 1988.
[15]. Wolinsky, L. C. *Los Angeles Times,* p.3, Dec.20, 1987.
[16]. *Consumer Reports,* p.542, Sept.1988.

CHAPTER 9: HOW TO REDUCE YOUR INTAKE OF TOXINS

[1]. Ershoff, B. H. *American Journal of Clinical Nutrition,* vol.27, p.1395, 1974; see also Ershoff, B. H., *Journal of Food Science,* vol.41, p.949, 1976.

2. Gunderson, E. L. *Journal of Association of Official Analytical Chemists,* vol.71, no.6, p.1200, 1988.

3. Zaridze, D. G., et al. *International Journal of Cancer,* vol.36, p.153, 1985.

4. National Research Council. *Regulating Pesticides in Food.* p.17. Washington, DC: National Academy Press, 1987.

5. Lecos, C. W. *FDA Consumer,* Dec.1986 & Jan. 1987.

6. National Academy of Sciences. *Alternative Agriculture.* National Research Council, Washington, DC, 1989.

7. Frons, M. *Business Week,* p.232, Sept.25, 1989.

8. Center for Science in the Public Interest. *Organic Agriculture: What the States Are Doing.* CSPI, 1501 16th St. NW, Washington, DC 20036.

9. *New York Times,* p.3, Dec.26, 1986.

10. Holehouse, D. *Edmonton Journal,* Oct.2, 1987.

11. Sheets, K. R., et al. *U.S. News and World Report,* p.53, Sept.18, 1989.

12. Kristof, K. M. *Glendale Daily News,* p.1, Mar.26, 1989.

13. Kendall, D., and Brusko, M. *The New Farm,* p.8, Feb.1988.

14. Sinclair, W. *Washington Post,* p.4, Mar.1, 1987.

15. *Nutrition Action Healthletter,* p.2, Jan.1985.

16. Thorndike, J. *Country Journal,* p.39, Apr.1982.

17. Creasy, R. *Edible Landscaping.* San Francisco: Sierra Club Books, 1982.

18. Fordham, J., et al. *Journal of Food Science,* vol.40, p.552, 1975.

19. Chen, L., et al. *Journal of Food Science,* vol.42, no.6, p.1666, 1977.

20. Chen, L., et al. *Journal of Food Science,* vol.40, p.1290, 1975.

21. Boyd, S., et al. (eds.) *Drinking Water: A Community Action Guide.* p.28. Washington, DC: Concern, Inc., 1986.

22. Sewell, B. H. *Business and Society Review,* no.59, p.46, Fall 1986.

CHAPTER 10: FOODS THAT INCREASE YOUR TOLERANCE OF TOXINS

[1]. Ames, B. N., et al. *Science,* vol.236, p.271, 1987.
[2]. Pendergrass, T. W. *Childhood Lymphoblastic Leukemia.* Pochedly, C. (ed.), p.11. Westport, CT: Praeger, 1985.
[3]. Epstein, S. S. *The Politics of Cancer.* San Francisco: Sierra Club Books, 1978.
[4]. Bailar, J. C., et al. *New England Journal of Medicine,* vol.314, p.1226, May 8, 1986.
[5]. Bartley, D. *Saturday Evening Post,* p.58, Nov.1989.
[6]. Lowe, J. *Glendale Daily News,* p.4, June 1, 1987.
[7]. Patterson, B. H., and Block, G. *American Journal of Public Health,* vol.78, p.282, Mar.1988.
[8]. Boyd, J. N., et al. *Food Chemistry and Toxicology,* vol.20, p.47, 1982.
[9]. Hitchins, A. D., and McDonough, F. E. *American Journal of Clinical Nutrition,* vol.49, p.675, 1989.
[10]. Niv, M., and Greenstein, N. M. *Clinical Pediatrics,* vol.2, p.407, 1963.
[11]. Salvador, P., and Salvadori, B. *Minerva Dietologica* (Italian), vol.14, p.8, 1973.
[12]. Mitchell, I. de G., and Kenworthy, R. *Journal of Applied Bacteriology,* vol.41, p.163, 1976.
[13]. Hitchins, A.D., et al. *American Journal of Clinical Nutrition,* vol.41, p.92, 1985.
[14]. Vesely, R., et al. *Journal of Immunology and Immunopharmacology,* vol.5, no.1, p.30, 1985.
[15]. Hitchins, A.D., et al. *Nutrition Reports International,* vol.31, p.601, 1985.
[16]. Yazicioğlu, A. von, and Yilmaz, N. *Milchwissenschaft* (German), vol.21, p.87, 1966.
[17]. Shahani, K. M., et al. *Society for Applied Bacteriology Symposium Series,* vol.11, p.257, 1983.
[18]. Shapiro, S. *Clinical Medicine,* vol.7, p.295, 1960.
[19]. Conge, G., et al. *Reproduction, Nutrition, Development* (French), vol.20, p.929, 1980.

[20]. DeSimone, C., et al. *Nutrition Reports International,* vol.33, p.419, 1986.

[21]. Ngumbi, P.M., and Nyakeri, L.N. *East African Medical Journal,* vol.61, no.5, p.372, May 1984.

[22]. Hitchins, A. D. and McDonough, F. E. *American Journal of Clinical Nutrition,* vol.49, p.675, 1989.

[23]. *Nutrition Reviews,* vol.42, no.11, p.374, Nov.1984.

[24]. Goldin, B. R., et al. *American Journal of Clinical Nutrition,* vol.39, p.756, 1984.

[25]. Gorbach, S. L. *Infection,* vol.10, no.6, p.379, 1982.

[26]. Le, M. G., et al. *Journal of the National Cancer Institute,* vol.77, p.633, 1986.

[27]. van Veer, P., et al. *Cancer Research,* vol.49, no.14, p.4020, July 15, 1989.

[28]. Friend, B. A., et al. *Journal of Applied Nutrition,* vol.36, no.2, p.125, 1984.

[29]. Shahani, K. M., et al. *Society of Applied Bacteriology Symposium Serial,* vol.11, p.257, 1983.

[30]. Bogdanov, I. G., et al. *Bulletin of Experimental Biological Medicine,* vol.84, p.1750, 1978.

[31]. Long, P. J., and Shannon, B. *Nutrition: An Inquiry into the Issues,* p.59. Englewood Cliffs, NJ: Prentice-Hall, 1983.

[32]. Kilara, A., and Shahani, K. M. *Journal of Dairy Science,* vol.59, p.2031, 1976.

[33]. Cochet, B., et al. *Gastroenterology,* vol.84, p.935, 1983.

[34]. Shashikanth, K. N., et al. *Folia Microbiologica,* vol.29, no.4, p.348, 1984.

[35]. Johnson, M. G., and Vaughn, R. H. *Applied Microbiology,* vol.17, p.903, 1969.

[36]. Fromtling, R. A., and Bulmer, G. S. *Mycologia,* vol.70, p.397, 1978: see also Delaha, E. C., et al. *Antimicrobial Agents and Chemotherapy,* vol.27, no.4, p.485, Apr.1985.

[37]. Amer, M., et al. *International Journal of Dermatology,* vol.19, p.285, 1980.

[38]. Adetumbi, M. A., and Lau, B. H. *Medical Hypotheses,* vol.12, no.3, p.227, 1983.

[39]. Prasad, G., and Sharma, V. D. *British Veterinarian Journal,* vol.136, p.448, 1980.

[40]. Tsai, Y., et al. *Planta Medica,* vol.5, p.460, Oct.1985.

[41]. Dept. of Neurology, *Chinese Medical Journal,* vol.93, p.123, 1980.

[42]. Delaha, E. C., et al. *Antimicrobial Agents and Chemotherapy,* vol.27, no.4, p.485, 1985.

[43]. *American Institute for Cancer Research Newsletter,* p.5, Fall, 1989.

[44]. Abdullah, T. H., et al. *Journal of the National Medical Association,* vol.80, no.4, p.439, Apr. 1988.

[45]. Belman, S. *Carcinogenesis,* vol.4, no.8, p.1063, 1983.

[46]. Kroning, F. *Acta Unio Intern.Contra.Cancrum,* vol.20, no.3, p.855, 1964.

[47]. You, W. C., et al. *Journal of the National Cancer Institute,* vol.81, p.162, Jan.18, 1989.

[48]. Ziment, I. *Practical Pulmonary Disease.* NY: John Wiley & Sons, 1983.

[49]. Fujiwara, M., and Natata, T. *Nature,* vol.216, p.84, 1967.

[50]. Nakagawa, S., et al. *Hiroshima Journal of Medical Science,* vol.34, no.3, p.303, Sept. 1985.

[51]. Lau, B. H., and Adetumbi, M. A. *Nutrition Research,* vol.3, p.119, 1983.

[52]. Morash, M. *The Victory Garden Cookbook.* NY: Alfred Knopf, 1982.

[53]. Walford, R. *Maximum Life Span.* NY: W. W. Norton, 1983.

[54]. Peto, R., et al. *Nature,* vol.290, p.201, Mar. 1981.

[55]. Norell, S. E., et al. *American Journal of Epidemiology,* vol.124, p.895, 1986.

[56]. Hennekens, C. H., et al. *Cancer,* vol.58, p.1837, 1986.

[57]. Mahmoud, L. A., et al. *International Journal of Cancer,* vol.30, p.143, 1982.

[58]. Stahelin, H. B., et al. *Journal of the National Cancer Institute,* vol.73, p.1463, Dec.1984.

[59]. Modan, B., et al. *International Journal of Cancer,* vol.28, p.421, 1981.

[60]. Magnus, K., (ed.) *Trends in Cancer Incidence.* Washington, DC: Hemisphere Publ., 1982.
[61]. LaVecchia, C. L., et al. *International Journal of Cancer,* vol.34, p.319, 1984.
[62]. Peto, R. *Cancer Surveys,* vol.2, p.327, 1983.
[63]. Blaun, R., and Belson, A. *Medical Month,* vol.1, p.53, 1983.
[64]. Micksche, M., et al. *Oncology,* vol.34, p.234, 1977.
[65]. Watson, R. R., and Moriguchi, S. *Nutrition Research,* vol.5, p.663, 1985; see also Watson, R. R. *Nutrition, Disease Resistance, and Immune Function.* NY: Maracel Dekker Pub., 1984.
[66]. Abraham, S. K., et al. *Mutation Research,* vol.172, p.51, 1986.
[67]. Park, Y. W. *Journal of Food Science,* vol.52, p.1022, 1987.
[68]. Bendich, A. *Federation of American Society of Experimental Biologists,* vol.3, p.1927, 1989.
[69]. Lourau, J., et al. *Experientia,* vol.6, p.25, 1950.
[70]. Spector, L., et al. *Proceedings of the Society for Experimental Biology and Medicine,* vol.100, p.405, 1959.
[71]. Wattenberg, L. W. *Cancer Research,* (sup.), vol.43, p.2488s, May 1983.
[72]. Graham, S., et al. *American Journal of Epidemiology,* vol.109, no.1, p.1, Jan.1979.
[73]. National Research Council. *Diet, Nutrition, and Cancer.* Washington, DC: National Academy Press, 1982.
[74]. Sugimura, T. *Science,* vol.233, p.312, July 1986.
[75]. Hoff, G., et al. *Scandinavian Journal of Gastroenterology,* vol.21, p.199, 1986.
[76]. Graham, S. *Cancer Research* (sup.), vol.43, p.2409s, 1983.
[77]. Marshall, J. R., et al. *Journal of the National Cancer Institute,* vol.70, p.847, 1983.
[78]. Ansher, S. S. *Federation of Chemistry and Toxicology,* vol.24, p.405, 1986.
[79]. Kensler, T. W., et al. *Cancer Research,* vol.47, p.4271, 1987.
[80]. Godlewski, C. E., et al. *Cancer Letters,* vol.28, p.151, 1985.
[81]. Tajima, K., and Tominaga, S. *Japanese Journal of Cancer Research,* vol.76, p.705, 1985.

[82]. Anderson, J. W. *American Journal of Clinical Nutrition,* vol.40, p.1146, 1984.

[83]. Graf, E., et al. *Journal of Biological Chemistry,* vol.262, p.11647, 1987.

[84]. Yavelow, J., et al. *Cancer Research* (sup.), vol.43, p.2454s, 1983.

[85]. Troll, W., et al. *Prostate,* vol.4, p.345, 1983.

[86]. Kennedy, A., and Little, J. B. *Cancer Research,* vol.41, p.2103, 1981.

[87]. Kennedy, A. *Carcinogenesis,* vol.6, p.1441, 1985.

[88]. Kennedy, A. R., and Billings, P. C., *Anticarcinogenesis and Radiation Protection.* Cerutti, P. A., et al. (eds), p.285. NY: Plenum Pub., 1987.

[89]. Beiler, J. M., et al. *Experimental Medicine and Surgery,* vol.11, p.179, 1953; see also Sanyal, S. N. *Science and Culture,* vol.25, no.12, p.661, June 1960.

[90]. Correa, P. *Cancer Research,* vol.40, p.3685, 1984.

[91]. Kronhausen, E., and Kronhausen, P. *Formula for Life,* p.401. NY: W. Morrow, 1989.

[92]. Teas, J. *Medical Hypotheses,* vol.7, p.601, 1981.

[93]. Teas, J. *Cancer Research,* vol.44, p.2758, 1984.

[94]. Reddy, B. S., et al. *Advances in Cancer Research,* vol.32, p.237, 1980.

[95]. Yamamoto, I., et al. *Japanese Journal of Experimental Medicine,* vol.44, p.543, 1974; see also Yamamoto, I., et al. *Cancer Letters,* vol.35, p.109, 1987.

[96]. Furosawa, E., and Furosawa S. *Oncology,* vol.42, p.364, 1985.

[97]. Story, J. A., and Kritchevsky, D. *American Journal of Clinical Nutrition,* vol.31, p.s199, 1978.

[98]. Raicht, R. F., et al. *Cancer Research,* vol.40, p.402, 1980.

[99]. Mautner, G. G., et al. *Journal of the American Pharmacology Association,* vol.42, p.294, 1953; see also Pratt, R., et al. *Journal of the American Pharmacology Association,* vol.40, p.575, 1951; see also Vacca, D. D., et al. *Journal of the American Pharmacology Association,* vol.43, p.24, 1954.

[100]. Kaneda, T. H. *Proceedings of the Seventh International Seaweed Symposium,* p.553. NY: John Wiley & Sons, 1972.

[101]. Sieburth, J. M. N. *Sciences*, vol.132, p.676, 1960.

[102]. McConnell, O. H. in *Marine Algae in Pharmaceutical Science*. Hoppe, H. A., et al. (eds.) NY: DeGruyter Pub., 1979.

[103]. Yosisige, K. *Herba Polonica*, vol.16, p.96, 1970.

[104]. Stara, J. F. *Abstracts of Symposium on Nuclear Medicine*. Omaha, NE, 1965.

[105]. Watanabe, Y. in *Advance in Phycology in Japan*. Tokida, H. (ed.), VEB Gustav Fischer Verlag Pub., 1975.

[106]. Konowalchuk, J., et al. *Applied and Environmental Microbiology*, vol.36, no.6, p.798, Dec.1978.

[107]. Konowalchuk, J., et al. *Journal of Food Science*, vol.41, p.1013, 1976.

[108]. Baig, M. M., et al. *ACS Symposium Series*, vol.143, p.25, 1980.

[109]. Ganguly, R., et al. *Indian Journal of Medical Research*, vol.66, no.3, p.359, Sept.1977.

[110]. Sobota, A. E. *Journal of Urology*, vol.131, p.1013, May 1984.

[111]. Moen, D. V. *Wisconsin Medical Journal*, vol.61, p.282, 1962; see also Der Marderosian, A. H. *Drug Therapy*, p.151, Nov.1977.

[112]. Surgeon General. *Nutrition and Health*, p.97, U.S. Dept. Health and Human Services, GPO# 017-001-00465-1, Washington, DC, 1988.

[113]. Robinson, C. H. *Fundamentals of Normal Nutrition*, p.86. NY: Macmillan, 1978.

[114]. Yolken, R. H. *New England Journal of Medicine*, vol.312, p.605, Mar.7, 1985.

[115]. Talbot, J. M. *Federation Proceeding*, vol.40, no.9, p.2337, July 1981.

[116]. Ershoff, B. H. *Journal of Food Science*, vol.41, p.949, 1976; see also Ershoff, B. H. *American Journal of Clinical Nutrition*, vol.27, p.1395, 1974.

[117]. Greenward, P., et al. *Contemporary Nutrition*, vol.11, p.1, 1986; or American Cancer Society, *Cancer*, vol.34, no.2, p.121, 1984; or McKeoun-Eyssen, G., et al. *Nutrition and Cancer*, vol.6, p.160, 1984; or Englyst, H. N., et al. *Nutrition*

and Cancer, vol.4, p.50, 1982; or Modan B., et al. *Journal of the National Cancer Institute,* vol.55, p.15, 1975.

[118]. Hughes, R. E. *Human Nutrition: Clinical Nutrition,* vol.40C, p.81, 1986.

[119]. Howie, B. J., et al. *American Journal of Clinical Nutrition,* vol.432, p.127, 1985.

[120]. Kochi, M., et al. *Cancer Treatments Report,* vol.69, no.5, p.533, May 1985; see also Takeuchi, S., et al. *Agricultural and Biological Chemistry,* vol.42, no.7, p.1449, 1978.

[121]. Karmali, R. S., et al. *Journal of the National Cancer Institute,* vol.73, p.457, 1984; see also Jurkowski, J. J., et al. *Journal of the National Cancer Institute,* vol.74, p.1145, 1985; see also Carroll, K. K., et al. *Nutrition and Cancer,* vol.6, p.254, 1984.

[122]. John, T. J., et al. *Indian Journal of Medical Research,* vol.69, p.542, Apr. 1979.

[123]. Tanizawa, H., et al. *Chemical and Pharmaceutical Bulletin,* vol.32, no.5, p.2011, 1984.

[124]. Wattenberg, L. W., *Cancer Research,* sup., vol.43, p.2488s, May 1983.

[125]. Kada, T., et al. *Mutation Research,* vol.150, p.127, 1985.

[126]. Stich, H. F., et al. *International Journal of Cancer,* vol.30, no.6, p.719, Dec.1982; see also Stich, H. F., et al. *Mutation Research,* vol.95, no.2, p.119, Aug. 1982.

[127]. Lai, D. Y. *The Nutrition Report,* vol.7, no.1, p.8, Jan.1989.

[128]. Majno, G. *The Healing Hand.* Cambridge, MA: Harvard Univ., 1975.

[129]. Bergman, A., et al. *American Journal of Surgery,* vol.145, no.3, p.374, Mar.1983.

[130]. Haffejee, I. E., et al. *British Medical Journal,* vol.290, p.1866, June 1985; see also Jedder, A., et al. *South African Medical Journal,* vol.67, no.7, p.257, Feb.1985.

[131]. Garland, C., et al. *Lancet,* p.307, Feb.9, 1985.

[132]. Yolken, R. H. *New England Journal of Medicine,* vol.312, p.605, Mar.7, 1985.

[133]. Takehara, M., et al. *Kobe Journal of Medical Science,* vol.30, no.3, p.25, Aug.1984.

[134]. Sugano, N., et al. *Cancer Letters,* vol.17, p.109, 1982.

[135]. Block, E. *Scientific American,* p.114, Mar.1985.

[136]. Sparnins, V. L., et al. *Carcinogenesis,* vol.9, no.1, p.131, Jan.1988.

[137]. You, W. C., et al. *Journal of the National Cancer Institute,* vol.81, no.2, p.162, Jan.18, 1989.

[138]. Lai, C. N., et al. *Mutation Research,* vol.77, p.245, 1980.

[139]. Barale, R., et al. *Mutation Research,* vol.120, p.145, 1983.

[140]. Marshall, J. R., et al. *Journal of the National Cancer Institute,* vol.70, no.5, p.847, May 1983.

[141]. Colkitz, G. A., et al. *American Journal of Clinical Nutrition,* vol.41, p.32, Jan.1985.

[142]. Mott, L., and Snyder, K. *Pesticide Alert.* San Francisco: Sierra Club Books, 1987.

[143]. Bernstein, J., et al. *American Journal of Clinical Nutrition,* vol.30, p.613, 1977.

[144]. Sanchez, A, et al., *American Journal of Clinical Nutrition,* vol.26, p.180, 1973.

[145]. Nalder, B.N., et al. *Journal of Nutrition,* Apr. 1972.

[146]. Bristol, JB, et al., *Proceedings of the American Association of Cancer Research,* vol.26, p.206, March 1985; or Bristol, JB *British Medical Journal,* vol.291, p.1457, 1985; or Seely, S., et al., *Medical Hypotheses,* vol.11, no.3, p.319, 1983; or Hoehn, SK, et al., *Nutrition and Cancer,* vol.1, no.3, p.27, Spring 1979.

CHAPTER 11: NUTRIENTS THAT INCREASE YOUR TOLERANCE OF TOXINS

[1]. Prasad, K. N., and Rama, B. N. in *Yearbook of Nutritional Medicine,* p.179. New Canaan, CT: Keats, 1985.

[2]. Surgeon General. *Nutrition and Health.* Dept. Health and Human Services, GPO# 017-001-00465-1, Washington, DC, 1988.

[3]. Newberne, P. M., and Conner, M. W. *Federation Proceedings,* vol.45, p.149, Feb.1986.

[4]. Ames, B. N. *Science,* vol.221, p.1256, Sept. 1983.
[5]. Machlin, L. J., and Bendich, A. *Federation of American Society for Experimental Biology,* vol.1, p.441, 1987.
[6]. Rao, A. V., et al. *Nutrition and Cancer,* vol.11, p.11, 1988.
[7]. Machlin, L. J. *Medical, Biochemical, and Chemical Aspects of Free Radicals,* p.351. NY: Elsevier Publ., 1989.
[8]. Machlin, L. J. *Nutrition,* p.51, 1987.
[9]. *Safety of Vitamins and Minerals.* Council for Responsible Nutrition, Washington, DC, 1986.
[10]. Kirn, T. F. *Journal of the American Medical Association,* vol.259, p.1296, Mar.4, 1988.
[11]. Pryor, W. A. *Free Radical Biology and Medicine,* vol.3, p.189, 1987.
[12]. Diplock, A. T. *Free Radical Biology and Medicine,* vol.3, p.199, 1987.
[13]. Bieri, J. G. *Free Radical Biology and Medicine,* vol.3, p.193, 1987.
[14]. Draper, H. H., and Bird, R. P. *Free Radical Biology and Medicine,* vol.3, p.203, 1987.
[15]. Worthington-Roberts, B., et al. *Journal of the American Dietetic Association,* vol.84, p.795, 1984.
[16]. Chandra, R. K. *Nutrition Research,* vol.8, p.225, 1988.
[17]. Craddock, V. M. *Lancet,* p.217, Jan.24, 1987.
[18]. Sugimura, T. *Science,* vol.233, p.312, July 1986.
[19]. Kune, G. A., and Kune, S. *Nutrition and Cancer,* vol.9, p.1, 1987.
[20]. Thorkild, I. A., et al. *New England Journal of Medicine,* vol.318, p.727, Mar.24, 1988.
[21]. Miyamoto, H., et al. *Cancer,* vol.60, p.1159, Sept. 1987.
[22]. Quillin, P. *Healing Nutrients.* NY: Vintage Books, 1987.
[23]. National Research Council. *Recommended Dietary Allowances,* p.1. Washington, DC: National Academy Press, 1989.
[24]. Hegsted, D. M., *Journal of Nutrition,* vol.116, p.478, 1986.
[25]. Golenski, J. D., and Blum, S. R. *Oregon Medicaid Priority-Setting Project.* Bioethics Consultation Group, Inc., Berkeley, CA (415-486-0626), Mar.1989.

[26]. Bendich, A. *Nutrition and Immunology,* p.125. NY: Alan R. Liss, 1988.

[27]. Horwitt, M. K. *American Journal of Clinical Nutrition,* vol.47, p.1088, June 1988.

[28]. Bendich, A., and Machlin, L. J. *American Journal of Clinical Nutrition,* vol.48, p.612, Sept.1988.

[29]. *Nutrition Research,* vol.7, p.801, 1987.

[30]. Machlin, L. J., and Bendich, A. *Federation of American Society for Experimental Biologists,* vol.1, p.441, 1987.

[31]. Stahelin, H. B., et al. *Journal of the National Cancer Institute,* vol.73, p.1463, 1984.

[32]. Orr, J. W., et al. *American Journal of Obstetrics and Gynecology,* vol.151, p.632, 1985; see also Romney, S. L., et al. *American Journal of Obstetrics and Gynecology,* vol.151, p.976, 1985.

[33]. Graham, S., et al. *American Journal of Epidemiology,* vol.113, no.6, p.675, 1981.

[34]. Fontham, E. T., et al. *Cancer,* vol.62, p.2267, Nov.15, 1988.

[35]. O'Connor, H. J., et al. *Carcinogenesis,* vol.6, no.11, p.1675, 1985; see also Wagner, D. A., et al. *Cancer Research,* vol.45, p.6519, 1985.

[36]. Greenblatt, M. *Journal of the National Cancer Institute,* vol.50, no.4, p.1055, 1973.

[37]. Bodo, M., et al. *Oncology,* vol.46, p.178, 1989.

[38]. Poydock, M. E., et al. *Experimental Cellular Biology,* vol.47, no.3, p.210, 1979.

[39]. Dowd, P.S., et al. *British Journal of Nutrition,* vol.55, p.515, 1986.

[40]. Bendich, A. *Food Technology,* p.112, Nov.1987.

[41]. Prinz, W., et al. *International Journal of Vitamin and Nutrition Research,* vol.47, no.3, p.248, 1977.

[42]. Kennes, B., et al. *Gerontology,* vol.29, no.5, p.305, 1983.

[43]. Cathcart, R. *Medical Hypotheses,* vol.14, p.423, 1984.

[44]. Martell, A. E. *Ascorbic Acid: Chemistry, Metabolism, and Uses.* Sieb, P.A. (ed.), p.153, American Chemical Society, Washington, DC, 1982.

[45]. Gerster, H., and Moser, U. *Nutrition Research,* vol.8, p.1327, 1988.

[46]. Peto, R., et al. *Nature,* vol.290, p.201, Mar.1981.

[47]. Bendich, A., et al. *Federation of American Society for Experimental Biologists,* vol.3, p.1927, 1989.

[48]. Heinonen, P. K., et al. *Archives of Gynecology and Obstetrics,* vol.241, p.151, 1987.

[49]. Brock, K. E., et al. *Journal of the National Cancer Institute,* vol.80, p.580, June 15, 1988.

[50]. Menkes, M. S., et al. *New England Journal of Medicine,* vol.315, p.1250, Nov.13, 1986.

[51]. Schwartz, J., and Shklar, G. *Nutrition and Cancer,* vol.11, p.35, 1988.

[52]. Lippman, S. M., and Meyskens, F. L. *Journal of the American College of Nutrition,* vol.7, p.269, 1988.

[53]. Stich, H. F., et al. *Cancer Letters,* vol.40, p.93, 1988.

[54]. Bendich, A. *Journal of Nutrition,* vol.119, p.112, 1989.

[55]. Alexander, M. A., et al. *Immunology Letters,* vol.9, p.221, 1985.

[56]. Chandra, R. K. *Contemporary Nutrition,* vol.11, p.11, 1986.

[57]. Alexander, M., et al. *Immunology Letters,* vol.9, p.221, 1985.

[58]. Bendich, A. *Clinical Nutrition,* vol.7, p.113, 1988.

[59]. Bendich, A., and Langseth, L. *American Journal of Clinical Nutrition,* vol.49, p.358, 1989.

[60]. Bendich, A. *Nutrition and Cancer,* vol.11, p.207, 1988.

[61]. Chen, L. H., et al. *Anticancer Research,* vol.8, p.739, 1988.

[62]. Knekt, P., et al. *American Journal of Epidemiology,* vol.127, p.28, Jan.1988.

[63]. Knekt, P. *International Journal of Epidemiology,* vol.17, p.281, 1988.

[64]. Wood, L. *New England Journal of Medicine,* vol.312, p.1060, 1985.

[65]. Bruce, W. R., et al. *American Journal of Clinical Nutrition,* vol.33, p.2511, 1980.

[66]. Stahelin, H. B., et al. *Journal of the National Cancer Institute,* vol.73, p.1463, 1984.

67. Wald, N.J., et al. *British Journal of Cancer,* vol.49, p.321, 1984.

68. Menkes, M. S., et al. *New England Journal of Medicine,* vol.315, p.1250, 1986.

69. Wagner, D. A., et al. *Cancer Research,* vol.45, p.6519, 1985.

70. Ingold, K. U., et al. *Archives of Biochemistry and Biophysics,* vol.259, p.224, Nov.1987.

71. Stahelin, H. B., *Recent Results in Cancer Research,* vol.108, p.227, 1988.

72. Bendich, A., et al. *Advances in Free Radical Biology and Medicine,* vol.2, p.419, 1986.

73. Beisel, W. R., et al. *Journal of the American Medical Association,* vol.245, no.1, p.53, 1981.

74. Bendich, A. *Oxygen Radicals in Biology and Medicine.* p.615. NY: Plenum Press, 1989.

75. Blumberg, J. *Medical Tribune,* Jan.8, 1986.

76. Lim, T. S., et al. *Immunology,* vol.44, p.289, 1981.

77. Bendich, A., and Machlin, L. J. *American Journal of Clinical Nutrition,* vol.48, p.612, 1988.

78. Budoff, P. W., *No More Hot Flashes.* NY: Warner Books, 1983.

79. Burney, P., et al. *American Journal of Clinical Nutrition,* vol.49, p.895, 1989.

80. Werbach, M. *Nutritional Influences on Illness.* p.112. Tarzana, CA: Third Line Press, 1987.

81. Willett, J. C., et al. *Lancet,* p.130, 1983.

82. Ip, C., and Sinha, D. *Carcinogenesis,* vol.2, no.5, p.435, 1981.

83. Kaskiewicz, K., et al. *Cancer,* vol.62, p.2635, Dec.15, 1988.

84. Clark, L. C., et al. *Journal of Nutrition,* vol.116, p.170, 1986; see also Schrauzer, G. N., et al. *Vitamins, Nutrition, and Cancer,* p.240, 1984.

85. Lawson, T., et al. *Chemico-Biological Interactions,* vol.45, p.95, 1983.

86. Watrach, A. M., et al. *Cancer Letters,* vol.25, p.41, 1984.

87. Gonzalez, M. J., et al. *Nutrition Reports International,* vol.37, no.1, p.41, Jan.1988.

88. Milner, J. A., et al. *Cancer Research,* vol.41, p.1652, 1981.

[89]. National Research Council. *Recommended Dietary Allowances*, p.284. Washington, DC: National Academy Press, 1989.

[90]. Spallholz, J. E., *Advances in Experimental Medicine and Biology*, vol.135, p.43, 1981.

[91]. Reffett, J. K., et al. *Journal of Nutrition*, vol.118, p.229, 1988.

[92]. Mulhern, S. A., et al. *Nutrition Research*, vol.5, p.201, 1985.

[93]. *Nutrition Reviews*, vol.34, p.347, 1976.

[94]. Orr, J. W. *American Journal of Obstetrics and Gynecology*, vol.151, p.632, 1985.

[95]. Butterworth, C. E. *American Journal of Clinical Nutrition*, vol.35, p.73, 1982.

[96]. Beisel, W. R. *American Journal of Clinical Nutrition*, vol.35, p.417, sup., 1982.

[97]. Prior, F. *Medical Hypotheses*, vol.16, p.421, 1985.

[98]. Ramaswamy, P., et al. *Nutrition and Cancer*, vol.6, p.176, 1984.

[99]. Axelrod, A. E., et al. *Vitamins and Hormones*, vol.22, p.591, 1964.

[100]. Talbott, J. *American Journal of Clinical Nutrition*, p.659, Oct.1987.

[101]. Cohen, M., and Bendich, A. *Toxicology Letters*, vol.34, p.129, 1986.

[102]. Williamson, J. M., et al. *Proceedings of the National Academy of Science*, vol.79, p.6246, Oct.1982.

[103]. Braverman, E. R., and Pfeiffer, C. C. *The Healing Nutrients Within*, p.98. New Canaan, CT: Keats, 1987.

[104]. Patt, H. M., et al. *Science*, vol.110, p.213, 1949.

[105]. Sprince, H., et al. *Agents and Actions*, vol.4, p.125, 1974.

[106]. Kronhausen, E., and Kronhausen, P. *Formula for Life*. p.119. NY: William Morrow, 1989.

[107]. Novi, A. M. *Science*, vol.212, p.541, 1981.

[108]. Meydani, M., et al. *Drug-Nutrient Interactions*, vol.2, p.217, 1984.

[109]. Barbul, A., et al. *Federation Proceedings*, vol.37, p.264, Apr.1978.

[111]. Barbul, A., et al. *Surgery,* vol.90, p.244, 1981.

[112]. Milner, J. A., et al. *Journal of Nutrition,* vol.109, p.489, 1979.

[113]. Phillips, R. L., et al. *Journal of the National Cancer Institute,* vol.74, p.307, 1985; see also Lew, E. A., et al. *Journal of Chronic Diseases,* vol.32, p.563, 1979.

[114]. Weindruch, R., et al. *Journal of Nutrition,* vol.116, p.641, 1986.

[115]. *American Journal of Clinical Nutrition,* vol.34, p.2756, 1981.

[116]. Mackie, B. S., et al. *Nutrition and Cancer,* vol.9, p.219, 1987.

[117]. Chandra, R. K. *Contemporary Nutrition,* vol.11, p.11, 1986.

[118]. *International Archives of Allergy and Applied Immunology,* vol.77, p.390, 1985.

[119]. Bennett, M., et al. *American Journal of Pathology,* vol.126, p.103, 1987.

[120]. Trocki, O., et al. *Journal of Parenteral and Enterological Nutrition,* vol.11, p.521, 1987; see also Pickett, J. D., et al. *Immunology,* vol.46, p.819, 1982.

[121]. Shu, X. O., et al. *Cancer,* vol.62, p.635, 1988.

[122]. Reddy, B., and Maruyama, H. *Cancer Research,* vol.46, p.3367, 1986.

[123]. Kaizer, L., et al. *Nutrition and Cancer,* vol.12, p.61, 1989.

[124]. McCarty, M. F. *Medical Hypotheses,* vol.22, p.97, 1987.

[125]. Reich, R., et al. *Biochemical and Biophysical Research Communications,* vol.160, p.559, 1989.

[126]. Karmali, R. A., et al. *Journal of the National Cancer Institute,* vol.73, no.2, p.457, Aug.1984.

[127]. Borgeson, C., et al. *Lipids,* vol.24, p.290, 1989.

[128]. Saynor, R. *Lancet,* vol.ii, p.696, Sept.22, 1984; see also Gunby, P. *Journal of the American Medical Association,* vol.247, p.729, Feb.12, 1982.

[129]. Das, U. N., et al. *Nutrition Research,* vol.5, p.101, 1985.

[130]. Dippenaar, N., et al. *South African Medical Journal,* vol.62, p.683, 1982; see also Booyens, J., et al. *South African Medical Journal,* vol.65, p.660, 1984.

[131]. Begin, M. E., et al. *Journal of the National Cancer Institute,* vol.77, p.1053, 1986.

[132]. Fujiwara, F., et al. *Prostaglandins and Leukotrienes in Medicine,* vol.23, p.311, 1986.

[133]. Karmali, R. A., et al. *Journal of Nutrition, Growth, and Cancer,* vol.2, p.41, 1985.

[134]. van der Merwe, C. F. *South African Medical Journal,* vol.65, p.712, 1984.

[135]. Levy, J. A. *Basic and Clinical Immunology.* p.297. Stites, D. P., (ed.), 4th ed. Los Altos, CA: Lange Medical Publ., 1982.

[136]. Foy, H., and Mbaya, V. *Progress in Food and Nutrition Science,* vol.2, p.357, 1977.

[137]. Shub, T., et al. *Antibiotiki,* vol.26, p.268, 1981; Miller, D. *Proceedings of the National Academy of Sciences,* vol.78, p.3605, 1981.

[138]. *International Agency for Research on Cancer (IARC),* vol.30-31, p.32, 1983.

[139]. Toss, G., and Symreng, T. *International Journal of Vitamin and Nutrition Research,* vol.53, no.1, p.27, 1983; see also Gray, T. K., et al. *Surveys in Immunological Research,* vol.43, no.3, p.200, 1985.

[140]. Sorenson, A. W., et al. *Nutrition and Cancer,* vol.11, p.135, 1988.

[141]. Newmark, H. L., et al. *Journal of the National Cancer Institute,* vol.72, no.6, p.1323, 1984; see also Sorenson, A. W., et al. *Nutrition and Cancer,* vol.11, p.135, 1988.

[142]. Wargovich, M. J., et al. *Carcinogenesis,* vol.4, no.9, p.1205, 1983.

[143]. Lipkin, M., and Newmark, H. *New England Journal of Medicine,* vol.313, p.1381, 1985.

[144]. Garland, C., et al. *Lancet,* vol.i., p.307, 1985.

[145]. *Science News,* p.141, Mar.2, 1985.

[146]. Blondell, J. M., *Medical Hypotheses,* vol.6, p.863, 1980.

[147]. Lin, H. J., et al. *Nutrition Reports International,* vol.15, p.635, 1977; Davies, I. J., et al. *Journal of Clinical Pathology,* vol.21, p.363, 1968; Habib, F. K. *Journal of Steroid Chemistry,* vol.9, p.403, 1978.

[148]. Papioannou, R., et al. *Journal of Orthomolecular Psychiatry,* vol.7, no.2, p.94, 1978.
[149]. Duncan, J. R., et al. *Journal of the National Cancer Institute,* vol.55, p.195, 1975.
[150]. *Nutrition Reviews,* vol.40, no.2, p.43, 1982.
[151]. Jackson, A., et al. *Teratology,* vol.19, p.341, 1979.
[152]. Chandra, R. K., *Journal of the American Medical Association,* vol.252, p.1443, 1984.
[153]. Wagner, P. A., et al. *International Journal of Vitamin and Nutrition Research,* vol.53, no.1, p.94, 1983.
[154]. *Federation for the American Society of Experimental Biology Abstracts,* Apr.1979.
[155]. Francis, A., et al. *Mutation Research,* vol.199, p.85, 1988.
[156]. Chandra, R. K., *Journal of the American College of Nutrition,* vol.4, no.1, p.5, 1985.
[157]. Eskin, B. A. *Biological Trace Element Research,* vol.5, p.399, 1983.
[158]. *Journal of Clinical Nutrition,* vol.35, p.442, 1982.
[159]. Thompson, H., et al. *Carcinogenesis,* vol.5, p.849, 1984.
[160]. Sinai, Y., et al. *Infection and Immunology,* vol.9, p.781, May 1974.
[161]. Se Simone, C., et al. *Acta Vitaminologica Enzymologica,* vol.4, p.135, 1982.
[162]. Graber, C. D., et al. *Journal of Infectious Diseases,* vol.143, no.1, p.101, 1981.
[163]. Masuda, M., et al. *Japanese Journal of Pharmacology,* vol.34, no.1, p.116, 1984.
[164]. Bliznakov, E. *Mechanisms of Ageing and Development,* vol.7, p.189, 1978.
[165]. Frank, B. *Nucleic Acid and Anti-Oxidant Therapy.* NY: Rainstone, 1977.
[166]. Rigby, P. G. *Cancer Research,* vol.31, p.4, Jan.1971.
[167]. Lacoue, L., et al. *Lancet,* p.161, July 26, 1980.
[168]. Visek, W. J., et al. *Journal of the American College of Nutrition,* vol.5, p.153, 1986.
[169]. Zhemkova, L. N., et al. *Radiobiologia,* vol.25, p.208, Mar.1985.

[170]. Michelson, R.A., et al. *Superoxide and Superoxide Dismutase.* p.496. NY: Academic Press, 1977.

CHAPTER 12: MIND AND EXERCISE TO INCREASE YOUR TOLERANCE OF TOXINS

[1]. Locke, S. *Foundations of Psychoneuroimmunology.* NY: Aldine Publ., 1985.

[2]. Green, E., and Green, A. *Beyond Biofeedback.* NY: Delta, 1977.

[3]. Ishigami, T. *American Review of Tuberculosis,* vol.2, p.470, 1918.

[4]. Cohen-Cole, S., et al. *Psychosomatic Medicine,* vol.43, p.91, 1981.

[5]. Kiecolt-Glaser, J. K., et al. *Psychosomatic Medicine,* 1987.

[6]. Locke, S., and Horning-Rohan, M. *Mind and Immunity: Behavioral Immunology.* NY: Institute for the Advancement of Health, 1983.

[7]. Barinaga, M. *Science,* vol.246, p.448, Oct.27, 1989.

[8]. Ornstein, R. E., and Sobel, D. S. *Healthy Pleasure.* NY: Addison-Wesley, 1989.

[9]. Hooper, J., and Teresi, D. *The Three Pound Universe.* NY: Dell, 1986.

[10]. Restak, R. *The Brain.* NY: Bantam, 1984.

[11]. Harrell, E., et al. *Physiological Psychology,* vol.9, no.2, p.193, 1979.

[12]. Selye, H. *The Stress of Life.* NY: McGraw-Hill, 1956.

[13]. Achterberg, J., et al. *Journal of Social Science and Medicine,* vol.12, p.135, May 1978.

[14]. Leaf, A. *National Geographic Magazine,* vol.143, p.93, 1973.

[15]. Gilman, S. C., et al. *Proceedings of the National Academy of Sciences,* vol.79, p.4226, July 1982.

[16]. Plotnikoff, M. E., et al. *Science News,* vol.122, July 24, 1982.

[17]. Wybran, J., et al. *Journal of Immunology,* vol.123, p.1068, 1979.

[18]. Ader, R., (ed.) *Psychoneuroimmunology.* NY: Academia Press, 1981.

[19]. Ader, R., and Cohen N. *Psychosomatic Medicine,* vol.44, p.127, 1982.

[20]. Hall, H. R. *Journal of Clinical Hypnosis,* vol.25, p.2, 1982; also vol.3, p.92, 1983.

[21]. Peavey, B. S. *Biofeedback Assisted Relaxation.* Ph.D. dissertation, North Texas State U., 1982.

[22]. Schneider, J., et al. Michigan State University, College of Medicine, East Lansing, MI, 1983.

[23]. Achterberg, J. *Imagery in Healing.* p.184. Boston: New Science Library, 1985.

[24]. Cousins, N. *Head First: The Biology of Hope.* NY: E. P. Dutton, 1989.

[25]. Elliott-Binns, C. P. *Journal of the Royal College of General Practitioners,* vol.35, p.364, Aug. 1985.

[26]. Lieber, D. B. *Dimensions of Critical Care in Nursing,* vol.5, p.162, May 1986.

[27]. Gawain, S. *Creative Visualization.* NY: Bantam, 1979.

[28]. Selye, H. *Stress without Distress.* NY: Signet, 1974.

[29]. Bortz, W. M. *Journal of the American Medical Association,* vol.248, no.10, p.1203, Sept.10, 1982.

[30]. Paffenbarger, R. S., et al. *New England Journal of Medicine,* vol.314, no.10, p.605, Mar.1986.

[31]. *Journal of Applied Physiology,* vol.61, p.1869, 1986; see also *Journal of Applied Physiology,* vol.59, p.426, 1985.

[32]. *Clinical and Experimental Immunology,* vol.45, p.351, 1981.

[33]. *Journal of Clinical Immunology,* vol.2, p.173, 1982.

[34]. *Medicine and Science in Sports and Exercise,* vol.20, p.s42, 1988.

[35]. Achterberg, J. *Imagery in Healing.* Boston: New Science Library, 1985.

Index